Man
Optics and

Manual of
Optics and Refraction

PK Mukherjee MS (Ophth)

Retired Professor and Head
Department of Ophthalmology
Pt Jawahar Lal Nehru Memorial Medical College
Raipur, Chhattisgarh, India

The Health Sciences Publishers

New Delhi | London | Philadelphia | Panama

Jaypee Brothers Medical Publishers (P) Ltd

Headquarters
Jaypee Brothers Medical Publishers (P) Ltd
4838/24, Ansari Road, Daryaganj
New Delhi 110 002, India
Phone: +91-11-43574357
Fax: +91-11-43574314
Email: jaypee@jaypeebrothers.com

Overseas Offices

J.P. Medical Ltd
83 Victoria Street, London
SW1H 0HW (UK)
Phone: +44 20 3170 8910
Fax: +44 (0)20 3008 6180
Email: info@jpmedpub.com

Jaypee-Highlights Medical Publishers Inc
City of Knowledge, Bld. 237, Clayton
Panama City, Panama
Phone: +1 507-301-0496
Fax: +1 507-301-0499
Email: cservice@jphmedical.com

Jaypee Medical Inc
The Bourse
111 South Independence Mall East
Suite 835, Philadelphia, PA 19106, USA
Phone: +1 267-519-9789
Email: jpmed.us@gmail.com

Jaypee Brothers Medical Publishers (P) Ltd
17/1-B Babar Road, Block-B, Shaymali
Mohammadpur, Dhaka-1207
Bangladesh
Mobile: +08801912003485
Email: jaypeedhaka@gmail.com

Jaypee Brothers Medical Publishers (P) Ltd
Bhotahity, Kathmandu
Nepal
Phone: +977-9741283608
Email: kathmandu@jaypeebrothers.com

Website: www.jaypeebrothers.com
Website: www.jaypeedigital.com

© 2015, Jaypee Brothers Medical Publishers

The views and opinions expressed in this book are solely those of the original contributor(s)/author(s) and do not necessarily represent those of editor(s) of the book.

All rights reserved. No part of this publication may be reproduced, stored or transmitted in any form or by any means, electronic, mechanical, photocopying, recording or otherwise, without the prior permission in writing of the publishers.

All brand names and product names used in this book are trade names, service marks, trademarks or registered trademarks of their respective owners. The publisher is not associated with any product or vendor mentioned in this book.

Medical knowledge and practice change constantly. This book is designed to provide accurate, authoritative information about the subject matter in question. However, readers are advised to check the most current information available on procedures included and check information from the manufacturer of each product to be administered, to verify the recommended dose, formula, method and duration of administration, adverse effects and contraindications. It is the responsibility of the practitioner to take all appropriate safety precautions. Neither the publisher nor the author(s)/editor(s) assume any liability for any injury and/or damage to persons or property arising from or related to use of material in this book.

This book is sold on the understanding that the publisher is not engaged in providing professional medical services. If such advice or services are required, the services of a competent medical professional should be sought.

Every effort has been made where necessary to contact holders of copyright to obtain permission to reproduce copyright material. If any have been inadvertently overlooked, the publisher will be pleased to make the necessary arrangements at the first opportunity.

Inquiries for bulk sales may be solicited at: jaypee@jaypeebrothers.com

Manual of Optics and Refraction

First Edition: **2015**

ISBN 978-93-5152-450-2

Printed at Rajkamal Electric Press, Plot No. 2, Phase-IV, Kundli, Haryana.

Preface

Errors of refraction are the most common ocular disorders for which people seek ophthalmic consultancy. The number of such persons is so high that WHO has put errors of refraction among the top six causes of blindness.

Errors of refraction cannot be cured, but only given palliation by a method as simple and cheap as spectacles or as complex and costly as refractive surgery. The latter is beyond the scope of this book. It has been given only a passing reference. The book mostly deals with spectacle, contact lenses and a lesser degree low vision aids. Contact lenses and low vision aids by their own merits are subspecialties for which to study them in detail larger books on specific subjects may be consulted.

The aim of prescribing spectacles is not only improving vision but also to give a useful and comfortable vision. The refractive errors and their management cannot be dealt without the knowledge of light, optics of various optical devices, and both physical optics and its pathological counterpart.

The present book is a compendium of physical properties of light, its modification as laser and fiberoptic devices, various types of optical devices, their optics, errors of refraction—their clinical presentation and management. The details of surgical procedures have been avoided. The book is illustrated with lots of colored and black/white diagrams, flow charts and tables. Appropriate photographs have also been provided wherever required.

There are many books available on the subject of errors of refraction. Some of these books are too large and cumbersome for undergraduates to comprehend. The postgraduates also sometimes try to avoid these due to sheer volume.

The students would prefer a handy book for ready-reference. The present book has been written not to do away with the classics, but to be used as a backup supplement. The book is written in simple language mostly for postgraduates, trainee and practicing optometrists, and medical teachers. The undergraduates will also find it useful.

PK Mukherjee

Acknowledgments

I express my heartfelt gratitude to Mr SL Adile, Director, Medical Education, Government of Chhattisgarh, India, and Mr AK Chandrakar, Professor and Head, Upgraded Department of Ophthalmology, Pt JNM Medical College, Raipur, Chhattisgarh, India, for going through the manuscript and their constructive suggestions. I am thankful to Prof ML Garg and Mrs Nidhi Pandey, Associate Professor, Department of Ophthalmology, Pt JNM Medical College, for all the help they have rendered to me by way of providing much needed reference, and Dr Santosh Singh Patel, Assistant Professor of the same department who provided me with the valuable photographs. I am thankful to all of them.

I am indebted to Dr Lalit Verma, General Secretary, All India Ophthalmological Society (AIOS), for his permission to use photographs and diagrams from the Continuing Medical Education (CME) books and the booklets published from time to time. I am thankful to Dr MD Singh for permitting to use figures from his article on Applanation Tonometers.

Shri Sravana, Local Representative of Appasamy Associates for his help to get approval of the firm to use the photographs from their books. I extend my thanks to Arvind Kasthuri and RK Narayanaswami, Executive Directors, Operations, Appasamy Associates, Chennai, Tamil Nadu, India for their permission to use the materials published in their books.

I am thankful to Shri Maneesh Dandekar of Hypersoft, Raipur, Chhattisgarh, India for all the trouble he has taken to hasten the preparation of the final manuscripts.

Young computer wizard Kumar Rahul (Anish) Ash, for all the trouble he has taken to draw the figures and diagrams as many times as required. He deserves a special mention and thanks.

My wife Protima was always there to collect, store and classify my ever-increasing correspondence. My two sons-in-law, Shri Satyadeep Sahukar and Dr Abir Bandyopadyay, and my two daughters, Dr Protima M Sahukar and Dr Preeti Bandyopadyay helped me to find the references from the Internet and drawing the figures on computer. Their efforts are duly acknowledged with thanks.

I am thankful to all the paramedics and the patients who have permitted to use their photographs in this book.

I wish to thank Shri Jitendar P Vij, Group Chairman, M/s Jaypee Brothers Medical Publishers (P) Ltd, New Delhi, for his suggestion, which motivated me to write this book. I am also thankful to him for the permission he has granted to use diagrams and figures published by Jaypee Brothers, in the books namely, *Principles and Practice of Refraction and Optics* by NC Singhal and *Ophthalmic Assistant* by me. Besides this, I am thankful to all the members of M/s Jaypee Brothers Medical Publishers (P) Ltd, New Delhi, especially Mr Ankit Vij (Group President), Mr Tarun Duneja (Director–Publishing), Ms Samina Khan (Executive Assistant to Director–Publishing) and the Bengaluru Branch for all the cooperation they have extended to me in writing this book.

Contents

1

Physical Properties of Light

Light, which is commonly referred as visible light, is a small, middle part of a large electromagnetic spectrum. On either side of this visible light are spectra that are not visible without special instrument.

The visible light is in fact polychromatic, i.e. it has seven colors of different wavelengths that are acronymed as VIBGYOR (Fig. 1.1). The white light will break into seven components when passed through a prism.

Wavelength of visible light extends between 400 and 700 nm = 4×10^{12} to 7×10^{12} Hz (to be precise, 3.97–7.23 THz).

The wavelengths less than 400 nm are called ultraviolet and more than 800 nm are called infrared.

One nanometer is one-billionth of a meter, i.e. 10^{-9} m = 1/1,000,000,000 m.

Mixture of seven colors of spectrum will result in white light as in Newton's disk (Fig. 1.2).

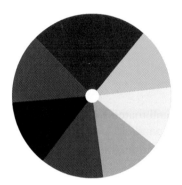

Figure 1.2: Newton's disk

By imposing a suitable interference filter between the source of light and a prism, the seven wavelengths can be separated in seven colors (Fig. 1.3). This phenomenon is used in production of laser.

Laser

The word laser is acronym for light amplification by stimulated emission of radiation.

Properties

1. Laser is monochromatic.
2. A particular laser has single wavelength.
3. This depends on the medium used.
4. It cannot be white.
5. It is always colored, i.e. green, blue-green, etc.
6. It is coherent, i.e. each wave (photon) is in the same phase as the next.

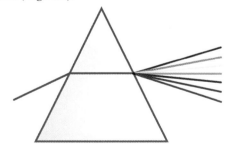

Figure 1.1: Breaking of white light into seven colors

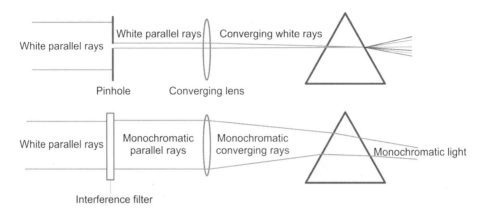

Figure 1.3: Passage of light through an interference filter

7. It is collimated, i.e. rays (photons) are exactly parallel.

8. Polarization: The photons vibrate in the same plane.

9. It produces bright light.

10. It produces intense heat and energy at short distance.

11. Laser can burn, coagulate, evaporate and disrupt.

12. It can be concentrated in a very small area.

Construction

Laser consists of a cylinder that may be solid or hollow; latter is filled with gas, liquid or a combination. These substances should have ability to absorb energy in one form and emit a new type of more useful energy. The energy can be thermal, mechanical, light or electrical. The process of conversion is called lasing. A cavity of the cylinder has two concave mirrors at each end (Fig. 1.4). One of them is fully reflective. The mirrors are coated with thin film of dielectric that reflects light close to the wavelength of the laser light. The other mirror is located on the other end of the tube. The focal length of each mirror almost

coincides with the center of the tube. The second mirror is partially reflective and is considered to be leaky. There are two slanting windows that close each end of the tube. The cavity or the rod is surrounded by source of energy that raises the energy level of the atoms within the cavity to a high level in a very unstable state. This is called population inversion. The next step is spontaneous decay of the energized atom to a lower energy level. This phenomenon is the basis behind the release of high energy in the form of light that is converted to suitable wavelength.

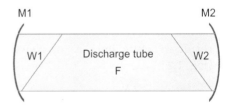

Figure 1.4: Optics of laser, M1 and M2 are two concave mirrors, focal length of which coincides with F, which is the center of the discharging tube. The concave mirrors are coated with dielectric film. M1 is fully-reflecting mirror and M2 is partially-reflecting mirror. M2 is considered to be leaky. W1 and W2 are two slanting windows to close each end of the tube separately.

Thus, to summarize, there are two steps:

1. Population inversion in active medium.
2. Amplification of appropriate wavelength.

The energy stored in the laser material, i.e. gas, liquid or solid, is released in a narrow beam of monochromatic light. This light is a source of high thermal energy, which is used in ophthalmology for various purposes.

There are two modes of laser delivery:

1. Continuous wave.
2. Pulse.

The beam is focused on a small spot, which is measured in millijoules (mJ).

Each spot is exposed for milliseconds and power is measured in megawatts.

Various types of laser available are:

1. Solid-state laser.
2. Gas laser.
3. Metal vapor laser.
4. Excimer laser.
5. Dye laser.
6. Diode laser.

The uses of laser in ophthalmology are enlisted in Table 1.1.

Commonly used lasers in ophthalmology are given in Table 1.2.

Mode of Delivery of Laser in Ophthalmology

• Slit lamp
• Indirect ophthalmoscope
• Operating microscope
• Endoscope
• Surface probe.

Changes on a Surface When Light Strikes

When light strikes a surface, following things can happen:

1. It is absorbed; hence the object looks gray or black.
2. All the rays go back, hence the surface looks white.
3. Only some waves are transmitted back; the object has a color of reflected ray only.
4. If the surface is polished, the rays will be reflected.
5. If the object is transparent, the rays will be refracted.
6. When a beam of light is reflected, its color does not change.
7. During refraction, the velocity of the light is hampered in denser medium.
8. The speed of light in a given medium is less than in vacuum.
9. Light can be polarized, partially polarized or remain non-polarized.
10. The beam of light cannot be deflected by change in electric or magnetic field.
11. Light can be made fluorescent by suitable exiting and barrier filters. This property is used in ophthalmology for fluorescein angiography.

Table 1.1: Uses of laser in ophthalmology

Mode	Lesion	Tissue treated
Photocoagulation	Thermal burn	Retina, trabecular meshwork
Photoablation	Breakdown of chemical bonds without thermal change	Cornea
Photodisruption	Breakdown to form plasma resulting in disruption of tissue	Posterior capsular opacity
Photovaporization	Vaporization of fluid from the tissue to cut	Small tumors

Fluorescence

Fluorescence is a phenomenon in which an object exposed to shorter wavelength emits light of longer wavelength. The character of reflected light is different from the original light. An object is said to be fluorescent when it has different colors, one by transmitted and other by reflected.

Outline of Fluorescein Angiography

The phenomenon of fluorescence is used to get a fluorescein angiograph of the retinal vessels. Fluorescein is used as aqueous solution of 2.5%, 5% and 10% as sodium fluorescein. Fluorescein has maximum absorption at 485 nm and peak fluorescence at 530 nm. To get a fluorescein photograph of the retinal vessels, 5 cm^3 of 10% aqueous solution of fluorescein is injected in the antecubital vein in a bolus. It takes 8 seconds to reach fluorescein from arm to retina. In this, 60%–80% of fluorescein becomes serum bound, mostly albumin, remaining staying free. To get fluorescence, white light is allowed to reach the retina via a blue excitation filter. This allows only blue light (490 nm) to reach the retina. Fluorescein in blood vessel absorbs the blue light and emits a yellow-green light in 530 nm wavelength. This contains reflected blue light as well and returns to camera passing through a blue-blocking filter as yellow-green light, to reach the camera. Photographs are taken by a special fundus camera at an interval of 1 second between 5 and 25 seconds (Fig. 1.5).

Table 1.2: Commonly used lasers in ophthalmology

Laser	Wave length	Effect
Argon laser Green Blue-green	514 nm 488 nm	Photocoagulation Photocoagulation
Nd:YAG* Single frequency Double frequency	1,064 nm 532 nm	Photodisruption Photocoagulation
Diode laser†	810 nm	Photocoagulation
Excimer laser‡	193 nm	Photoablation
Ruby laser	550 nm	Photocoagulation
Krypton laser Red Yellow	647 nm 568 nm	Photocoagulation Photocoagulation

*ND:YAG, neodymium-doped yttrium aluminum garnet; †Diode laser is a semiconductor crystal; ‡Excimer laser is a dimer.

Fluorescein angiogram consists of:

1. Prearterial phase (choroidal phase): This consists of fluorescein circulating in the choroidal circulation without reaching the retinal arteries.
2. Arterial phase: This starts 1 second after the choroidal phase and lasts till all the retinal arterioles are filled.
3. Arteriovenous phase:
   a. This is a transit phase.
   b. It consists of filling of retinal arterioles.
   c. The capillaries are also filled.
   d. The retinal veins show lamellar flow.

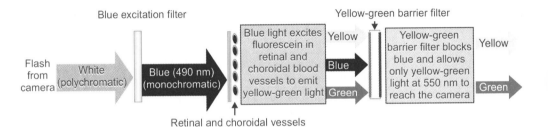

Figure 1.5: Diagrammatic representation of fluorescein angiography

4. Venous phase: In this phase, the fluorescein is draining out of the retinal circulation. It comprises of emptying of arterioles and complete filling of the veins.

Measurement of Light

Light is measured by two methods:

1. Radiometry.
2. Photometry.

Radiometry measures total power of the light in watt. Photometry measures in candela, lumen, lux, foot-candle and apostilb. Lumen measures total amount of visible light emitted by a source of light. Lux (LX) is lumen per square meter.

Nomenclature of units for measurement of light:

1. Candle and candela: Candle is the old term used to measure light in units based on the response to light. It has been replaced by a more precise term, candela.
2. Luminance refers to the amount of reflected or emitted light by a cool surface. It is depicted by number of lumens per square meter incident on a given surface. A candela is equivalent to 4π lumens.
3. Apostilb is defined as luminance of a surface that emits 1 lumen per square meter. The term apostilb is widely used in automated perimetry.
4. The objects that cause luminance are called luminescent. There are two types of luminescent objects depending on duration of light emission after source of excitation is removed. They are fluorescents and phosphorescents. Light emitted from cool object is called luminescence. For example, fluorescein light, clock dials, glowing watches, television, etc.

GEOMETRICAL OPTICS

Properties of Light

1. Light travels in a straight line.
2. Its path can be reflected or deviated, but not bent.
3. It comprises of many rays put together.
4. A bunch of rays is called pencil of rays.
5. The rays of light can be parallel to each other; they can diverge from a point or may converge to a point (Figs 1.6A to C).
6. Divergence is referred to as negative convergence.
7. Rays coming from infinity are considered parallel. They will not come to pinpoint focus unless passed through an optical system.
8. For all practical purposes, rays coming from 6 m are considered to be parallel. Rays coming from a point less than 6 m are considered to be divergent. Shorter the distance; more is the divergence.
9. When light strikes a surface, following things can happen:
   a. The light is completely absorbed and the object looks dark.
   b. Rays of some wavelength are reflected back. The reflected wavelengths impart color to the object.
   c. The rays are partially reflected back and partially pass through the medium. The medium is called translucent.
   d. If all the rays pass through the medium, the medium is called transparent.

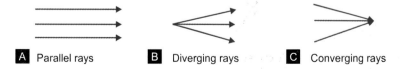

| A | Parallel rays | B | Diverging rays | C | Converging rays |

Figures 1.6A to C: Behavior of light rays. **A.** Parallel rays; **B.** Diverging rays; **C.** Converging rays.

e. If the surface of the object is bright, almost all the rays go back, the phenomenon is called reflection.

f. If the rays change direction, while passing through the medium, the phenomenon is known as refraction.

Fiberoptic Cable

Light travels in a straight line. It does not follow an angular or curved pat, but its direction can be changed in linear fashion with the help of multiple mirrors or prisms, or along the curve by fiberoptic cable also known as optical fiber.

This is a flexible, thin, cylindrical, dielectric waveguide that transmits light along its axis by using property of total internal reflection. A typical fiber consists of a core and a protective coat called cladding. Both are made of dielectric material. The cladding is surrounded by buffer, which in turn is surrounded by outer jacket. The refractive index of the core is more than the cladding. The light passing through the fiberoptic cable is not influenced by electromagnetic field (Figs 1.7A to E).

Effect of Light on the Eye

Interaction of energy of light with the retina creates neurochemical change that gives the sensation of sight. Before reaching the retina, the light passes through successive media of different density, each differing from the other.

Ocular Media

The various ocular media are:

- Tear film
- Cornea
- Aqueous humor
- Lens
- Vitreous humor.

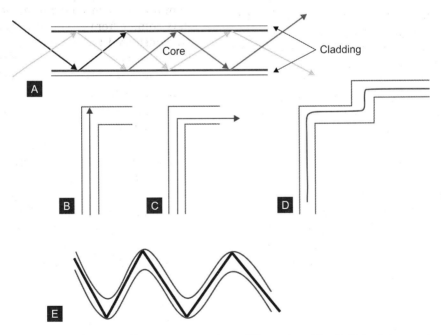

Figures 1.7A to E: Optics of fiberoptic cables. **A.** Outline of fiberoptic cables; **B.** Light does not circumvent the bend; **C.** Light is reflected by 90° by mirror (not obstructed by bend); **D** and **E.** Light negotiating multiple bends through fiberoptic cables.

Ocular Surfaces

The various ocular surfaces that have optical effect on the eye are:

1. Anterior and posterior surface of the cornea.
2. Aqueous.
3. Anterior and posterior surfaces of the lens.
4. Anterior surface of the vitreous.

Absorption of Light in Different Media

The absorption of light in different media is variable:

1. Rays with wavelength less than 295 nm are absorbed by cornea.
2. Rays between 295 and 600 nm will pass through the cornea to reach the lens.

3. Rays shorter than 350 nm are absorbed by lens.
4. Rays between 350 nm and 600 nm will reach the retina. This is applicable only to phakic eyes.
5. In the absence of lens, the rays between 295 nm and 600 nm will reach the retina.
6. All the media of the eye put together are uniformly permeable to wavelength between 390 nm and 600 nm.
7. Eyes with clear media are more sensitive to wavelength 550 nm that represent yellow-green spectrum.
8. The eyes are less sensitive to ultraviolet and infrared rays.
9. Rays beyond ultraviolet and infrared are invisible to normal eye, requiring special devices to be perceived.

2

Reflection

Reflection is defined as the change of path of light without any change in the medium. All the reflections end up in producing images of the object kept in front of the reflecting surface. There are two types of images formed by mirrors. They are:

1. Virtual image.
2. Real image.

VIRTUAL IMAGE

a. Virtual image cannot be focused on a screen.
b. It is always upright.
c. No light is really passing through the apparent location of the image.
d. The virtual image formed by plane mirror is laterally inverted.

REAL IMAGE

a. Real image can be focused on a screen.
b. It is always inverted.
c. The light passes through the location of the image.

Any polished surface can reflect light; the mirrors are the best reflector. There are two types of mirrors:

1. Plane mirror.
2. Spherical mirror.

In spherical mirror, there are two types:

a. Concave mirror.
b. Convex mirror.

LAWS OF REFLECTION

1. Light rays falling on the surface are called incident rays.
2. Light rays traversing back are called reflected rays.
3. A line at right angle to the reflecting surface is called normal.
4. Light traveling along the normal is reflected back along the normal.
5. The angle formed by the incident ray and the normal is called angle of incidence.
6. The angle formed by the reflected ray and the normal is called angle of reflection.
7. The angle of incidence and the angle of reflection are equal.
8. The incident ray, the reflected ray and the normal are in the same plane.
9. The line joining the center of curvature to any point on the curved mirror is the normal of that mirror.
10. The focal length of the plane mirror is infinity.

Diagrammatic Explanation for Laws of Reflection

In the Figure 2.1:

- PM is a plane mirror
- NN_1 is normal at N_1 on plane mirror PM
- IN_1 is ray of incidence
- N_1R is the reflected ray
- $< IN_1N$ is angle of incidence ($\angle a$)
- $< NN_1R$ is the angle of reflection ($\angle b$)

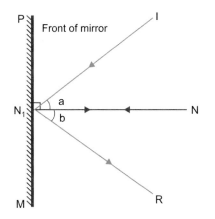

Figure 2.1: Diagrammatic representation of laws of reflection

- $< IN_1N = NN_1R$
- Lines IN_1, NN_1 and N_1R are in the same plane.

PLANE MIRROR

Image Formation by a Plane Mirror

In the Figure 2.2:
- PM is the plane mirror
- O is the object
- AN is the normal at A on PM

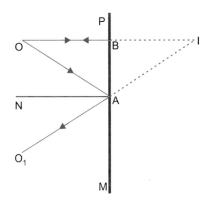

Figure 2.2: Image formation by a plane mirror

- OA is the incident ray
- AO_1 is reflected ray
- $< OAN$ is angle of incidence
- $< NAO_1$ is the angle of reflection
- $< OAN = < NAO_1$
- I is the virtual image
- OB is also normal to PM; hence OB is reflected back along the same line
- OB = BI
- $< OAB$ and $< BAI$ are equal
- Ray O_1A, when extended back, meets BI at I forming virtual image.

Characteristics of Image Formed by a Plane Mirror

1. Image is virtual and erect.
2. It is of same size as the object.
3. It has the same distance as object to the mirror.
4. It is laterally reversed.
5. The image moves twice the angle through which the mirror is rotated.

   If the plane mirror is rotated by 10°, then the image moves by 20°.
6. The minimum length (Fig. 2.3) of the mirror required to form full size image of the object is half the size of the object, i.e. if an object of 1 meter tall is kept in front of half a meter long plane mirror, it will be sufficient to accommodate the image of the object.

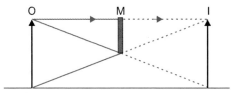

Figure 2.3: Relation between length of the plane mirror, object and image. O is the object of 2 m high, M is plane mirror of 1 m high and I is the image of 2 m high.

Number of Images

From the description given above, it is clear that a single plane mirror will form a single image, if an object is kept in front of it, at any distance. If there is more than one mirror, there will be more than one image, depending upon the angle of the two adjoining mirrors with each other. The number of images formed by two plane mirrors inclined to each other is calculated by the formula:

$$n = \frac{360}{\theta} - 1$$

where, n is the number of images formed and θ is the angle between two mirrors.

Thus, an object kept in between two mirrors, at right angles (90°) to each other, will have 3 images, at 60° will have 5 images, while 45° will have 7 images.

Less the angle between two mirrors, more the number of images.

$$n = \frac{360}{90} - 1 = 4 - 1 = 3$$

$$n = \frac{360}{60} - 1 = 6 - 1 = 5$$

$$n = \frac{360}{45} - 1 = 8 - 1 = 7$$

An object placed between two parallel plane mirrors will form infinite number of images.

This is true only for mirrors kept at right angles or less than that.

This property of image formation in plane mirrors is used to manufacture kaleidoscopes (Fig. 2.4).

Uses of Plane Mirror in Ophthalmology

1. In a small clinic, a plane mirror is used at a distance of 3 m with a reverse Snellen's

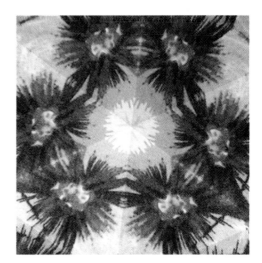

Figure 2.4: A typical kaleidoscope image

chart kept at little higher position than patient's head.

2. As a plane mirror of half the size of the object is required for full length image, a mirror half the height of Snellen's chart will be sufficient.

3. Used in plane mirror retinoscope.

4. Used in various ophthalmoscopes, both direct and indirect.

5. Other instruments where the plane mirrors are used include—slit lamp, synaptophore, stereoscope—to change the direction of rays and save space.

SPHERICAL MIRROR

Spherical mirrors are part of a hollow sphere, one surface of which is silvered (polish), the other surface is reflecting. The rays falling on the reflecting surface do not pass through the substance of the mirror, which is mostly made up of glass.

There are two types of spherical mirrors:

1. Concave mirror.

2. Convex mirror.

In the concave mirror, the inner surface of the hollow sphere is the reflecting surface. In convex mirror, the outer surface of the hollow sphere is the reflecting surface.

Nomenclature in Spherical Mirror Image

1. Pole: It is the vertex of the mirror.
2. Center of curvature: It is the center of curvature of the sphere, out of which the mirror is fashioned (Fig. 2.5).
3. Radius of curvature: It is the line joining the center of curvature to the pole.
4. Principal axis: It is the line joining center of curvature and the vertex.
5. Principal focus of the mirror: It is a point on the principal axis, where parallel rays either meet (concave mirror) or seem to meet (convex mirror).
6. Normal in a spherical mirror: It is a line that joins any point of the mirror to the center of curvature.
7. All the measurements are valid from the pole of the mirror.
8. By convention, all the incident rays are taken to travel from left to right.
9. Focal length of a concave mirror is taken as negative.
10. Focal length of a convex mirror is taken as positive.
11. R and V are sides of the mirror:
    a. The side of the mirror on which the incident rays fall is called R side of the mirror because the real image R will be formed on this side. Position of object, image, radius of curvature and focus on this side are taken as positive.
    b. The region behind the mirror is called the V side because, the virtual image is formed on this side and all the measurement on this side are negative (refer Fig. 2.5).

Behavior of Images in Relation to Position of the Object

Plane Mirror

The image of an object kept at any distance in front of the mirror will be formed behind the mirror. The image thus formed is virtual, erect and of the same size as the object. The distance between the object and the mirror is equal to distance between mirror and image. The image is laterally reversed (Fig. 2.6).

Concave Mirror

The nature of image is real/virtual and size is magnified/minified.

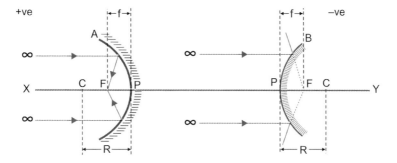

Figure 2.5: Nomenclature in spherical mirrors. A is a concave mirror, B is a convex mirror, XY is the principle axis, P is the pole of the mirror, C is the center of curvature, f is the focus of the mirror, CP is the radius of curvature (R) and PF is the focal length (F).

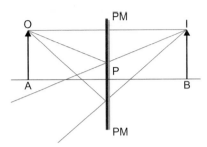

Figure 2.6: Image formation in a plane mirror. PM is a plane mirror, OA is an object in front of the plane mirror, IB is the image of the OA behind the plane mirror, AP = PB, OA = IB.

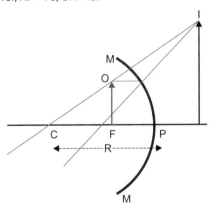

Figure 2.7: Image formation by a concave mirror. MM is a concave mirror, P is the pole, F is the focus, C is the center of curvature of the mirror, O is the object and I is its image. The distance CP represents the radius of curvature (R) of the mirror MM.

Distance of the image from the mirror, position of the image in front/back will depend on the position of the object in relation to the mirror.

The image I of the object O kept between center of curvature C and mirror M is formed behind the mirror, it is erect, virtual and magnified. The distance between the object O and mirror is less than mirror and the image (Fig. 2.7).

This is only applicable when the object is between F and P. The image is virtual, erect and magnified; and on the other side of the mirror. Images formed by other positions are illustrated in Figures 2.8A to F.

This is applicable only when the object is very near to the mirror. The position and nature of the image in relation to concave mirror are given in Table 2.1.

Convex Mirror

The image of an object kept in front of the mirror is formed behind the mirror. It is smaller than the object, erect and virtual. The distance between the image and the mirror is less than between the object and the mirror (Fig. 2.9 and Box 2.1).

Box 2.1: Behavior of image in relation to position of object

The image formed by convex and plane mirrors are virtual
Image formed by concave mirror can be real or virtual
The distance between mirror and the image is least in convex mirror, most in concave mirror and equal in plane mirror

It has been noted earlier that the position, size and nature of the image in concave mirror depends on the distance of the object from the mirror. Object of same size, when moved through different distances, form images of different size at different positions. All the images are real, hence inverted except when the object is between focus and the mirror.

Uses of Concave Mirror in Ophthalmology

1. Mirror retinoscope: To find out high error of refraction.

2. In indirect ophthalmoscope.

Uses of Convex Mirror in Ophthalmology

1. Convex mirror per se does not have any use in ophthalmology.

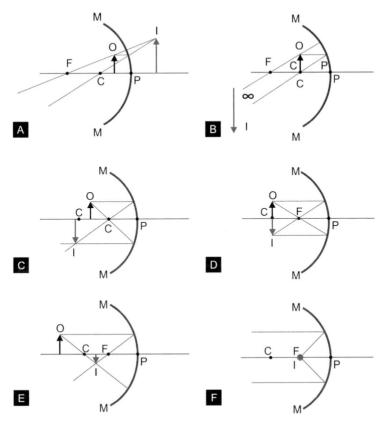

Figures 2.8A to F: Image formation by concave mirror when the object is kept at various distances from the pole. **A.** Virtual, erected and magnified image; **B.** Real, inverted and highly magnified image; **C.** Real, inverted and little magnified image; **D.** Real, inverted and same size image; **E.** Real, inverted and diminished size image; **F.** Real, inverted and very small size image (C, center of curvature; F, focus; I, image; MM, concave mirror; O, object; P, pole).

Table 2.1: Position and nature of the image formed by a concave mirror in relation to distance of the object from the mirror

Position of the object	Position of the image	Nature of the image	Inverted/ Erect	Size	Figure reference
Between focus and pole	Behind the mirror	Virtual	Erected	Magnified	Figure 2.8A
At focus	Infinity	Real	Inverted	Highly magnified	Figure 2.8B
Between focus and curvature	Beyond center of curvature	Real	Inverted	Little magnified	Figure 2.8C
Center of curvature	Same place	Real	Inverted	Same size	Figure 2.8D
Beyond the center of curvature	Between focus and center of curvature	Real	Inverted	Diminished	Figure 2.8E
At infinity	At focus	Real	Inverted	Very small	Figure 2.8F

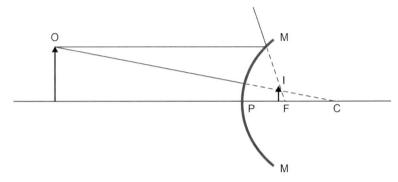

Figure 2.9: Image formation by convex mirror. MM is the convex mirror, P is the pole, C is the center of curvature, F is the focus, O is the object and I is the image of O formed behind the mirror; I is minified, virtual, erect and behind the mirror. *Note:* Character of image in convex mirror will be the same as above irrespective of position of the object.

2. The anterior surface of the cornea, which acts as a convex mirror is used to determine the curvature of the cornea (keratometer) and irregularity of the corneal surface (keratoscope).

3. Purkinje images 1, 2 and 3 are formed by anterior and posterior surface of the cornea and anterior surface of the lens, all of which act as convex polished surfaces.

Calculation of Position of the Image

Calculation of position of image in spherical mirror is done by given formula:

$$\frac{1}{v} + \frac{1}{u} = \frac{1}{f} = \frac{2}{r}$$

where, u is distance of the object from the mirror, v is the distance of image from the mirror, f is the focal length of the mirror and r is the radius of the curvature.

Calculation of Magnification

Calculation of magnification of image in concave mirror:

$$m = \frac{I}{O} = -\frac{v}{u}$$

where, m is the magnification of the image, I is the size of the image, O is the size of the object, u is distance of the object from the mirror and v is the distance of image from the mirror.

3

Refraction

Previously, it has been discussed that when light strikes a surface, it may be absorbed, reflected or refracted.

Refraction of light is a phenomenon of change in the path of light when it passes from one medium to another due to change in velocity. The phenomenon of altering the path of light by an optical device is called vergence (this is not to be confused with convergence, which is part of near reflex).

There are three types of optical vergence:

1. Convergence = plus vergence = positive vergence (Fig. 3.1A).
2. Parallel = zero vergence (Fig. 3.1B).
3. Divergence = minus vergence = negative vergence (Fig. 3.1C).

Vergence denotes power of the optical device.

REFRACTION AT TWO INTERFACES

To be refracted, the light should strike the interface between two media in an angular direction. Light striking the interface at right angles does not change its path and passes unrefracted (Fig. 3.2).

Terms Used in Refraction

1. Normal: This a line at right angles to the interface (Fig. 3.3).
2. Incidence ray: The ray that strikes the interface at the base of the normal in an angular fashion.

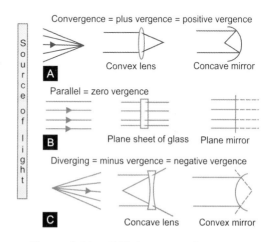

Figures 3.1A to C: Various types of vergence

3. Refracted ray: This is the deviated ray in the second medium.
4. The angle between the normal and the incident ray is called angle of incidence.
5. The angle between the refracted ray and the normal is called angle of refraction.
6. The incidence ray is at the other side of the refracted ray. If the incidence ray is on the left side of the normal, then the refracted ray will be on the right side of the normal.
7. The two angles are never equal.

When light travels in different media, following happen:

1. The velocity and wavelength change.
2. Denser the medium, lesser will be the velocity.

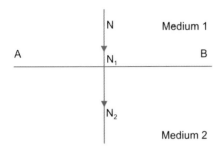

Figure 3.2: Refraction of light at two interfaces passing through normal. AB is the interface between mediums 1 and 2; N, N_1 and N_2 are normal at AB; the ray N, N_1 and N_2 passes unrefracted.

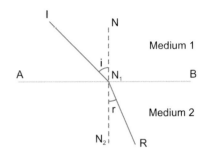

Figure 3.3: Terms used in refraction of rays at an interface. AB is the interface between the mediums 1 and 2; medium 2 is denser than medium 1; N, N_1 and N_2 are the normals to the interface; IN_1 is the ray of incidence; N_1R is the ray of refraction; $\angle IN_1N$ is the angle of incidence; $\angle RN_1N_2$ is the angle of refraction. The angle of incidence is denoted by i and angle of refraction by r.

3. In case of normal, the velocity is reduced, but the direction is unchanged.
4. Color of the light does not change by refraction in a clear medium.
5. The frequency of light is unchanged by refraction.

Laws of Refraction or Snell's Law of Refraction

1. The incident ray, the normal to the interface and the refracted ray lie on the same plane.
2. Incidence ray and the refracted rays are on either side of the normal. The ratio of sine of angle of incidence to sine of angle of refraction is constant and called the refractive index of the second medium with respect to the first medium.

It is denoted by 'n'. The angle of incidence is denoted by 'i'. The angle of refraction is denoted by 'r'.

Thus,

$$n = \frac{\sin i}{\sin r}$$

The refractive index is not absolute, it is only a ratio.

The refractive index is inversely proportional to the velocity of light in the medium.

Critical Angle

Critical angle is the angle of incidence above which total internal reflection occurs. It is defined as the angle when the incidence ray is of such an angle that the refracted ray is at right angles to the normal (Fig. 3.4).

Total Internal Reflection

Total internal reflection is an optical phenomenon that happens when a ray of light strikes a medium at an angle larger than a particular critical angle with respect to the normal to the surface.

REFRACTION OF LIGHT THROUGH A SLAB OF GLASS WITH AIR ALL ROUND

Critical angle of glass is 48.6°, diamond is 24° (refractive index is 2.42) and water is 48.75°. An incident ray when passing through a slab of glass with air on either side will exit the slab as refracted ray and will be parallel to incident ray (Fig. 3.5).

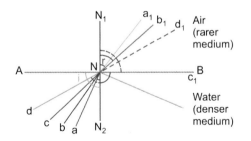

Figure 3.4: Critical angle and total internal reflection, AB is the interface between two media (air and water). Air is rarer than water. N_1, N and N_2 is normal at N on AB. a, N and a_1 is a ray passing from denser medium to the rarer medium and is refracted as Na_1. The angle of incidence is $\angle aNN_2$ and the angle of refraction is $\angle N_1Na_1$. bN is another ray that makes an angle of incidence $\angle BNN_2$, which is more than $\angle aNN_2$ and is refracted as Nb_1. The $\angle N_1Nb_1$ is larger than N_1Na_1, but $\angle 90°$. Similarly, cN, a ray that is refracted along Nc_1. The $\angle N_1Nc_1$ is 90°. The angle cNN_2 is called critical angle. Now, is the incident ray moves away from the normal N_1N and N_2, as dN, the angle of refraction will be more than 90°. The ray will not emerge on interface AB, but will be reflected as Nd_1. This phenomenon is called total internal reflection.

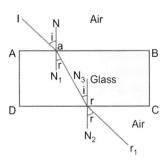

Figure 3.5: Refraction of light through a glass slab with air all around. ABCD is a glass slab with air on both sides. Ia is the incident ray, ar is the first refracted ray and rr_1 is the second refracted ray. N, a and N_1 is the normal at AB and N_3, r and N_2 is the normal at CD. $\angle$ IaN is the first angle of incidence on AB; $\angle N_1ar$ is the angle of refraction on AB; $\angle arN_3$ is the angle of incidence at CD and $\angle N_2rr_1$ is the angle of refraction on CD. Ia is the incident ray at AB, if extended will leave CD parallel with rrl.

The phenomenon of total internal reflection is used in many ophthalmic instruments like gonioscope and fiber optic cables that have many medical as well as non-medical uses.

REFRACTION ON TWO SURFACES INCLINED TO EACH OTHER

Till now, we were discussing refraction on two surfaces, parallel to each other. Let's consider refraction on two surfaces that are inclined to each other.

An optical medium that has three surfaces, two inclined to each other, meeting at a point and a broad base opposite is called prism (Fig. 3.6A).

The point where the two surfaces meet is the apex of the prism and the angle between the two inclined planes is called the prism angle. The surface opposite the apex is the base. The line passing from the apex to the base at right angles is called the axis of the prism (Fig. 3.6B).

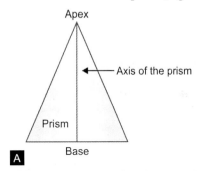

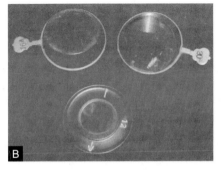

Figures 3.6A and B: A. Nomenclature of prism; **B.** Large angle prisms available in usual trial boxes.

Refraction by a Prism

1. The refraction by prism follows Snell's law of refraction.

2. The ray striking the surface of the prism (incident ray) is deviated toward the base and runs parallel to the base to exit at the other surface of the prism (Fig. 3.7).

3. Thus the ray arising from object O is refracted as I and seems to deviate towards the apex when seen from the opposite side.

4. Greater is the angle formed at the apex, stronger is the effect on light.

5. The prisms alter the direction of the light rays, but not the vergence. When white light passes through the prism, it is broken into seven components of vibgyor.

6. A line parallel to the base of the prism, when viewed through the prism is displaced toward the apex, but not when at right angles to the base (axis) (Figs 3.8A to C and 3.9).

7. A prism does not change the focus.

8. A prism does not alter the size of the object.

9. Prisms kept side-by-side with apices on the same side have an additive effect (Fig. 3.10).

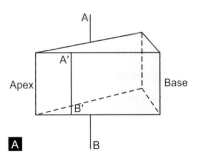

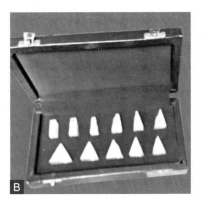

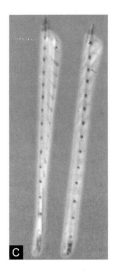

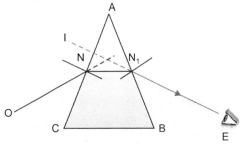

Figure 3.7: Refraction through a prism ABC is a prism with A as apex and BC as base. ∠ CAB is called angle of prism. A ray ON is refracted as NN₁, which is parallel to the base BC and exits from the prism on the plane AB at N₁ to reach E. If the line EN₁ is extended to I, the object O seems to be coming from I, i.e. the image of the object is shifted toward the apex of the prism.

Figures 3.8A to C: Behavior of a line passing parallel to the base. **A.** The image of the line shifts toward the apex of the prism, i.e. when the line AB is seen through the prism, it is shifted to A′B′ toward the apex of the prism; **B.** Loose prisms; **C.** Prism bar [*Courtesy:* Dr Vipul Mandaviya (with permission)].

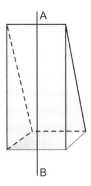

Figure 3.9: Behavior of light rays when passing parallel to the axis of prism. When the line AB is seen through axis of the prism, it does not deviate.

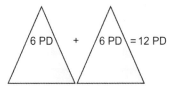

Figure 3.10: Additive effects of two prisms with apices on the same side

10. Prisms kept with apices in opposite side have diminutive effect (Fig. 3.11).

11. If two prisms of same power are put in such a way that their apices are opposite to each other, the resultant device will behave like a plate of glass (Fig. 3.12).

    Features 9, 10 and 11 are the basis of Risley's prism that is used in diagnosis of squint (Fig. 3.13).

    A prism bar consists of a battery of prisms of increasing strength arranged in a flat mount. It is moved in front of the eye, either vertically or horizontally. It is used for cover test and to measure fusional response. The prism bar can be replaced by loose prisms in increasing strength (refer Figs 3.8B and C).

12. The strength of prism is measured in prism diopters (Box 3.1). A prism diopter gives an apparent displacement of 1 cm of an object kept at 1 mm away from the prism. Prism diopter is referred as

PD/Δ. The displacement increases proportionately to the power of the prism. More is the power, larger is the deviation.

Box 3.1: Prism measurement units

It should be remembered that 10Δ is not 10 times 1Δ
1° of decentering of corneal reflex in Hirschberg test is 2Δ of ocular deviation
Other units used in the past were apical angle, angle of deviation and centrad
The unit centrad is used for strong non-ophthalmic prisms

13. Two prisms kept with their bases against each other will act as a converging optical device and with their apices against each other will act as a diverging optical device (Fig. 3.14). The lenses are nothing, but stacks of prisms (Fig. 3.15). Individual prisms do not have any convergence.

14. A prism diopter is a unit of measurement of strength of a prism (Fig. 3.16).

Prentice's Position

When one surface of the prism is at 90° and the other is inclined to it. Light falling on the surface at right angles will go undeviated, but when it emerges on the inclined surface, it will deviate towards the base (Fig. 3.17).

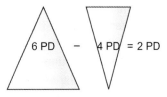

Figure 3.11: Diminutive effects of two prisms when their apices are kept opposite to each other

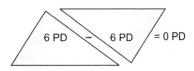

Figure 3.12: Effect of two prisms of same strength with apices in opposite directions

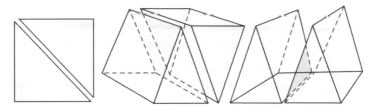

Figure 3.13: Principle of Risley's rotating prism

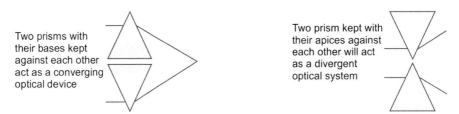

Two prisms with their bases kept against each other act as a converging optical device

Two prism kept with their apices against each other will act as a divergent optical system

Figure 3.14: Depicting optical systems formed by prisms

Prentice's Rule

According to Prentice's rule, the prismatic displacement produced by a spherical glass when not looking through the optical center is equal to dioptric power of the lens multiplied by the distance from the optical center in meters. The formula for Prentice's rule is:

$$p = c \times F$$

where p, is the amount of prism correction, c is the decentration in centimeters and F is the power in diopters.

This is applicable when not looking through the center of the lens. The rule is used to decenter a spherical lens.

The total internal reflection by a prism depends on Prentice's position (Fig. 3.18). The image formed by a prism is real. As the prisms have no vergence, they do not have any focus or any focal length. Hence, they do not form the image. The hypothetical image is real image.

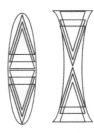

Figure 3.15: Construction of spherical lenses by a stack of prisms. Individual prisms do not have any convergence.

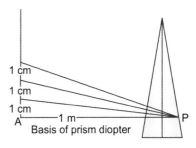

1 cm
1 cm
1 cm
A ——1 m—— P
Basis of prism diopter

Figure 3.16: Basis of prism diopter (PD), P is the prism. A is the object at 1 m from P. When viewed through the prism, it will seem to come from a point, which is 1 cm deviated toward the apex. If the power of the prism is increased, the deviation will increase proportionately.

USES OF PRISMS IN OPHTHALMOLOGY

In clinical optics, the prisms are made of glass/plastic with small refracting angle.

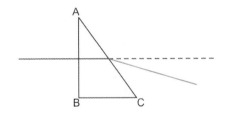

Figure 3.17: Prentice's position. The light falling on surface AB at right angles is not deviated, but when it exits through inclined plane AC, it is deviated.

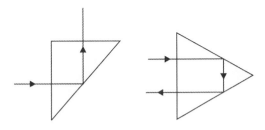

Figure 3.18: Total internal reflection by prisms

The prisms can be used for therapeutic or diagnostic purpose. They are also used in optical instruments to deviate the ray. For therapeutic purposes, prisms are included in spectacles. They can be:

1. Ground on the spherical correction after due decentration in ametropes.
2. Only prism in emmetropes.
3. The prisms can be clip in prisms or Fresnel membrane.

Fresnel Prisms

These are series of small prisms kept adjacent to each other with their base on the same plane on a thin adhesive membrane. The total powers of the prisms are the sum of strength of all the prisms put together. In section, they have a serrated look. On front and back view, they look like series of parallel lines (Fig. 3.19). They are available in two forms, a more common adhesive patch and less common clip on. They are available between 1Δ and 40Δ. The patches are applied on the back surface of the spectacle correction in front of the non-deviating eye.

They reduce the vision slightly. Reduction in vision increases after 12Δ. They may produce a feeling a loss of field of vision. The Fresnel prism is an excellent device in treating diplopia in adult patients.

Prescription of Prisms

1. Prisms do not improve vision.
2. The power of prism cannot be determined by retinoscopy.
3. The strength of prism to be prescribed depends on angle of squint.
4. To find out the power of the prism, prisms are added till diplopia disappears or corneal reflex is brought to the center.
5. Base out prisms are prescribed for esodeviation and base in prisms are prescribed for exodeviation.
6. The strength of the prism is equally divided between two eyes with identical base.

The mnemonic used in prescription of prism—ATP where A stands for apex, T for toward and P stands for phoria. This also holds good for tropia as well.

Uses of Prism in Clinical Optics

Prism can be divided into following groups:

1. Diagnostic.
2. Therapeutic.
3. Part of optical instruments.
4. Miscellaneous.

Diagnostics

1. Measurement:
   a. Prism can be used objectively or subjectively to measure the deviation in squint of both the types, i.e. tropia or phoria. The objective measurements are Krimsky test and prism cover test. The subjective measurements are determination of angle of deviation along with Maddox rod.

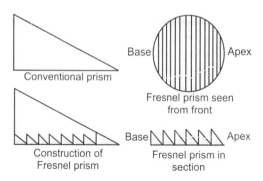

Figure 3.19: Construction of Fresnel prism

b. Measurement of fusional reserve.

2. Conformation of presence of microtropia with 4Δ.

For diagnostic purposes, prisms can be used in various forms:

1. Prism bars: Horizontal and vertical (refer Fig. 3.8C).
2. Loose prisms (refer Fig. 3.8B).
3. Prism in trial frame (refer Fig. 3.6B).

Some Diagnostic Tests with Prism

Prism cover test

Prism cover test is used both for phorias and tropias to measure total deviation. To perform the test an alternate cover test is performed in which the recently uncovered eye moves to make a movement of redress opposite the direction of the deviation, i.e. if the eye was turned nasally, it will move laterally and vice versa. Prisms of increasing strength are put in front of eye till all the movements are stopped. The strength of the strongest prism that stops movement denotes deviation in prism diopter. In case of esodeviation, the prism is put base out and in case of exodeviation, the prism is put base in.

Maddox rod test

Maddox rod (groove): The original device was a hemicylinder that produced a line parallel to

its long axis (Fig. 3.20). The present day Maddox rod, which is also called Maddox grooves is a small, handy, cheap optical device to detect and measure muscle imbalance in both phoria and tropias. The device cannot be used to differentiate between latent and manifest squint. The device is of the size of ususal glasses used in trial sets. It consists of six red hemicylinders put parallel to each other. The back surface of the device is flat and the front surface is corrugated. The hemicylinders are housed in a metal frame. The disk can be rotated through 360° (Figs 3.21A and B).

The patient sits with best correction to look at a white light kept at 6 m. A trial frame is put on. If the patient has any error of refraction, the power is put in the trial frame. A Maddox rod is put with its axis horizontal in front of the right eye by convention. The left eye is left open, which sees the illumination as white light. The right eye that is seen through the Maddox rod sees a vertical streak of red light.

The Maddox rod test finds out presence of deviation, direction of deviation and type of diplopia.

Interpretation: As follows:

1. If the red streak passes through the bulb, the patient is orthophoric (Fig. 3.22).
2. If the streak does not pass through the white light, the eye behind the Maddox rod is deviated.

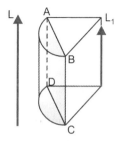

Figure 3.20: Optics of Maddox rod a simple cylindrical lens ABCD produces a line L₁, which is the image of light L.

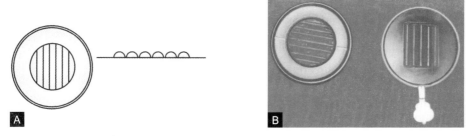

Figures 3.21A and B: Maddox rod. **A.** Construction; **B.** Photograph.

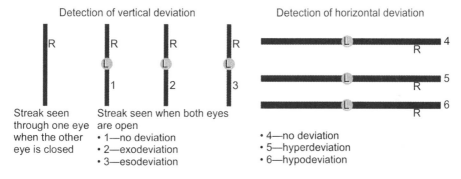

Detection of vertical deviation

R

R
L
1

R
L
2

R
L
3

Streak seen through one eye when the other eye is closed

Streak seen when both eyes are open
• 1—no deviation
• 2—exodeviation
• 3—esodeviation

Detection of horizontal deviation

L
R
4

L
R
5

L
R
6

• 4—no deviation
• 5—hyperdeviation
• 6—hypodeviation

Figure 3.22: Detection of horizontal and vertical deviation. L is white light and R is streak seen through Maddox rod.

3. If the red streak passes on the same side as the Maddox rod, the eye has uncrossed diplopia and the eye is esophoric.

4. If the light passes on the other side, the eye has crossed diplopia and the eye is exophoric.

5. Now loose prisms of increasing strength are put in front of the eye without Maddox rod with apex toward the red line, i.e. in case of esodeviation, the prism is put with base out and in exodeviation, the prism is put with base in. The power of the prism that brings back the red light to the center of the white light denotes deviation in prism diopter.

6. For vertical squint, the Maddox rod is put vertically and prisms are put with base up or down.

7. The deviation can directly be measured on Maddox tangent without using prism.

Two Maddox rod test: The test is used to detect and measure cyclodeviation (Fig. 3.23).

Requirements: As follows:

1. Two Maddox rods, one white and the other red of same strength.

2. A 6Δ prism.

3. A white fixation light.

4. A good sturdy trial frame.

Performing the test: Procedure as follows:

a. Test is preferably done in dark room.

b. Do cover test to find out the eye suspected to have cyclodeviation.

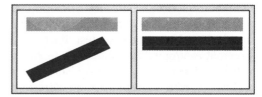

Figure 3.23: Two Maddox rod test

c. Put the trial frame.

d. Put the red Maddox rod in front of the eye suspected to have cyclodeviation at 90° (vertical).

e. The eye with red Maddox rod will see a red streak.

f. Put the white Maddox rod in front of the other eye at 90°.

g. A white Maddox rod will see a white streak.

h. The 6Δ prism is put behind the white Maddox rod to separate two images.

i. In orthophoria, two parallel lines will be seen.

j. In case of cyclophoria, the red line will be inclined to the white line, which can be made parallel by rotating 6Δ prism. This will give the magnitude and direction of cyclophoria.

k. The test cannot differentiate between phoria and tropia.

Maddox double prism: This consists of two transparent prism of 4Δ mounted in a rim with their base against each other, making the device thickest in the center and thinner on the periphery. The posterior surface is flat. The device is used to detect cyclophoria. To use the device, the patient looks at a line, one eye is occluded, the prism is put in front of the non-occluded eye. The line breaks into two parallel to each other, one seen through each prism. The next step is to open the other eye. The patient sees a third line in between the first two, but parallel to them, if no cyclophoria is present. In case of cyclophoria, the line will become oblique (Figs 3.24A to C–3.26).

Detection of microtropia: This test finds presence of microtropia. It also denotes presence of monofixation/bifixation. The microtropia is a small angle tropia, which is difficult to diagnose by Heirshberg and cover test. The eyes are generally esotropic. The condition is unilateral with small central scotoma, anisometropic, amblyopia, with abnormal retinal correspondence. The test is called 4Δ base out test.

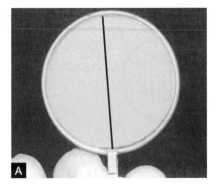

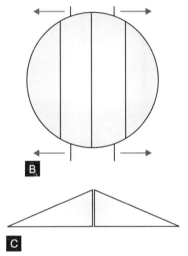

Figures 3.24A to C: Maddox double prism. **A.** Photograph; **B.** Optics; **C.** Construction.

To perform the test:

1. Vision is noted.

2. The amblyopic eye is identified. The amblyopic eye is generally non-fixing.

3. Both eyes are kept open.

4. The patient is asked to look straight ahead.

5. A fixation light is put in front of the eye as in Heirshberg test and the position of corneal reflex is noted.

6. A prism 4Δ base out is put alternatively in front of each eye in succession, first in front of the fixing eye.

7. If both eyes move and stay moved, microtropia is confirmed.

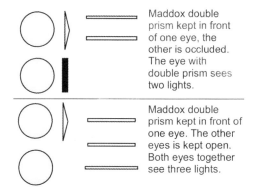

Maddox double prism kept in front of one eye, the other is occluded. The eye with double prism sees two lights.

Maddox double prism kept in front of one eye. The other eyes is kept open. Both eyes together see three lights.

Figure 3.25: Maddox double prism test

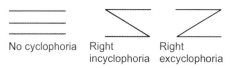

No cyclophoria   Right incyclophoria   Right excyclophoria

Figure 3.26: Results of Maddox double prism test

As has been discussed earlier, a cylinder deviates the rays at right angle to its axis, it does not bring the rays to a pinpoint focus, but forms a line instead. This optical phenomenon is used in construction of Maddox rod. Logically, a single strong plus cylinder of any color should serve the purpose, but for the convenience, this has been modified by a stack of strong plus red colored hemicylinders. The device has to be kept near the eye, i.e. at the anterior focal plane. The optics involved has two parts:

1. When the rod has been placed close to the eye, the incident parallel rays are brought to the focus as real inverted image parallel to the axis of the cylinder.
2. The real image is formed too close to the eye to be focused. Hence, is ignored and the eye instead sees virtual image at right angles to the axis of the cylinder.

Measurement of fusional reserve

There are two types of fusional reserves:

1. Divergence reserve.
2. Convergence reserve.

These tests are done in heterophoria and microtropia, which may be asymptomatic due to presence of relative fusional reserve.

They differ for distance and near. The normal ranges are:

1. Divergence reserve:
   a. Distance: 6Δ–8Δ with rapid recovery.
   b. Near: 14Δ–18Δ.
2. Convergence reserve:
   a. Distance: 20Δ–30Δ with rapid recovery.
   b. Near: 25Δ–35Δ.

To measure the divergence reserve, base in prism is put in front of any eye and the strength is increased gradually till the patient complains of diplopia.

To measure convergence reserve, base out prism of increasing strength are used till diplopia occurs. For vertical fusional reserves, the prisms are used base up or down. The vertical reserves are 3Δ–4Δ for both near and distance.

Therapeutic

The therapeutic uses of prism are to relieve diplopia in:

1. Recent paralytic squint in primary position. When the patient does not like to use patch for cosmetic and social cause.
2. Decompensated phoria.
3. Increased fusional reserve.

Prisms Used in Optical Instruments

Prisms are used in many optical devices. They range from commonly used binomag to highly sophisticated instruments like slit lamp, gonioscopes, applanation tonometer, keratometer, binocular indirect ophthalmoscope, direct ophthalmoscope, etc.

Binomag: It is a low powered binocular magnifier used for examination of anterior segment of the eye. It can be handheld or worn on the head leaving both hands free to manipulate the lids. It is not self-illuminated, hence required a separate source of illumination. The power of the magnifier is +6D that gives a magnification of 1.5X. It has an addition 4Δ prism, basein, incorporated in the spherical lens to relax the convergence of the examiner.

Miscellaneous

In case of uniocular malinger, the patient claims loss of vision in one eye. Generally total or severe loss is claimed. To do the test, the visions in two eyes are noted separately. If there is any error of refraction, it is found out by retinoscope and corrected. Now the patient is made to sit in front of the Snellen's chart at 6 m with both eyes open and a 6Δ prism is put in front of so called blind eye. If the patient complains of diplopia, he/she has vision in the so called blind eye.

4 Refraction Through Curved Optical Devices

So far, we have either studied refraction through flat surfaces parallel to each other or inclined to each other in the form of slab or prism, respectively. Now, we would consider refraction through curved surfaces called lenses.

LENS

A lens is a transparent optical device, which has at least one curved surface. The lenses are made of either glass or plastic.

Types

Lenses are of three types (Fig. 4.1):

1. Spherical lenses.
2. Cylindrical lenses.
3. Spherocylinder.

The spherical lenses are cut out of a sphere and the cylindrical lenses are part of a cylinder, both can be pure convex, pure concave or mixed.

All the lenses obey law of refraction as any flat refractive medium.

The spherical lenses have a single power in all meridians and bring the parallel rays to a pinpoint focus that may be real or virtual (Figs 4.2A and B).

A cylindrical lens has power only in one axis, which is at right angles to the long axis and forms a line of parallel rays, parallel to the axis of the cylindrical lens (Fig. 4.3).

Parts of the spherical lens (Fig. 4.4):

1. Pole.
2. Curvature.
3. Radius of curvature.
4. Center of curvature.
5. Axis.
6. Optical center.
7. Geometrical center.

Curvature

1. The lenses have two surfaces, unlike prisms that have three surfaces. Both the surfaces of the spherical lenses are not always of same curvature. The other surface can be less curved, flat or of opposite sign (Fig. 4.5).

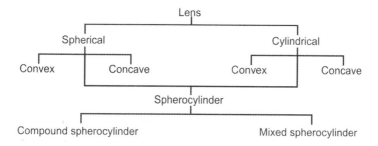

Figure 4.1:Types of lenses

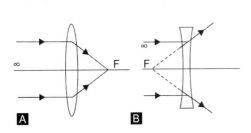

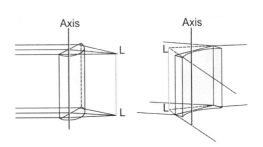

Figures 4.2A and B: Spherical lenses. **A.** Behavior of parallel rays in convex spherical lenses; **B.** Behavior of parallel rays in concave spherical lenses with pinpoint focus at F (∞ = Infinity).

Figure 4.3: Behavior of parallel rays in cylindrical lenses. Parallel rays at right angles to the axis are brought to focus in a line LL.

2. Even the two meridians of the same surface can have different curves like a teaspoon. Such surfaces are called toric surfaces (Figs 4.6 and 4.7). The curvatures have different focal lengths.

3. Though the lenses are part of a sphere, they behave as if they were made up of a stack of prisms, either with their bases against each other and apices away or with their apices against each other and bases away. The former are convex lenses and the latter are concave lenses (Fig. 4.8).

4. The convex lenses are also called plus lenses, converging lenses, positive lenses or magnifying lenses.

5. The concave lenses are also known as minus lenses, diverging lenses, negative lenses or minifying lenses.

6. The convex lenses are thick in the center. The image moves against the movement of the lens (Fig. 4.9). The images are real and inverted except when the object is very near the lens, between the focus and the lens.

7. The concave lenses are thick at the periphery and thin at the center. The image of the object moves with the movement of the lens (Fig. 4.10). All images irrespective of distance from the lens are virtual, hence erect. The images are minified.

How to Identify Spherical Lenses?

Thick lenses can be identified by their physical shapes. Difficulty arises with the thin lenses in the spectacles. Only the thick lenses like aphakic lenses or myodisk can be identified by their shape. To find out if a lens in spectacle is convex or concave, two steps are required as given below.

First step requires seeing a distant object:

1. Hold the spectacle by the frame.

2. Bring it near the eye with the side arms of the spectacle away and look at a distant object, better if it is a vertical linear object like a door frame or vision drum is seen (Fig. 4.11).

3. If there is magnification of the object, the lens is convex (Fig. 4.12A); if the object looks smaller, it is a concave lens

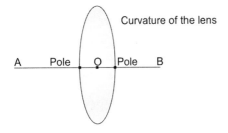

Figure 4.4: Various parts of spherical lens. O is optical center and AB is principal axis.

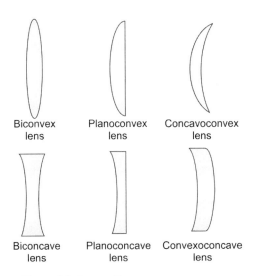

Biconvex   Planoconvex   Concavoconvex
lens   lens   lens

Biconcave   Planoconcave   Convexoconcave
lens   lens   lens

Figure 4.5: Types of lenses as per curvatures

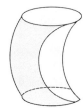

Figure 4.6: A torus

(Fig. 4.12B). In case of plain glass, there will be no change in the size of the object (Fig. 4.12C).

4. In none of the cases, there will be a change in the shape of the object.

5. Move the lens from side to side:

   a. If the image does not move, the device is plain glass.

   b. If the image moves with the movement of the lens, the lens is concave.

   c. If the image moves against the lens, the image is convex.

6. The observer holds the spectacle as shown, but away from the eyes and looks at a near object like wristwatch; and moves the lens in anteroposterior direction. In case of plain glass, there will be

no change in the size of the object. In case of convex lens, the object will look larger as the object is brought near the eyes of the observer. In case of minus lenses, the object will look small and smaller, if the object is brought near the eyes of the observer (Fig. 4.13).

The second step consists of rotating the lens to find out distortion. Distortion in the object denotes presence of cylindrical component. The better method is the use of a lensometer or Geneva lensometer.

Lensometer

Lensometer is also known as lensmeter or focimeter (Fig. 4.14). It is a small table-mounted optical instrument that looks more or less like a monocular clinical microscope, which it is not. In fact, it is a telescope. It is used mostly by opticians. It has many uses pertaining to manufacture of spectacles or verifying the power of lenses alone or in spectacle. During manufacturing of lens, it properly orients the lens block (uncut lens) and checks the power after the lens has been fashioned. The lensometer is used to find out the following:

1. Type of lens.

2. Spherical power.

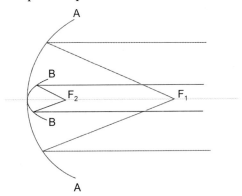

Figure 4.7: Optics of toric surfaces. The surface AA is less curved than the surface BB. The parallel rays falling on surface AA are brought to focus at F_1 and parallel rays falling on surface BB are brought to focus on F_2.

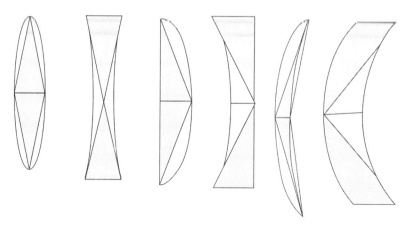

Figure 4.8: Construction of spherical lenses

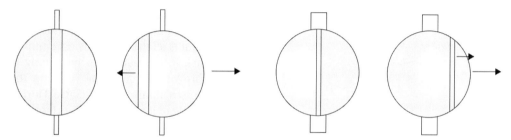

Figure 4.9: Movement of image in convex lens. The image moves against the movement of the lens.

Figure 4.10: Movement of image in concave lens. The image moves with the movement of the concave lens.

3. Cylindrical power.
4. Axis of cylinder.
5. Power added for near vision.
6. Presence of prism.
7. Orientation of prism.
8. Accuracy of progressive lens, which are otherwise difficult to neutralize manually.
9. Optical and geometrical centers of the lens.
10. Specially designed lensometer with support can measure power of the contact lens.

The present age lensometers are computerized with a digital display. They give a digital printout without going through usual focusing of optical instrument.

Geneva Lensometer

Geneva lensometer is an outdated mechanical device also called lens clock or lens gauge. It is a spherometer that physically measures

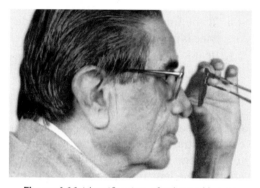

Figure 4.11: Identification of spherical lenses

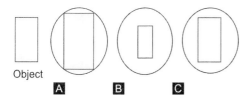

Object

A   B   C

Figures 4.12A to C: Change in size of the same object when seen through. **A.** Plain sheet of glass; **B.** Convex lens; **C.** Concave lens.

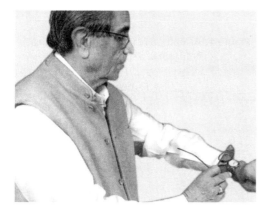

Figure 4.13: Identification of spherical lens by looking object like a wristwatch

the sagital depth (curve) of refractive surface and calculates the refractive power on the basis of refractive index of the glass used in the spectacles. Generally, the instruments are calibrated with assumed refractive index of the glass as 1.53 (crowned glass) with scope of adjustment for other glasses.

Geometrical and Optical Centers of the Lens

A spherical lens has two centers, i.e. a geometrical center and an optical center. Geometrical center is the center of the sphere, out of which the lens has been carved out. In fact, the geometrical center may be outside the lens. The two centers generally do not coincide. The spectacle should be so made that the optical center should come in front of the

pupil and fall on the optical axis. The phenomenon is explained in Figures 4.15A to C.

LS is a smaller lens, cut out of the large lens.

O is the geometrical center of L and OS is the optical center of the smaller lens LS.

Thus, the two do not coincide.

The optical center may need to be decentered to coincide with the pupil and optical axis as per Prentice's rule. In thin lens, the optical and geometrical centers are very near. The optical center of a complex lens may or may not be inside the lens.

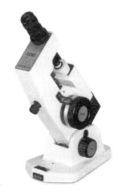

Figure 4.14: A lensometer
[*Courtesy:* Appasamy Associates (with permission)]

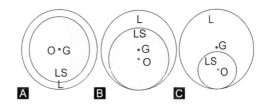

A   B   C

Figures 4.15A to C: Relation between geometrical center and optical center of spherical lenses. **A.** Geometrical and optical centers coincide and are inside the lens; **B.** Geometrical and optical centers do not coincide and are inside the lens; **C.** Geometric and optical centers do not coincide and the geometrical center is outside the lens (O is optical center; G is geometrical center of a large spherical lens out of which a small lens has been carved out).

How to Find Out the Optical Center of a Given Lens?

Hold the lens as shown in Figure 4.11 and look at a vertical line, if the image of the vertical line in the lens and the lines above and below are in one line, the line has optical center somewhere along it. Draw the line. If the image is shifted, move the lens to bring the image in alignment with the line above and below. Now, draw a line passing through the three parts. Rotate the lens by 180°, repeat the procedure and draw the line as above. The intersection of the two lines is the optical center of the lens (Fig. 4.16). The same results can be obtained by looking at a vertical and horizontal line separately.

Some commonly used terms in image formation by spherical lenses (Figs 4.17 and 4.18A and B):

1. Pole: This is the highest point on the curvature of the lens. There are two poles, anterior and posterior.

2. Center of curvature: The center of curvature represents the center of the sphere, out of which at least one surface of the lens has been cut. In case of biconvex and biconcave lenses, there will be two centers of curvature, one for each surface. It is denoted by letter c.

3. Radius of curvature: Radius of curvature is the radius of the sphere from which the spherical lens has been cut. It is denoted by letter R.

4. Optical center: The optical center of the lens (O) is the principal point = nodal point of the lens. It is situated on the principal axis of the lens. Rays passing through this is not refracted. The optical center need not be inside the lens. In meniscus lens, it is outside the substance of the lens. The principal axis and the principal plane of the lens cut each other on the nodal point.

5. Principal axis: Principal axis is the line joining the center of curvature (c) to the surface of the lens.

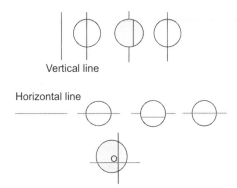

Figure 4.16: Method of finding out the optical center (O) of a spherical lens

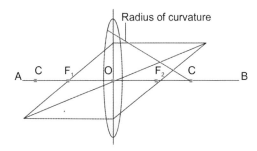

Figure 4.17: Terms used in image formation by spherical lens. AB is the principal axis; C, C are the two centers of curvature; F$_1$ and F$_2$ are the two foci; F$_1$ is the principal focus; O is the optical center.

6. Secondary axis: Any of the several hypothetical lines passing through the optic center of the lens is known as secondary axis (Fig. 4.19).

7. The foci of the lens:

    a. Principal focus: This is a point on the principal axis where the parallel rays either converges as in convex lens and meet or seem to diverge as in concave lens (Figs 4.20A and B).

    b. First principal focus: The first principal focus is point on the principal axis. By convention, it is taken to be situated on the left side of the lens. Rays arising from this point after refraction through the rays become parallel to the principal axis (F$_1$ in Fig. 4.20).

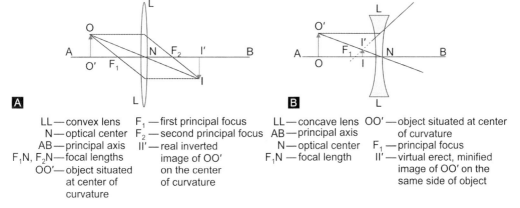

A	**B**
LL—convex lens F₁—first principal focus	LL—concave lens OO'—object situated at center
N—optical center F₂—second principal focus AB—principal axis	of curvature
AB—principal axis II'—real inverted	N—optical center F₁—principal focus
F₁N, F₂N—focal lengths image of OO'	F₁N—focal length II'—virtual erect, minified
OO'—object situated on the center	image of OO' on the
at center of of curvature	same side of object
curvature	

LL—convex lens   F₁—first principal focus
N—optical center   F₂—second principal focus
AB—principal axis   II'—real inverted
F₁N, F₂N—focal lengths   image of OO'
OO'—object situated   on the center
   at center of   of curvature
   curvature

LL—concave lens   OO'—object situated at center
AB—principal axis   of curvature
N—optical center   F₁—principal focus
F₁N—focal length   II'—virtual erect, minified
      image of OO' on the
      same side of object

Figures 4.18A and B: Image formation by spherical lens in relation to various parts of the lens. **A.** Image formation by convex lens; **B.** Image formed by concave lens.

c. Second principal focus: It is a point on the principal axis on the right side of the lens, where rays parallel to the principal axis converge in convex lens and seem to diverge as in concave lens (F_2 in Fig. 4.20).

d. Focal length: It is the distance between the optic center and the principal focus. In the Figure 4.20 F_1N and F_2N are the two focal lengths of a biconvex lens respectively. It is obvious that when a lens has two principal foci, it should have two focal lengths.

e. The first focal length: It is the distance between F_1 and N.

f. The second focal length: It is the distance between F_2 and N.

g. When medium as well as curvature on each side of the lens are the same, then $F_1 = F_2$. If the media on two sides of the lens differ, F_1 and F_2 will be separate as happens with contact lens, i.e. air with refractive index 1 on one side and cornea with refractive index 1.37 on the other side.

Strength of Lens

Strength of lens is the measurement of converging or diverging power of the lens. It is measured in diopter.

A diopter is a unit of measurement of convergence (positive/negative) of an optical device. It is reciprocal of focal length in meters. Shorter the focal length more is the power. It is denoted by letter D.

The relation between diopter and focal length is detailed in Table 4.1.

Image Formation by Lenses

Images formed by two main types of lenses, i.e. spherical and cylindrical differ. The spherical lenses bring parallel rays to a pinpoint focus. The cylindrical lenses convert parallel rays in a line.

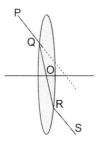

Figure 4.19: Secondary axis of a spherical lens. PQ is a ray that strikes the lens at Q obliquely and passes through optical center O to emerge as RS. The line QR is the secondary axis. The ray QR when extended forward becomes parallel to RS.

Table 4.1: Relation between diopters and focal length of a spherical lens

Diopter	Focal length
1D	1 m = 100 cm
2D	0.5 m = 50 cm
4D	0.25 m = 25 cm
5D	0.20 m = 20 cm
10D	0.10 m = 10 cm

Image Formation by Spherical Lenses

The characteristic of images formed by convex spherical lens in relation to position of the object is detailed in Table 4.2.

Points to be remembered regarding formation of the images by spherical lenses (Figs 4.21A to F):

1. It is presumed that all lenses under consideration are coaxial and homocentric.
2. The lenses are infinitely thin.
3. The object and the images are conjugate.
4. Each optical system has infinite number of conjugate planes.
5. For calculation, the lens is represented by a single line, which is considered the principal plane of the lens.
6. The line cuts the principal axis at the nodal point, which becomes the optic center of the lens (Fig. 4.22).
7. Rays passing through the nodal point are undeviated.
8. The point on the principal axis where an object kept, forms an image at infinity is called primary focal point (Fig. 4.23A).
9. The secondary focal point (Fig. 4.23B) is a point on the principal axis, where the

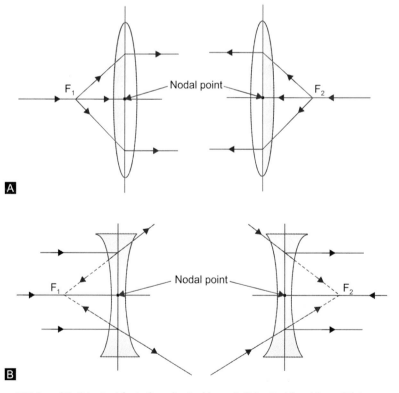

Figures 4.20A and B: Principal foci of a spherical lens. **A.** Principal focal F$_1$ and F$_2$ in convex lens; **B.** Principal focal F$_1$ and F$_2$ in concave lens.

Table 4.2: Characteristic of images formed by convex spherical lens in relation to position of the object

Position of the object	Position of the image	Nature of image	Size of image	Figure 4.22
Between F_1 and N	Between F_1 and F_2, nearer to F_2	Virtual and erect	Magnified	A
At focus F_1	At infinity	Real and inverted	Magnified	B
Between F_1 and $2F_1$	Beyond F_2	Real and inverted	Magnified	C
At $2F_1$	At $2F_2$	Real and inverted	Same	D
Beyond $2F_1$	Between F_2 and $2F_2$	Real and inverted	Minified	E
At infinity	At focus F_2	Real and inverted	Minified	F

parallel rays will come to focus. It will be on the opposite side of the primary focal point.

10. If the media on each side of the lens is same, if provided that the lens has equal curvature on both sides, the distance between the optical center and the focal points will be same and conjugate.

11. The distance between the optical center and the primary focal plane is the focal length of the lens.

12. Converging or diverging power of the lens is measured in diopters.

13. The dioptric power of the lens is reciprocal of the focal length of the lens in meters:

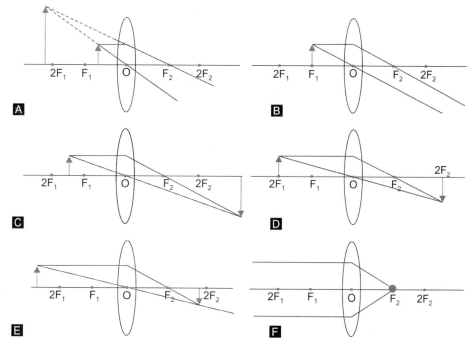

Figures 4.21A to F: Principal foci of a spherical lens. **A.** When position of object is between F_1 and N; **B.** At focus; **C.** Between F_1 and $2F_1$; **D.** At F_1; **E.** Beyond $2F_1$; **F.** At infinity.

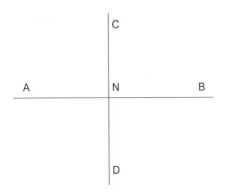

Figure 4.22: Relation of nodal point to principal axis. AB is the principal axis of the lens. CD is the principal plane of the lens. CD cuts AB at N, which is the nodal point and is considered to be the optical center.

a. Diopter is the unit of measurement of vergence—positive/negative—convergence/divergence of the optical device.

b. It is measured as reciprocal of focal length of the device in meters. $D = 1/f$ or $f = 1/D$, where D is the diopter and f is the focal length in meters.

c. Diopter is represented by the letter D. Depending on the nature of the device, a spherical lens is denoted as Dsph and cylindrical lens is denoted by Dcyl.

d. A convex sphere or cylinder is prefixed by sign plus and a concave sphere or cylinder by sign negative. The axis of the cylinder is suffixed by a degree.

e. A diopter can also be measured as difference between the reciprocal of the image to optical center and reciprocal of object to optical center.

f. $D = 1/v - 1/u$ or $D = (n' - n)/r$ where, n' is the refractive index of lens, n is the refractive index of air and r is the radius of curvature of the lens.

14. A lens that refracts more is more powerful than less refracting lens.

15. The focal length depends on:
    a. Curvature of the lens.
    b. Refractive index of the lens.
    The refractive index of air is taken as 1.

16. The ratio between the size of the image and distance of the image is equal to ratio between size of the object and distance of the object.

17. An image can be erect or inverted. The erect images are virtual and the inverted images are real.

18. An image can be of the same size as the object, magnified or minified (refer Figs 4.21A to F).

19. An image can be on the same side of the object or on the opposite side.

Various Foci and Axis in Convex Lens

Principal Focus of a Convex Lens

When parallel rays pass through a convex lens, they converge to meet at a point on the principal axis and it is called principal focus (Fig. 4.24). The diverging rays arising from

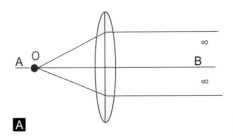

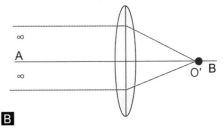

Figures 4.23A and B: Primary and secondary focal point of a convex lens. O is the primary focal point and O' is the secondary focal point of the convex lens. O and O' will be opposite to each other.

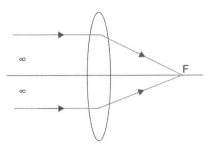

Figure 4.24: Principal focus of a lens. Parallel rays from infinity after passing through a convex lens are brought to focus at F (the principal focus).

the principal focus become parallel on the opposite side.

Principal Axis of a Convex Lens

The central part of the convex lens through which the principal axis is supposed to pass is considered a plate of glass with parallel side and not curved as may seem to be logical. As this is a plate with parallel sides, rays passing through this are not refracted and the line is called principal axis (Fig. 4.25). The rays passing through the principal axis go undeviated.

Secondary Axis

Let us consider I as a convex lens on AB as its principal axis. O is the optical center on axis AB. PO is a ray that strikes the lens at O on the left surface and pass through O, the optical center to reach the other surface at R and leave the lens as RS. The ray, PQRS passing through O is supposed to pass through a plate, thus PO becomes parallel to RS and OR becomes secondary axis (Fig. 4.26).

Conjugate Foci

1. Rays emitting from a distance less than infinity are divergent.
2. When they pass through the lens, they are brought to focus at a point B away from the principal focus (Fig. 4.27).

3. If the direction of rays is reversed, the rays coming from B will come to focus at A (refer Fig. 4.27).
4. A and B are called conjugate foci.
5. Rays arising from principal focus will become parallel and will form an image at infinity (Fig. 4.28).

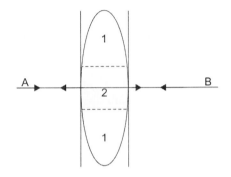

Figure 4.25: The concept of principal axis in a convex lens. 1 is a convex lens, 2 is a hypothetical glass with parallel surfaces and AB, the principal axis, passes through 2 without deviation.

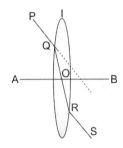

Figure 4.26: Concept of secondary axis

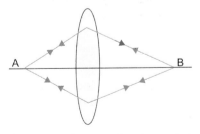

Figure 4.27: Concept of conjugate foci, A and B are conjugate to each other

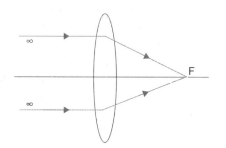

Figure 4.28: Rays arising from focus become parallel when passing through the convex lens

6. If the object A is brought nearer the lens, the rays will remain divergent and leave the lens as divergent to meet hypothetically at a point beyond infinity and these divergent rays when traced back to B, will form a virtual image behind A (Fig. 4.29). This virtual image cannot be seen on a screen. It can be seen from the opposite side. This concept of virtual image is utilized in optics of simple magnifier.

Spherical Lenses

Features of Image Formed

Type, size and location of the image depend on the position of the object in relation to type of the lens, i.e. convex or concave and distance from the lens. There are six possible variations in convex lens, while there is only one type of image in concave lens. The images formed by spherical lenses are of two types, i.e. real and virtual. The images can be erect or inverted. They can be magnified or minified.

Real Image

An image is said to be real when formed on the opposite side of the lens. It may be inverted; it may be very small or very large in size and can be focused on a screen. All the images formed by convex lenses in reference to position of the object form real image except when the object is between F_1 and optic center (simple magnifier).

Virtual Image

Images formed by concave lenses are virtual. They are erect, small, on the same side as the object and cannot be focused on the screen.

Types of Spherical Lenses

Spherical lenses can be convex or concave. The convex lenses can be biconvex, planoconvex or concavoconvex. In biconvex lens, both the surfaces are spherical. They can be of equal curvature or different curvature (Fig. 4.30).

The power of the spherical lenses depends upon the algebraic sum of the power on the two surfaces (Fig. 4.31). The planoconvex has

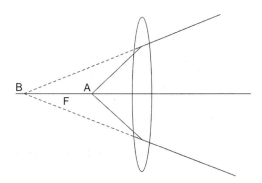

Figure 4.29: Concept of virtual image

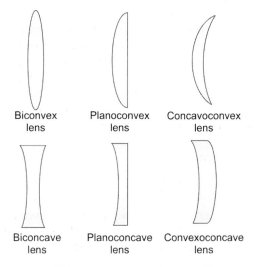

Biconvex lens   Planoconvex lens   Concavoconvex lens

Biconcave lens   Planoconcave lens   Convexoconcave lens

Figure 4.30: Different types of spherical lenses

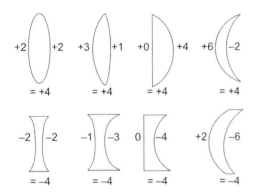

Figure 4.31: Power of the lenses as per curvatures

one spherical and the other plane surface. The concavoconvex have both the surfaces curved; one is more than the other is. The more curved surface has more plus power than the other does, which has minus power. Overall, the result is that there are converging lens.

The concave lenses can be biconcave, planoconcave or convexoconcave.

The suffix denotes the converging behavior of the lens. Thus, the term concavoconvex will denote a converging lens, while convexoconcave denote a diverging lens.

Uses of Spherical Lenses in Ophthalmology

Spherical lenses are used to correct hypermetropia, aphakia and presbyopia. They are used in corneal loupes, condensing lens in indirect ophthalmoscope, various telescopes and indirect examination of the fundus +78D to +90D.

Cylindrical Lenses

Cylindrical lenses are a cut from a cylinder (Fig. 4.32). The outer surface of the cylinder gives the lens plus power, while the inner surface gives minus power.

The cylindrical lens has an axis and a meridian. The axis of the lens is the axis of original cylinder out of which the lens has been fashioned. The meridian is at right angles to the axis.

The cylindrical lens has no power along the axis. The power is in the meridian. Hence, the cylindrical lens cannot bring parallel rays to a pinpoint focus like a spherical lens, but to a line called focal line that represents the focal length of the curve surface (Fig. 4.33). The presence of cylinder in a lens becomes obvious, if there is a distortion in shape of the image on rotating the lens.

Uses of Cylinder in Ophthalmology

Cylindrical lens are used to correct astigmatism. They are used in cross cylinder and Maddox rods.

Spherocylinders

When cylindrical component is added to the spherical value, the resultant lens is called spherocylinder. The spherocylinders are of following types:

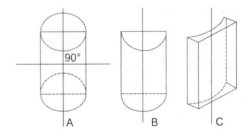

Figure 4.32: Fashioning of convex and concave cylinders. A is a cylinder out of which convex cylinder B and concave cylinder C have been carved.

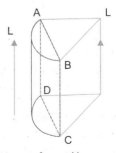

Figure 4.33: Image formed by a convex cylinder

1. Sphere and cylinder of the same sign:
   a. Plus cylinder added to a plus sphere.
   b. Minus cylinder added to minus sphere.
2. Sphere and cylinder of opposite sign:
   a. Plus cylinder added to minus sphere.
   b. Minus cylinder added to plus sphere.

In the first two instances, the value of the sphere is enhanced by the value of the cylinder at right angles to its axis. In the second instance, the value of the sphere is reduced by the value of the cylinder. For example, if a +1D cylinder at 180° is added to +2D sphere, the value of the vertical meridian will become +3D. The horizontal value will remain +2D.

Similarly, when a –1D cylinder at 180° is added to +2D sphere, the value of the vertical meridian will be reduced by +1D, but the horizontal power will remain +2D.

If two cylinders of same diopter are added to one another with axis at right angles to each other, the resultant value will be that of a sphere. For example, a +2D cylinder at 180° is added to a +2D cylinder at 90°, the resultant value will be +2D sphere.

TORIC SURFACES

A surface is said to be toric (refer Figs 4.6 and 4.7), if the curvature of the two surfaces are different and at right angles to each other with different dioptric value. The best example is a teaspoon. The practical example is a combination of a sphere and cylinder, the effect of toric surface is that rays from more curved surface come to focus earlier than that of less curved surface.

Let us consider a spherocylinder with power +2D and +4D with axes at right angles to each other. Parallel rays passing through spherocylinder will be focused at different distances from the lens, light passing through +4D part will come to focus at 25 cm as a vertical line and the rays passing through the +2D will form a horizontal line at 50 cm from the spherocylinder.

The line can be real or virtual. In between the first focal line and the lens, the image formed will be vertical ellipse, while the figure beyond second focal line will be horizontal ellipse. Midway between the vertical and horizontal ellipse at 33 cm, will be a circle. This is called circle of least confusion (CLC) or diffusion. The ellipse between the CLC and first focal line will be a vertical ellipse that will be the smaller than the ellipse formed between the lens and the first focal plane. Similarly, the horizontal ellipse formed between the CLC and second focal plane will be smaller than the horizontal ellipse formed beyond the second focal line. The diameter of the CLC gradually diminishes as the focal line gets nearer and a situation will arise, when the two focal lines will coincide and the circle will be converted in a pinpoint denoting equal refractive power in all meridians.

STURM'S CONOID

Sturm's conoid is a three dimensional geometric figure formed by rays passing through a spherocylinder (Figs 4.34A and B). The curvatures of the two surfaces of a spherocylinder are different. One surface is more curved than the other. The long axes of the two meridians are at right angles to each other. The rays after being refracted by more curved surface will come to focus on the principal axis earlier than less curved surface. The other will come to focus at a point farther away on the principal axis. The focus will be lines and not points. The lines will be at right angles to each other and separated by a distance. The distance between the two lines is called Sturm's interval. This represents the power of the cylinder. The distant half between the two lines is the spherical equivalent of the spherocylinder. To complete the picture, if the converging rays are traced further, they would diverge and following possible images will be formed.

At a certain position, the divergence of the vertical rays is same as the convergence of the horizontal rays. This will produce a circle, this

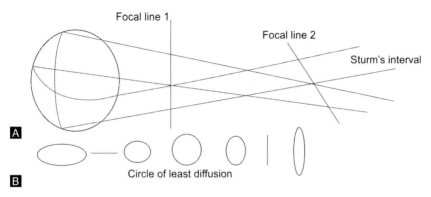

Figures 4.34A and B: Strum's conoid. **A.** The blue lines represent less curved surface and the red lines represent more curved surface; **B.** Circle of least diffusion.

is called circle of least diffusion. The figure between the circle of least diffusion and the toric surface will be horizontal, ellipse and those opposite to these will be vertical ellipses.

Practical Implication of Sturm's Conoid

1. Sturm's interval is the difference between two meridians at right angle.
2. Sturm's interval represents the cylindrical value of the astigmatism.
3. Lesser the length of the Sturm's interval, smaller will be the astigmatism.
4. By abolishing the Sturm's interval, the astigmatism will be abolished.
5. The midpoint in the Sturm's interval represents the spherical equivalent of spherocylinder (Figs 4.35A to C).
6. If some of the Sturm's interval is left, the astigmatism will persist in proportion to residual distance.
7. Hence, astigmatism can neither be undercorrected, nor overcorrected.
8. Plus lens contracts the Sturm's interval and move focal line to the left (Fig. 4.35D).
9. A minus lens expands the Sturm's interval and shifts the focal length to the right (Fig. 4.35E).

10. Similarly, a plus cylinder 90° will move the vertical focal line and CLC left and a minus cylinder to right.
11. Is not sharp throughout the lens. It is more blurred at the periphery and sharper at the center. The sharpest central area is called CLC.

Let us consider a spherocylinder that has power +2D at horizontal plane and +4D at vertical plane. The parallel rays passing through the spherocylinder will be focused at different distances. The rays passing through +2D will focus at 50 cm from the spherocylinder and the rays passing through +4D will converge more and come to focus at 25 cm and will be called first focus, while the rays passing through +2D will be called second focus.

The image formed at first focus will be horizontal and second focus will be vertical. In between the first focal line and the lens, the image formed will be a horizontal ellipse, while image formed beyond second focus will be vertical ellipse. Midway between the vertical and horizontal ellipse will be positioned at 33 cm that will be forming a small circle called CLC. The ellipse formed between the CLC and the first focal line will be horizontal and smaller than ellipse formed between

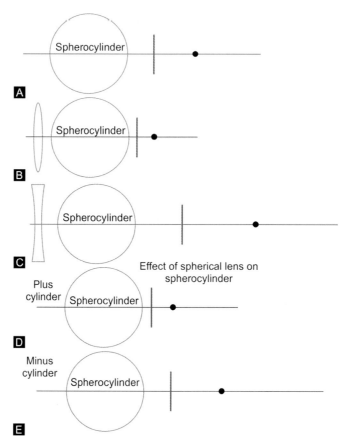

A

B

C

D

Minus
cylinder

Plus
cylinder

Effect of spherical lens on
spherocylinder

E

Figures 4.35A to E: Effects of cylindrical lenses on spherocylinder

the lens and first focus. Similarly, the ellipse formed between the CLC and second focal plane will be smaller than the vertical ellipse formed beyond the second focus. The diameter of CLC gradually diminishes as the focal lines get nearer and a situation will arise when the two focal lines coincide and the circle will be converted into pinpoint denoting equal refractive power in all meridians.

ASTIGMATIC CROSS

Astigmatic cross is a diagrammatic representation of power at two principal meridians (Fig. 4.36). The difference between the two meridians is value of the cylinder. The lower

power is the spherical equivalent. The spherical and cylindrical values are attained by retinoscopy. Let us consider a situation, where the horizontal meridian has a power of +2D and the vertical power is +3D. Thus, the value of the sphere will be +2D and the value of the cylinder will be difference between power in two meridians, i.e. +3D − (+2D) = +1D.

This can be written as any of the following:

1. +2D sphere with +1D cylinder at 180°.
2. +2 X 90° +3D X 180° where, X denotes axis and combination.
3. +3D with -1D cylinder at 90°.

In another case (Fig. 4.37), the horizontal power is −1D and the vertical power is +2D.

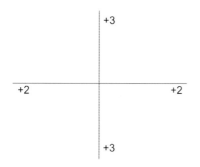

Figure 4.36: Astigmatic cross

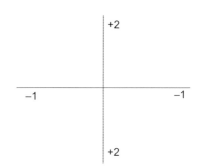

Figure 4.37: Another type of astigmatic cross

The value of the cylinder will be +3D and the spherical value can either be –1D sphere with +3D cylinder at 180°. This can also be written as +1D sphere with –2D cylinder 90°.

The toric prescriptions are written differently. This process of changing the signs of cylinder and sphere; and axis of cylinder is called transposition. While transposing spherocylinders, the power of the cylinder does not change, but the sign and the axis change. The change in the axis is through 90°.

This is also applicable in near addition. Thus, any spherocylinder can be written as:

1. Combination of two cylinders.
2. A sphere with additional plus cylinder.
3. A sphere with additional minus cylinder.

The other method of transposing is:

$$S + C \times a = (S + C) - C \times a \pm 90°$$

where,

S is the value of sphere,

C is the value of cylinder,

a is the axis of the cylinder.

Image Formation by Concave Lens

The image formed by concave lens differs from convex lens. The images are always virtual, erect, small and on the same side (Figs 4.38 and 4.39).

Parallel rays when meet the lens L diverge on the other side and appear to come from a point on the side of the object to meet the principal axis AB at F_1, which is the principal focus.

AB is the principal axis of a concave lens L. N is the optical center of the lens L. OO' is an object placed beyond principal focus F_1 on the left side. II' is a virtual, erect, minified image of OO' on the principal axis between F_1 and the lens.

Image Formation by Cylinders

Cylinders do not bring the parallel rays to a pinpoint focus. Instead, they form a focal line, which is parallel to the long axis of the cylinder (Figs 4.40 and 4.41).

Image Formation by Combination of Lenses

In a combination of lens, the final image is formed by the total diopters of all the lenses, put together.

In a combination of lenses, the image of an object produced by the first lens acts as object for the second and image formed by the second lens acts as a object for third lens. Such additions can go on indefinitely (Figs 4.42A and B).

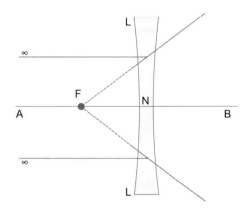

Figure 4.38: Behavior of parallel rays in a biconcave lens. LL is a biconcave lens; AB is its principal axis; N is the nodal point. Parallel rays on meeting the lens become divergent and when traced back appear to come to focus on a point F on the principal axis, which is the principal focus of the lens.

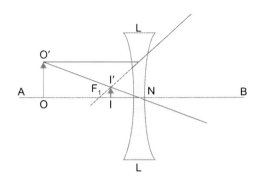

Figure 4.39: Example of image formation by concave lens. LL is a concave lens; N is the optical center; AB is the principal axis; F_1N is the focal length OO' is the object; F_1 is the principal focus II' is the virtual, erect, minified image of OO' on the same side of the object.

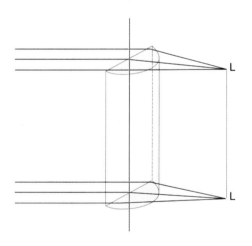

Figure 4.40: Refraction through a convex cylinder. Rays entering the cylinder at right angles to its axis are refracted to form a line LL. The line LL is on the opposite side of the object and is real.

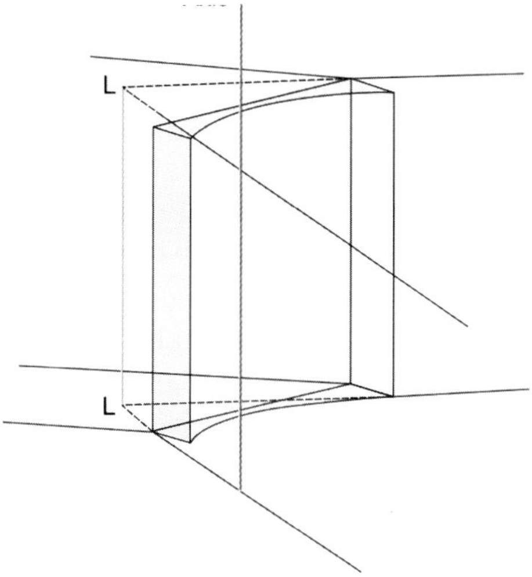

Figure 4.41: Refraction through a concave cylinder. The line striking the cylinder perpendicular to its axis become divergent and seem to be brought to a line focus that is virtual in nature and on the same side as the object.

If two extremely thin, coaxial homo-centric lenses are put against each other, with minimum distance between the two lenses, they will behave like the following Figure 4.43.

In practice, the total power of multiple lenses is algebraic sum of power of all the lenses. Thus, when +1Dsph is added to a lens of –1Dsph will act as a plain glass neutralizing each other (Fig. 4.44).

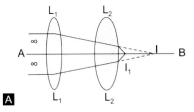

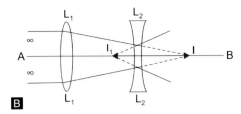

A		**B**

Let L_1L_1 is a convex lens, the principal axis of which is AB. Normally, in a single plus lens, the parallel rays should meet at I on the principal axis AB, but as a second lens L_2L_2 is interposed, the total power of the lens is enhanced and the rays converge more and come to focus at I_1.

L_1L_1 is a convex lens, the principal axis of which is AB. Normally, in a single plus lens, the parallel rays should meet at I on the principal axis AB, but the second concave lens L_2L_2 is interposed, the total power of the lens is decreased and the rays diverge and appear to meet at I_1.

Figures 4.42A and B: Image formation in combination of lenses

If +2Dsph is added to +1Dsph will have power of +3Dsph. Similarly, if –3Dsph is added to +2Dsph will have total power of –1Dsph.

Power of the cylinder added to cylinder can be:

1. If the axes are parallel, the power will be enhanced as cylinder, i.e. +1Dcyl at 90° added to a lens of +2Dcyl at 90° will act as a +3Dcyl at 90°.

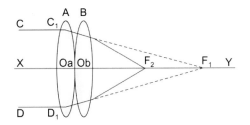

Figure 4.43: Image formation in combination of two convex lenses. XY is a line on which two extremely thin convex lenses, A and B are put against each other in such a way that they are homocentric. They have Oa and Ob as their optical centers. Let us consider CC_1 and DD_1 as two rays parallel to XY, the principal axis. The ray CC_1 meets the first lens A at C_1 and the ray DD_1 meets the second lens B at D_1. If the lens A was alone, the parallel rays should have come to focus at F_1, but a second lens B is interposed between F_1 and A. Hence, the rays CC_1 and DD_1 will come to focus at F_2.

2. If the cylinder of the same value is added with axes at right angles to each other, the combination will act as sphere of the same power.

   This is applicable in case of sphere and cylinder of the same sign as well. When the sign on the sphere and the cylinder are different, the resultant power is no doubt the algebraic sum, but the axes and the sign changes (Figs 4.45 and 4.46).

3. Let us consider a combination of lenses of different signs. The power of the first lens is +2D, the second is +5D and the third is –5D (Fig. 4.47).

   The first and the second lenses are separated by a distance of 50 cm.

   The second and third lenses are separated by a distance of only 5 cm.

   The position of the image can be calculated by following observations:

   1. The image formed by the first lens, which has power of +2D and focal length of 25 cm. Thus, the image will be formed at 25 cm in front of the first lens.

   2. This image acts as object for second lens, which has power of +5D and focal length of 20 cm. The object will be 100 cm or 1 m in front of the second lens.

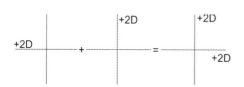

Figure 4.44: Power of lenses

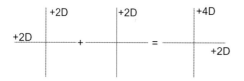

Figure 4.45: Algebraic sum of power lens

3. The image produced by the second lens will be located 25 cm behind the second lens.

4. This image will act as object for the third lens that lies 25 cm behind the third lens.

5. The final image will be at infinity.

From the above observation, it is obvious that such calculations will go on with increase in number of lenses, requiring tedious calculation. Fortunately, Gauss and Listing simplified the calculation. This is generally referred to as theorem of Gauss.

The Gauss's theorem postulates that a homocentric coaxial system of lenses can be considered as a whole, if the object and image distances are measured from two theoretical principal planes. The whole system will have six cardinal points.

This dictum is applicable only, if the lenses are infinitely thin, infinitely near and accurately centered on the same axis.

Cardinal Points

1. Two principal foci F_1 and F_2 (Fig. 4.48).
2. Two principal points H_1 and H_2 (refer Fig. 4.48).
3. Nodal points N_1 and N_2 (refer Fig. 4.48).

First principal focus F_1: This is a point on principal axis. It is taken to be at left side of the lens. The rays emanating from F_1 become parallel to the principal axis.

Second principal focus F_2: The second principal focus F_2 is point on the right side of the lens. The parallel rays after passing through the lens either converge or diverge from it on the principal axis.

Principal points: There are two principal points, H_1 and H_2. They are conjugate to each. They are situated at a point where the principal plane and principal axis intersect. The light passing through the first principal point passes through second principal point after refraction.

Nodal points: There are two nodal points, N_1 and N_2 situated on the principal axis. They are such that a ray directed toward the first nodal point before refraction, comes out of the second nodal point after refraction, making the incident and refracted rays parallel.

Calculation of Position of Image

Calculation of position of image formed by spherical lens is done by the following formula:

$$\frac{1}{F_2} = \frac{1}{V} - \frac{1}{u}$$

where,

F_2 is the second focal length of the lens.

u is the distance between the principal point and the object.

v is the distance between the image and principal point of the lens.

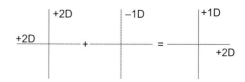

Figure 4.46: Algebraic sum of different sign lens

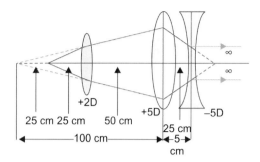

Figure 4.47: Pathway of light through multiple lenses of different signs and power

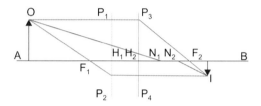

Figure 4.48: Cardinal points of a compound homocentric system as per Gauss's theorem. AB is the lens on which the two principal planes. P_1P_2 and P_3P_4 are placed at right angles. O is the object; I is the image; F_1 and F_2 are two principal foci; H_1 and H_2 are two principal points; N_1 and N_2 are two nodal points.

MAGNIFICATION

Magnification is the ratio between size of the image to the size of the object, which is equal to ratio between image to object distance. There are two types of magnification:

1. Linear.
2. Angular.

Linear Magnification

Linear magnification is the ratio between the heights of the image to the height of the object. This is true only for an infinitely thin lens surrounded by air. This ratio is also equal to ratio of the distance of the image from the lens to the distance of the object from the lens. Linear magnification is also referred to as transverse or lateral magnification. The square of

transverse magnification is also called axial magnification (Fig. 4.49). Also refer Chapter 10, Low Vision Aids as well.

Calculation of linear magnification of image formed by spherical lenses as follows:

$$lm = \frac{i}{o} + \frac{v}{u}$$

where, lm represents linear magnification.

i is the size of the image.

o is the size of the object.

v is the distance between the image and the lens.

u is the distance between object and lens.

The linear magnification discussed above is not used in ophthalmic practice.

Angular Magnification

Magnification used in ophthalmic practice or a system of lenses is called angular magnification. This is applicable to optical devices like simple magnifier to combination of lenses used in astronomical telescope (refer Fig. 7.7), galilean telescope and microscopes. The astronomical telescope has a combination of convex lenses, the galilean telescope (refer Fig. 7.5) and microscope have a combination of convex and concave lenses.

To produce angular magnification, an optical device (magnifier) is interposed between the eye and the object. The object is kept at fixed position, the lens moves to and fro to change the desired magnification. Best magnification is obtained by keeping the object within the anterior focal plane of the magnifier. The commonest example is simple magnifier like a corneal loupe that gives an erect, virtual and magnified image of the object when kept within focal length of the magnifier (refer Fig. 7.17).

The angular magnification is more than linear magnification. Relation between the linear and the angular magnification of the same object at the same distance is explained in Figures 4.50A and B.

To simplify the matters, the magnification by an optical device is calculated as:

$$M = \frac{\text{Size of the image}}{\text{Size of the object}}$$

$$= \frac{\text{Distance of the image}}{\text{Distance of the object}}$$

If the distance between the object and the lens changes, the effective power of the lens will also change.

The commonly used magnifiers with their magnification are shown in Table 4.3.

Magnification of a Simple Magnifier

A simple magnifier consists of a strong plus lens, commonly used for hand magnifier is +10D, which has a focal length of 10 cm and still stronger combination of lenses are used for monocular corneal loupe with a dioptric power of +40D and focal length of 2.5 cm.

Magnification in a Handheld Magnifier of +10D

If the object of interest is held at a fixed distance from the eye and the magnifier is interposed between the eye and the object, which is within the focal length of the lens, i.e. less than 10 cm. A real, magnified and erect image will be formed toward the object, but farther away from the object from the eye (Fig. 4.51). Hence, the magnification will be:

Tangent IEI'/Tangent OEO'

II'/I'E/OO'/O'E

= (II'x O'E)/(I'E x OO')

Table 4.3: Commonly used magnifiers with their magnification

Instrument	Power	Magnification
Monocular corneal loupe	+40D	10X
Binocular corneal loupe	+6D	1.5X
Condensing lens of indirect ophthalmoscope	+20D +30D +60D +90D	3X 2X 1X <1
Direct ophthalmoscope		15X
Slit lamp	Variable	10X–25X
Operating telescope	Variable	2.5X–6X
Operating microscope	Variable	Variable

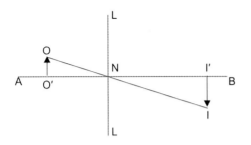

Figure 4.49: Linear magnification. AB is the principal axis; LL is the infinitely thin lens with air all around; N is the nodal point; OO' is the object; II' is the image of OO', which is inverted, magnified and real. O'N is the distance between the object and the lens; I'N is the distance between the image and the lens. So, O'N / I'N = OO' / II'.

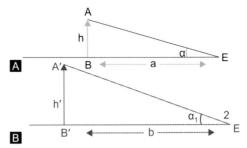

Figures 4.50A and B: Concept of angular magnification. A. AB represents an object seen without magnification of height h; angle formed by AB at E is α; distance between B and E is a; B. A'B' represent an object seen through a magnifier of height h' forms an angle of α₁ at E; distance between B' and E is b; tangent of angle α is h/a; tangent of the angle α₁ is h'/b; thus, angular magnification is tangent α₁/tangent α.

A handheld magnifier gives maximum magnification when the object is kept at focus of the lens (Fig. 4.52). This will give so large image that the image will look blurred. The image will be real and inverted. It can be derived as follows.

An object OO is kept at the anterior focal point of the lens of +10 D, i.e. at 100 mm = 10 cm = 0.1 m from the lens. The lens itself is at 150 mm = 15 cm = 0.15 m from the eye (E). The object O forms an angle of α on the eye. Its image forms an angle of α_1 (Fig. 4.53).

Angular magnification is $1 + (0.15 \times 10) = 1 + (1.5) = 2.5X$.

Let us consider an object AB kept at a distance of D from the eye to subtend an angle α on the eye E. Now, this is moved to a distance D′, which subtends an angle α'. The tangent of α is AB/D and of α' is A′B′/D′. We also know that AB = A′B′. The tangent α'/tangent α, becomes D/D′ = Magnification M_1. To increase the magnification, a plus lens is interposed between A′B′. Let us call this second magnification as M_2. The final magnification is given by product of two magnifications that is M_1 and M_2 and referred to as M. Thus, $M = M_1 \times M_2$ (Fig. 4.54).

We have seen,

$M_1 = D/D'$

$M_2 = D/D'(1 + 150/100)$

And $D' - 1/f = 150$ mm

$M = D/D'(1 + 150 \times F)$

$M = D/D'(1 + D' \times F - 1)$

Finally, M = tangent α/tangent $\alpha' = D/D'$

For ease of calculation, the distance D′ is taken as 25 cm = 250 mm = ¼ m. Thus, M = F/4 where F is the power of the magnifier, hence a lens of +40D will give a magnification of 40/4 = 10X. This is called effective angular magnification.

This is applicable to both galilean as well as astronomical telescope.

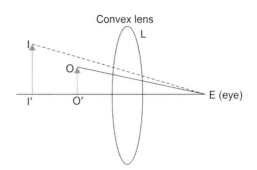

Figure 4.51: Optics of a simple magnifier. L is the convex lens; OO is the object; II′ is the virtual, erect and magnified image of OO′ and E is the eye.

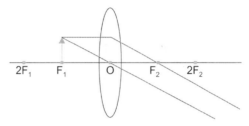

Figure 4.52: Maximum magnification in a convex lens

The galilean telescope needs only two spherical lenses:

1. Convex (converging).
2. Concave (diverging).

The galilean telescope gives moderately flat field without astigmatic distortion.

TELESCOPES

Telescopes are optical devices that enlarge the angle subtended by a distant object larger than subtended by the same object at same distance without the device.

There are two types of telescopes:

1. Those using lenses also known as refracting telescopes.
2. Those using concave mirrors also known as reflecting telescopes. They do not have any medical use.

The former has two types (Table 4.4):

a. Galilean telescopes.
b. Astronomical telescopes.

Table 4.4: Difference in properties between galilean and astronomical telescope

Telescopes	Galilean	Astronomical
Eyepiece	Concave	Convex
Objective	Convex	Convex
Image	Magnified and erect	Magnified and inverted

1. Both have:
   a. An eyepiece each (oculus toward the observer).
   b. An objective (oculus toward the object).
2. Magnification in both the types is given by the formula:

   Diopter eyepiece/Diopter objective

3. In both the types, the objective is fixed; only the eyepiece can be moved forward or backward to focus.

The galilean telescope is a terrestrial telescope, while astronomical is celestial telescope.

Galilean Telescope

The galilean telescope is a terrestrial telescope, while astronomical is celestial telescope.

Clinical applications of galilean telescopes are:

1. While seeing through direct ophthalmoscopes, the myopic addition acts as a galilean telescope with a minus lens. Minus lens in the ophthalmoscope acts as an eyepiece and patients own lens as objective. Hence, myopic disks look larger.
2. Hypermetropic correction gives a reverse galilean effect.
3. Aphakic correction acts as a galilean telescope. The spectacle or contact lens act as an objective and a hypothetical –12.5D in aphakic eye as eyepiece. Thus, a +10D gives a magnification of 1.25X or 25%.

In galilean telescope, the focal length of the eyepiece is shorter than the focal length of the objective. The two lenses are separated by the sum of the algebraic sum of their focal lengths. For example, if the focal length of the eyepiece is –4 cm and that of the objective is +12 cm. They will be separated by a distance of 8 cm. The anterior focal plane of the objective coincides with the posterior focal plane of the oculus. This makes the rays parallel both ways, entering or exiting.

Let us consider AB to be the convex objective of a particular galilean telescope with a focal length of 12 cm and power of +8D and CD a the concave oculus with focal length of –4 cm and power –25D. XY is the image of an object at infinity. N is the nodal point of AB and N' is the nodal point of CD. NX is the positive focal plane of convex lens AB.

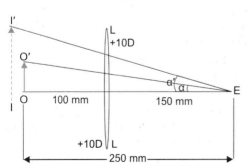

Figure 4.53: Derivation of angular magnification

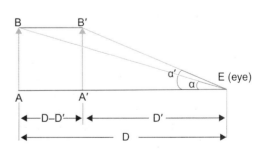

Figure 4.54: Increase in magnification as the object moves nearer the eye

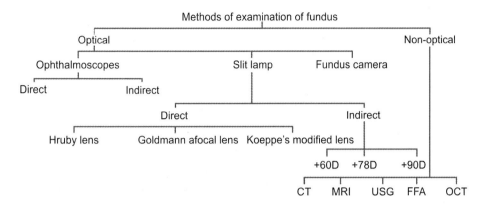

Figure 4.55: Various devices available to examine fundus (CT, computed tomography; FFA, fundus fluorescein angiography; MRI, magnetic resonance imaging, OCT, optical coherence tomography; USG, ultrasonography).

The tangent α = XY/XN and tangent α1 = XY/XN'.

The angular magnification tangent α1/ tangent α = 12/4 = 3X.

IMAGE CHARACTERISTICS

Characteristics of image in various types of appliances are shown in Figure 4.55.

Ophthalmoscope

1. Direct: Image is virtual, erect, magnified and behind the eye.

2. Indirect: Image is real, inverted, magnified and infront of the eye.

Slit Lamp

1. Direct: Image is virtual, erect, magnified and in the eye.

2. Indirect: Image is real, inverted, magnified and infront of the eye.

Application

1. Direct ophthalmoscope.
2. Indirect ophthalmoscope.
3. Hruby lens.

5

Optics of Normal Eye

The purpose of the eye is visual. Clear vision requires three independently acting components. They are:

1. Optical—comprising of cornea, aqueous, lens and vitreous.
2. Neurochemical—brought about by retina.
3. Neural.
   a. Anterior: Accommodation.
   b. Posterior: Extending from retina to the visual cortex.

Characteristics of Optical Components

The optical components should have following qualities:

1. It should have a short focal length.
2. Optical components should be coaxial.
3. Their center of curvature should be on the same axis.
4. The curved surface of different optical components especially cornea should be spherical.
5. The component should be able to focus distance as well as near objects effortlessly.
6. It should have good depth of focus.
7. It should have the ability to resolve the combination into six cardinal points.

Limitations of Optical Components

However, optical system is not as ideal as expected to be. It has following shortcomings:

1. The surfaces of the cornea and lens are more aspheric than perfect sphere.
2. The lens is not homogeneous.
3. Its refractive indices vary in cortex and nucleus. It is different in different locations. In the peripheral cortex, it is 1.386, while in the nucleus it is 1.41 with a mean of 1.39. Actual value is taken as 1.42. This is thought to be due to the complex architecture of the lens.
4. Though the lens is biconvex spherical, its two surfaces are not equal. The anterior surface is flatter than the posterior surface.
5. The lens is slightly decentered in relation to the optical axis.
6. All the refracting surfaces are not isotropic.
7. The dioptric power is variable. It is maximum when fully accommodated.

OPTICAL CONSTANTS

To counteract the shortcomings of optical components, there are four optical constants. They are:

1. Refractive indices of various optical media.
2. Radii of curvatures of refracting surfaces.
3. Diopters of optical element.
4. Cardinal points.

Refractive Indices of Various Optical Media

Refractive indices of various optical media are given in Table 5.1.

Table 5.1: Refractive indices of various optical media

Sl No	Optical media	Refractive index
1.	Cornea	1.377
2.	Aqueous	1.337
3.	Lens: a. Anterior capsule b. Anterior cortex c. Nucleus d. Posterior cortex	1.42 1.359 1.387 1.406 1.385
4.	Vitreous	1.336

Radii of Curvature of Various Optical Surfaces

Radii of curvature are variable for distant and near. The variables are applicable only to the lens as it is only optical system that can change its focus in the form of accommodation. The curvature of the cornea is non-changeable, hence constant for distant as well as near (Table 5.2).

Diopters in Optical Element

Power of various optical components is given in Table 5.3.

Cardinal Points

Measurement of cardinal points from the cornea is given in Table 5.4 and Figure 5.1.

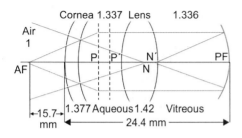

Figure 5.1: Cardinal points of the eye. AF is the anterior principal focus, 15.7 mm in front of the cornea; PF is the posterior principal focus, 24.4 mm behind the cornea; N and N' are the two nodal points in the posterior part of the lens; P and P' are the two principal points in the anterior chamber.

Like radii of curvature and dioptric power, the cardinal points also differ for distant and near. There are six cardinal points for each eye based on Gauss's theorem (refer Table 5.4); to them, two focal lengths are added.

Table 5.2: Radii of curvature of various refracting surfaces for near and distance

Sl No	Refractive surface	Radius of curvature	
		Distant	Near
1.	Anterior lens capsule	10.0 mm	5.33 mm
2.	Posterior lens capsule	6.0 mm	5.3 mm
3.	Cornea	7.8 mm	7.8 mm

Table 5.3: Power of various optical components for near and distance

Sl No	Optical component	Power (in diopters)	
		Distant	Near
1.	Cornea	+43D	+43D
2.	Lens	+20D	+33D
3.	Total	+60D	+70D

Table 5.4: Measurement of the cardinal points of the accommodated and non-accommodated eye

Sl No	Cardinal point	Distance of apex from cornea	
		Distant	Near
1.	Principal point a. First b. Second	 1.5 mm 1.6 mm	 1.8 mm 2.0 mm
2.	Focal point a. First b. Second	 15.2 mm 22.3 mm	 12.3 mm 18.9 mm
3.	Nodal point a. First b. Second	 6.3 mm 7.3 mm	 6.5 mm 6.9 mm
4.	Focal length a. First b. Second	 16.7 mm 22.3 mm	 14.1 mm 18.9 mm

From early discussion, it is obvious that it requires repeated and complicated calculations to find out the cardinal points of the eye. Hence, over the years, many physicist and ophthalmologists have worked out a simple way and constructed reduced/schematic eyes for easy calculations.

REDUCED/SCHEMATIC EYES

Chief among them were—Gullstrand, Listing, Donders, Tshering and Helmholtz. Out of all of them, Gullstrand's model is taken as most authentic. Schematic eye of Donders has oversimplified this concept and called it reduced eye. Comparison of Gullstrand's schematic eye and Listing's reduced eye is shown in Figure 5.2 and Table 5.5.

Allvar Gullstrand (1862–1930) was awarded noble prize for 'work in diffraction of light by lens as applied to the eyes' in 1911.

Donders Simplified Reduced Eye

Donder thought of eye as single unit of curved surface with following features:

1. It is a perfect sphere.
2. Its power is +60D.
3. The curvature of the anterior surface is 5.75 mm in between two media; air and

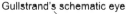
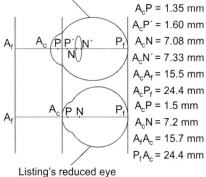

Figure 5.2: Comparison of schematic eye and the reduced eye. A_f is the anterior focal plane; A_c is the anterior corneal surface; P_f is the posterior focal plane; P is the principal point; N is the nodal point; P and P' are two focal points; N and N' are two nodal points.

cornea with refractive indices of 1 and 1.33 respectively.

4. The plane of curved surface is situated behind the cornea; 1.33 mm from the anterior surface.
5. There is single nodal point.
6. The nodal point is situated 7.08 mm behind the anterior surface of cornea.
7. The anterior focal length of the curved surface is 17.05 mm, which is 15.7 mm in front of the cornea.

Table 5.5: Comparing Gullstrand's schematic eye and Listing's reduced eye

Features	Gullstrand's schematic eye	Listing's reduced eye
Principal focus F_1 F_2	15.7 mm in front of the cornea 24.4 mm behind the cornea	17 mm in front of the cornea 24.4 mm behind the cornea
Principal points P_1 P_2	1.3 mm behind the cornea in anterior chamber 1.60 mm in the anterior chamber	1.5 mm behind the cornea in anterior chamber Nil*
Nodal points N_1 N_2	7.08 mm from the cornea 7.33 mm from the cornea in the lens	7.2 mm from the cornea 7.22 mm from the cornea in the lens

*There is only one principal point in Listing's reduced eye

8. The corresponding posterior focal lengths are 22.78 mm and 24.4 mm.

9. The refractive index is 1.336.

Calculation of Retinal Size in Reduced Eye

To calculate the retinal size in reduced eye, following measurements are taken into consideration (Figs 5.3 to 5.5):

1. The nodal point N is taken as center of curvature of the single anterior refracting surface.

2. Anterior focal plane is 17.2 mm in front of the cornea (refer Fig. 5.4).

3. Posterior focal plane is 22.9 mm from the anterior corneal plane.

4. The distance from the nodal point to the posterior focal plane is 17.2 mm.

5. A ray from the top of an object O passes through the nodal point N to form an image I on the retina (refer Fig. 5.3).

6. As the ray passes through the nodal point, it does not bend.

7. As there is no bending of the ray after passing through the nodal point, the angle subtended by the object is equal to the angle subtended by the image.

8. The size of the retinal image is found out by multiplying distance from nodal point to retina, which is 17.2 mm by angle subtended by the object. The angle is measured in radians and not in degrees. Thus, if an object subtends an angle of 0.1 radian at the nodal point, the size of the retinal image will be 17.2 × 0.1 = 1.72 mm.

9. The axial hypermetropia has smallest retinal image because, the retina is nearest to the nodal point.

10. The axial myopia has the largest retinal image because the retina is farthest from the nodal point.

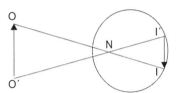

Figure 5.3: Formation of retinal image in reduced eye. N is the nodal point of the reduced eye, which in fact is the optical center. OO′ is the object and I′I is its inverted image on the retina. The rays passing through N are undeviated. The ∠ONO′ and ∠I′NI are equal and represent the visual angle.

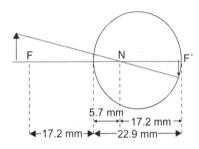

Figure 5.4: Retinal image size in a reduced eye. F is the anterior focal plane; N is the nodal point; F′ is the posterior focal plane on the retina.

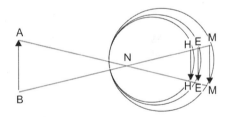

Figure 5.5: Relative size of the retinal image on different dimensions of the eye. MM is the image on myopic eye, which is longer than the emmetropic EE and the hypermetropic HH. The hypermetropic eye has the shortest axial length. AB is the object. N is the nodal point.

11. The emmetropic size is in between because, the retina is 17.2 mm away from the nodal point, which is physiological (refer Fig. 5.5).

REFLECTION BY OPTICAL COMPONENTS OF THE EYE AND THE PURKINJE'S IMAGE

From the previous discussion we have seen that the two optical components of the eye are cornea and lens. They act as converging lens with short focal length. The cornea acts as a +40D lens, while the lens in situ acts as +17D lens and both combine to form a +60D lens.

Purkinje's Image

Besides acting as converging lenses, the optical system has another clinically important function, i.e. they also function as mirrors. The anterior surface of the cornea, the posterior surface of the cornea and anterior surface of lens act as convex mirrors forming a small, virtual, erect images, which move with the movement of the object (light) (Fig. 5.6 and Table 5.6).

The posterior surface of the lens act as a concave mirror forming an inverted, real, small image that moves against the movement of the object.

The images collectively are called Purkinje-Sanson images. The image formed by the anterior surface of the cornea is called the first image; the second is formed by the posterior surface of the cornea and the third by anterior surface of the lens. The first and the third images are bright and are separated by a distance that is sum of thickness of cornea

and depth of AC. The second image is faintest of the four and very near to the first; may be missed unless looked for. The fourth is also bright, smaller than the third image and moves faster than the third against it. This phenomenon is explained on the basis of the fact that the posterior surface is more curved than the anterior surface of the lens. During accommodation when the curvature of the lens increases, the third and the fourth images become smaller, but retain their character.

With advent of better illumination system, the Purkinje-Sanson images have lost their clinical importance and treated as of academic interest only. However, when slit lamp is not available, a simple bright torch elicits some important clinical findings like presence or absence of lens.

Note: If the intraocular lens (IOL) is biconvex, the Purkinje's images will behave similar

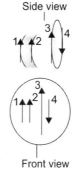

Side view

1, 2 and 3 are the virtual images formed on the convex (mirror) surface on the anterior and posterior surface of the cornea and anterior surface of the lens
4 is the real, inverted and minified image on the posterior concave (mirror) surface of the lens

Front view

Figure 5.6: Purkinje's images

Table 5.6: Significance of various Purkinje's image

Sl No	Image	Present	Absent
1.	First	Bright, clear anterior surface of cornea	Opaque cornea
2.	Second	Clear cornea from epithelium to endothelium	Posteriorly placed corneal opacity
3.	Third	Presence of lens, clear or opaque and intraocular lens (IOL)	Aphakia
4.	Fourth	Clear lens	Opaque lens or aphakia

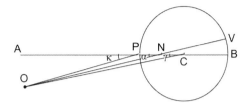

Figure 5.7: Visual axes of the eye and angles. O is the point of fixation; OP is the line joining center of the cornea and the point of fixation; P is the center of the cornea; AB is the optical axis; ONV is the visual axis; AP is the pupillary axis; OC is the axis of fixation; ∠ONA is ∠α, ∠OPA is ∠κ and ∠OCA is ∠γ.

to clear lens except that it will be brighter than the normal clear lens in situ. If the lens is planoconvex, with plain surface posteriorly, the fourth image will act as if formed by a plain mirror that is erect and virtual.

The other uses based on principal of Purkinje's image are Placido's disk, keratometer and Hirschberg's corneal reflex.

Axes of the Eye in Relation to Refraction

So far we have discussed about only the principal axis that passes through the optical center of an artificial lens outside the eye. The two principal foci of which are situated on each side of the optical device (lens) on the principal axis (Fig. 5.7).

This is not applicable to eye because the eye is not a fixed optical device like an artificial lens. It has following axes:

1. Visual axis: This is an imaginary line that joins the fixation point to the nodal point and when extended back meets the retina at the fovea.

2. Optical axis: This is a line that joins the center of cornea and nodal point. This when extended back meets the retina on the nasal side of the fovea.

3. Axis of fixation: A line that joins fixation point to center of curvature. From the above description, it is obvious that the three axes do not overlap each other, but form different angles between them, out of which only angle kappa (∠ κ) has clinical importance. The other two angles are angle alpha (∠ α) and angle gamma (∠ γ).

Angle Kappa

Angle kappa is formed between the two lines, i.e. the line perpendicular to the center of cornea and the visual axis (refer Fig. 5.7).

Logically, they should coincide, but like other normal phenomena this is not so. The two lines meet to form the angle. The angle kappa is called positive, if the reflex is formed on the nasal side of the cornea and when it is formed on the temporal side, it is called negative. The positive angle kappa gives a false impression of exodeviation and esodeviation when the angle is negative. In emmetropia, the angle is positive, but less than 5°.

6

Errors of Refraction

Errors of refraction are the commonest ocular disorders for which people seek ophthalmic consultation. About 20%–25% of populations have some error of refraction or the other. It inflicts all the races and both the sexes. Different age groups have predilection for different types of errors of refraction. Children under 15 are more likely to have myopia while persons above 40 are more prone to get hypermetropia unmasked. Generally, errors of refraction are bilateral and almost equal in two eyes, gradually developing and progressing slowly. It is not uncommon to have difference in diopter or type in two eyes, i.e. spherical/astigmatism, myopia/hypermetropia. Rapid change in power requires investigation to exclude central nuclear sclerosis, hyperglycemia, neglected blunt trauma, chronic simple glaucoma.

The commonest symptom of error of refraction in the eye inflicted is diminished distant vision, which is inevitable in myopia. No myopic eye can have normal vision. However, it may be normal or subnormal in hypermetropia. With proper treatment, distant vision improves to 6/6–6/9 and near vision improves to n/6.

Absence of error of refraction is called emmetropia and presence of error of refraction is called ametropia, which can be spherical or astigmatic. Both eyes can be myopia, hypermetropic or may have different types of error of refraction.

EMMETROPIA

In emmetropia, the parallel rays of light are brought to pinpoint focus on the photosensitive layer on the retina, when accommodation is at rest (Fig. 6.1).

If the eye accommodates, the retinal image in emmetropia moves forwards away from the retina resulting in a circle of blur on the retina (Fig. 6.2).

This produces mild to moderate myopia, diminishing distant vision. An emmetropic eye accommodates for near as per age and distance of the near point from the retina (refer 'Accommodation' in Chapter 8). Lesser is the age, more is the accommodation. Similarly, shorter the near point more is accommodation required.

Features of an Emmetropic Eye

1. The anteroposterior length from anterior surface of the cornea to retina is 24 mm.

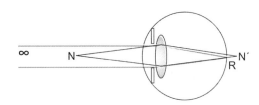

Figure 6.1: Emmetropia rays from infinity are brought to focus on the retina (R) and the rays from near point (N) are brought to focus behind the retina at N' when accommodation is at rest.

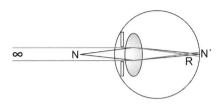

Figure 6.2: Accommodation in an emmetropic eye

2. The average diameter of cornea is 11 mm vertically and 12 mm horizontally.
3. This makes cornea more curved in vertical meridian.
4. The curvature of the cornea is 7.8 mm.
5. The central 3 mm of the cornea is more spherical than the periphery.
6. The total dioptric power of an emmetropic eye is +60D with anterior focal length of 15 mm and posterior focal length of 24 mm.
7. The parallel rays are focused on the photosensitive layer of the retina when accommodation is at rest.
8. The unaided vision in an emmetropic eye is 6/6 provided, the media are clear and the fundus is normal.
9. In an emmetropic eye, the angle kappa is 5° positive.
10. An emmetropic eye is generally orthophoric, but can be heterophoric or heterotropic.
11. The accommodation of an emmetropic eye varies with age. It is more in young people as compared to old people.
12. Near point also varies with age. In pre-presbyopic adult, it is about 30 cm and gradually increases with age.

AMETROPIA

Ametropias are a group of refractive disorders of the eye where the parallel rays are not brought to pinpoint focus on the retina when accommodation is at rest. Accommodation worsens myopia and astigmatism facultative hypermetropia is corrected by accommodation.

In compound hypermetropic astigmatism, the error is partially abolished because, the refraction in all meridians shifts toward the retina, reducing the circle of blur.

Ametropia can be divided into two types:
1. Spherical.
2. Cylindrical.

Both spherical and cylindrical errors can either be myopic, corrected by minus lens and hypermetropic, corrected by plus lens.

Etiology

The following are the ways by which ametropia can be produced:
1. Abnormal axial length of the eyeball.
2. Change in curvature of the ocular media:
   • Cornea:
     – Steep
     – Flat.
   • Lens:
     – Increased
     – Decreased.
3. Alteration in refractive index of ocular media:
   • Lens:
     – Increased
     – Decreased
     – Absent.
   • Cornea: Increased.
4. Position of the ocular media: This is seen only in lens:
   • Move forwards
   • Move backwards
   • Tilt
   • Absent.

Abnormal Axial Length of the Eyeball

The normal adult emmetropic eye is 24 mm long. 1 mm of change in axial length produces an ametropia of 3D, i.e. if the eyeball is 25 mm long, it will become myopic by 3D and if it is 23 mm long, it will become hypermetropic by 3D. The axial length may be as less as 20 mm or as much as 30 mm. Thus, making them hypermetropic by (24 – 20) × 3 = 4 × 3 = 12D or myopic by (30 – 24) × 3 = 6 × 3 = 18D respectively. Such a high hypermetropia is infrequent except in aphakia. Changes in the axial length are the commonest cause of ametropia as compared to other causes.

Change in Curvature of the Ocular Media

The change is more marked and frequent in cornea. The change in lenticular curvature is relatively rare and seen only in congenital conditions of lenticonus.

For all clinical purposes, the corneal curvature is taken as 8 mm. An increase in 1 mm curvature will produce 6D–7D of myopia, while flattening of curvature by same degree will produce hypermetropia of 6D–7D. The example of increased corneal curvature, resulting in myopia is keratoconus. Flattening of corneal curvature is of less clinical importance. It can be seen in microphthalmos, microcornea and cornea plana. The cornea in a soft eye is relatively flatter. Irregular change in corneal curvature induces astigmatism.

Alteration of Refractive Index of Ocular Media

Abnormality of refractive index of lens is very common acquired cause of ametropia. Less common is change in the refractive index of cornea. Refractive indices of aqueous humor and vitreous humor are not known to change.

The normal refractive index of a clear lens is 1.337. If it becomes more as seen in central nuclear sclerosis, early concussion cataract and hyperglycemia, the error of refraction shifts toward myopia. This change in myopia may be very little or may be as much as –3D. In contrast to this, if the refractive index becomes less

than 1.337, the ametropia shifts toward hypermetropia. The commonest cause of such shift is drug-induced hypoglycemia following initiation of antidiabetic treatment or steep increase in dose of antidiabetic drug in patient already under treatment for diabetes or skipping the diet. This can also happen following switching to unaccustomed exercise regime. Some other drugs like acetazolamide and its derivatives are known to cause mild to moderate myopia.

Corneal edema also produces moderate myopia.

Position of Ocular Media

Out of four components of the ocular media, i.e. cornea, aqueous humor, lens and vitreous humor, only lens can undergo displacement. Posterior shift of the whole lens can cause hypermetropia, anterior shift of the whole lens causes myopia. Tilting of the lens induces astigmatism.

CLASSIFICATION OF AMETROPIA

Ametropia is mainly classified into myopia, hypermetropia and astigmatism (Fig. 6.3).

MYOPIA

Myopia is that error of refraction where parallel rays are brought to focus in front of the retina when accommodation is at rest (Fig. 6.4). Accommodation worsens myopia (Figs 6.5A and B). The myopic far point is at a finite distance in front of the eye.

Myopia is the commonest form of error of refraction all over the world. Primary myopia is more common in children. Central nuclear sclerosis is the common cause of acquired secondary myopia after 50 years of age.

In myopia, parallel rays are brought to focus in front of the retina at the secondary focal point of the eye forming a circle of blur on the retina. More is the myopia, larger is the circle of blur and farther is the image from the retina.

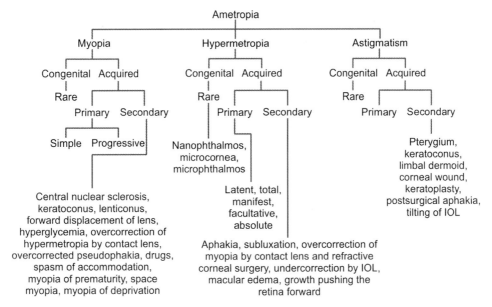

Figure 6.3: Outline of classification of ametropia (IOL, intraocular lens)

The far point of the myopic eye is between cornea and infinity from where the rays arise to behave like parallel rays. The far point is equal to a concave lens, the focal point of which coincides with it. The near point of the myopia of the 4D is 25 cm.

Accommodation worsens the myopia as it shifts the image forward making the circle of blur larger (refer Figs 6.5A and B).

The commonest form of myopia is axial myopia, followed by index myopia. Myopia is prevalent world over; some races are more prone than others. It is equal in both sexes. It is generally bilateral and almost equal in both the eyes. Most of the time, myopia is gradual in onset, when acute, the causes other than axial myopia should be sought. Most of the myopias stabilize after few years. It has strong genetic influence. 20% of myopic children are born to parents who are myopes. If one parent has myopia, this figure drops to 10%. Rest of the myopias are sporadic who may pass the tendency to the coming generations. It is common to see many of the siblings to have myopia.

Clinical Types of Myopia/ Classification of Myopia

Myopia has been classified variously. The most comprehensive classification is shown in Figure 6.6.

Congenital Myopia

Congenital myopia is rare. The exact cause, especially in unilateral cases, which is otherwise more common than bilateral, is not well understood. In bilateral cases, the cause may be some unknown factors, which influence the growth of the sclera in utero. The congenital myopia, unilateral or bilateral is present at birth, but missed unless fundus has been

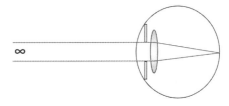

Figure 6.4: Emmetropia when accommodation is at rest

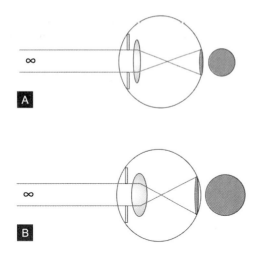

Figures 6.5A and B: Myopia with or without active accommodation. **A.** Myopia without accommodation (small circle of blur); **B.** Myopia with active accommodation (large active of blur).

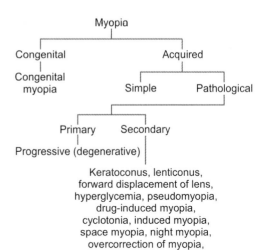

Figure 6.6: Classification of myopia

examined for some reason. In bilateral cases, its presence becomes obvious by 2–3 years when parents become aware of poor vision in the child. Unilateral cases go unnoticed unless the child starts squinting. Squint is generally esotropia, as the eye converges to see clearly at far point that may be as short as 12–15 mm in front of the eye. The eye in unilateral myopia may be large enough to draw parent's attention. The congenital myopia is generally 8–10 diopters, which invariably does not progress much. The fundus changes are similar to that seen in progressive myopia. In unilateral cases, the eye with myopia is generally amblyopic due to prevailing anisometropia and changes in the fundus. The congenital myopia may be associated with other congenital anomalies like cataract, aniridia, megalocornea, Marfan's syndrome and homocystinuria.

Management: The management of congenital myopia consists of:

1. Early diagnosis.
2. Full cycloplegic refraction with special reference to associated astigmatism, which is common.
3. Little under correction to give comfortable near correction.
4. Management of amblyopia when present by usual antiamblyopic treatment.
5. Contact lenses are given when the child is old enough to manage the contact lenses.
6. Refractive surgery after 21 years of age.
7. Regular yearly examination of fundus under full mydriasis by indirect ophthalmoscope for any degeneration.
8. Peripheral degenerations when present should be managed by the standard procedures.
9. These patients are prone to develop rhegmatogenous retinal detachment in spite of fairly good visual correction.
10. The best corrected vision in congenital myopia is seldom better than 6/12.
11. Clear lens extraction is a viable option.
12. The eyes are prone to develop posterior subcapsular opacity, open angle glaucoma, macular degeneration and macular hemorrhage.

Acquired Myopia

Acquired myopia is difficult to classify satisfactorily. It can roughly be divided into primary myopia where no specific causative factor can be found to correlate with the condition and secondary where, the condition can be attributed to some ocular or systemic cause.

Primary myopia

Primary myopia can be divided into two classes:

1. Simple myopia.
2. Progressive myopia.

Features of the two may overlap.

Simple myopia

Simple myopia is the commonest type of myopia. There are two age groups that are inflicted by this refractive disorder. They are:

1. Simple myopia in children.
2. Simple myopia in young adults.

The etiopathogenesis is same in both. The former is more frequent than the latter. As the former is seen between 6 and 12 years that corresponds to school age, it is also called school myopia (Table 6.1).

It has been amply proved that near work in school has no effect on progress of school myopia.

The latter is seen between 15 and 20 years of age when a person reaches high school or college, so it is called college myopia, refer Table 6.1. It is less in diopters as compared to school myopia, but is more often associated with moderate amount of astigmatism. The glasses required to give best vision, rarely exceeds –2D to –2.5D. Prognosis in both is good and vision can be improved to 6/6 with correction. Both the conditions stabilize after few years. The school myopia stabilizes in about 5–6 years with increment of 0.5D–1.00D every year. The college myopia stabilizes in about 2–3 years with little increase in power.

The commonest cause of simple myopia is disparity between dioptric power of the eye and the axial length. The axial length in simple myopia is in excess to axial length of an emmetropic eye. The exact cause of simple myopia is not well elucidated. It is thought to be a condition of overshooting the physiological limits of growth of the eyeball. At birth, all eyes except congenital myopia have short axial length, hence are hypermetropic. As the child grows, over next years the axial length increases reducing axial hypermetropia. By the age of 5–6 years, the axial length becomes almost 24 mm that is equal to axial length in adult and the child becomes emmetropic. Only about 10%–15% of the eyes will keep on growing beyond stipulated 24 mm and become myopic. Like all primary myopias, simple myopia too has genetic predisposition. Exact mode of inheritance is not clear. There are two theories, one feels that it is autosomal dominant and the other feels it to be recessive. The exact genetics behind the condition

Table 6.1: Comparison between school myopia and college myopia

Features	School myopia	College myopia
Type of myopia	Simple	Simple
Age of onset	First decade	Second half of second decade
Increment in power	0.5D–1.00D yearly	Not much
Final power after stabilization	–5D to –6D	–2D to –2.5D
Associated astigmatism	Less common	Frequent
Stabilized by	17–18 year	22–25 year

can only be reached by mapping the myopic gene marker, which is being awaited.

Symptoms: The symptoms are mostly visual, which manifests as diminished distant vision, with normal near vision, hence, it is also called nearsightedness. The term nearsighted is relevant when referred to myopia in contrast to farsightedness used for hypermetropia because myopia is always associated with diminished distant vision and normal near vision, while hypermetropia may have diminished distant vision need not have diminished near vision.

The child may not be aware of diminished vision, but the parents realize that the child does not recognize far objects as other children. The child moves too close the television or the teacher complains that the child does not comprehend writings on the blackboard. The diminished vision is gradual, painless and almost equal in both eyes. It rarely causes headache or asthenopia.

Signs: There are hardly any external signs in simple myopia of moderate degree except deliberate narrowing of the interpalpebral aperture, phorias that may break into tropias. The child narrows the interpalpebral aperture to produce a pinhole effect that increases the vision by few lines.

The fundus changes are minimal that include:

1. Disk larger than emmetropia and hypermetropia.
2. Paleness of disk.
3. Temporal crescent (rare).

Complications: In simple myopia are few under 40 years of age. The complications become evident by 4th–5th decade and include:

1. Early development of central nuclear sclerosis.
2. Chronic simple glaucoma.
3. Lattice degeneration of the peripheral retina.

4. Rhegmatogenous retinal detachment.
5. Rhegmatogenous detachment is more frequent in simple myopia as compared to emmetropia and hypermetropia, but less common than in progressive myopia.

Diagnosis: As follows:

1. History of bilateral, gradual, diminished distant vision in a child is strongly suggestive of simple myopia.
2. Positive family history of myopia in parents and siblings point toward presence of myopia.
3. Narrowing of interpalpebral aperture—improvement of vision by pinhole to almost 6/6.
4. Subjective improvement with minus glasses.
5. The confirmatory diagnosis is reached by retinoscopy under cycloplegia that automatically eliminated pseudomyopia in the child.
6. The retinoscopy reading can be arrived at either by mirror retinoscope or streak retinoscope.
7. Autorefractometers are handy tools in screening myopia in large number of children.

Autorefractometer (Figs 6.7 and 6.8): It is a computerized digital instrument that is used to find out the error of refraction quickly as is required in mass screening of errors of refraction or in non-communicative, non-verbal or illiterate persons. It can be done under both cycloplegia or without cycloplegia. One eye at a time is examined. The machine contains a picture that moves in and out of focus when the patient looks at it and multiple readings are taken, which are computerized to give an average power along with its axes.

Treatment (Figs 6.9A and B):

1. There is no medical treatment available for myopia.
2. Diets do not have any role to play in improving vision.

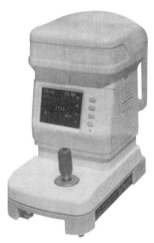

Figure 6.7: Autorefractometer

3. No vitamin can stop the progress of myopia.

4. Exercise and yoga have no role in management of myopia.

5. The definitive treatment is optical by spectacle.

Optical treatment is not curative, it is only palliative. Optical treatment does not stop progression of myopia; neither does it reduce the power.

6. The optical treatment consists of prescribing full correction in children and young adults and under correction over 30 years.

Myopes over 40 years do require near correction. They develop habit of removing the spectacle to do near work. This has led to misconception that presbyopia does not develop in myopes.

7. Older children who can manage contact lenses will prefer contact lenses over spectacles due to cosmetic reasons. Contact lenses in no way lead to reduction of myopia. The hypothesis that constant use of contact lens reduces or stabilizes myopia is called orthokeratology.

Orthokeratology: This is a technique used in myopia where a flat hard contact lens is prescribed for constant use. The contact lens should be flatter than the corneal curvature. The reduction of progression, if at all, is transient. This method is no more in vogue.

8. Refractive surgery is not indicated unless the patient has reached the age of 20 years

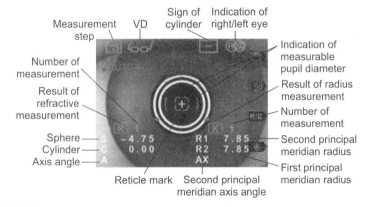

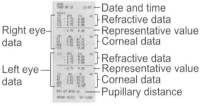

Figure 6.8: Autorefractometry. **A.** Various readings that can be taken by an autorefractometer; **B.** A typical reading [*Courtesy:* Appasamy Associates (with permission)].

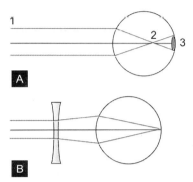

Figures 6.9A and B: Correction of myopia. **A.** Myopic eye; **B.** Myopic correction by concave lens, it brings the posterior focal plane on the retina, eliminating the circle of blur (**1.** Parallel rays brought to focus in front of the retina; **2.** It is posterior focal plane of the myopic eye; **3.** Circle of blurred vision).

and there is no increase in the power for at least 1 year.

9. The aim of treatment of myopia is not only improving vision, but also to bring back disparity between accommodation and convergence within physiological limits to make an eye orthophoric for distance and near. This will also eliminate any asthenopia when present.

Progressive myopia

Progressive myopia is also known as degenerative or pathological myopia. The optics involved in progressive myopia is same as simple myopia, i.e. increased axial length that brings the far point nearer than infinity, very close to eye forming a large circle of blur on the retina. It may be considered as exaggerated form of simple myopia with rapid progression and degenerative changes in posterior segment. Progressive myopia may begin at birth or first few years of life and increase relentlessly. The age of first presentation is little less than found in simple myopia. The extent of myopia at the first presentation may be as much as –3D or –4D, which progresses faster than in simple myopia. The progression may

be as much as –1D to –2D per year and reach the maximum by age of 12–15 tears. The maximum power may be as much as –20D to –25D. This fast progression differentiates it from congenital myopia, which rarely progresses beyond 8D–10D. Progressive myopia like simple myopia is a bilateral condition with strong hereditary tendency. It is mostly recessive trait. Both the parents are found to have some degree of axial myopia. Association of low degree of astigmatism is common. The power of the cylinder in progressive myopia does not follow the progression of the spherical power. Due to some unexplained factors, progressive myopia is more common in women. Some races are more prone to develop progressive myopia than others.

The exact cause of axial enlargement of the eye in progressive myopia not well understood. It is postulated that stretching of sclera is secondary to abnormal retinal growth. The choroidal changes are however, consequent to sclera stretching. The stretching of sclera is mostly posterior to equator. This is in contrast to stretching of sclera in buphthalmos where stretching is seen all over the globe, including the cornea.

Symptoms:

1. The commonest symptom for which the person seeks medical help is gross diminished distant vision that is not corrected much by narrowing the interpalpebral aperture. The vision may be as low as 2/60 to 3/60 without much improvement with pinhole even.

2. The best corrected vision fails to reach 6/6, which is rule in simple myopia. Nonimprovement of vision is due to changes in the retina in the posterior pole.

3. The patient keeps the book very near to read.

4. The patient may complain of glare due to relatively large and sluggish pupil.

5. Some patients may complain of large floaters in field. These are called muscae

volitantes. They are due to liquefaction of the vitreous.

6. Patients have diminished dark vision and prolonged dark adaptation due to peripheral chorioretinal degeneration.

7. Flashes of light are ominous sign of impending retinal detachment.

8. Squint: Commonest type of squint is esotropia. Sometimes there may be esotropic strabismus fixus due to degenerative changes in extraocular muscle.

Signs in progressive myopia can be divided into two groups such as:

1. Involving the anterior segment.
2. Involving the posterior segment.

1. **Signs in anterior segment:**

   a. The eyes have a bulging appearance due to posterior elongation of the globe. In case of unilateral high myopia, the affected eye may really bulge forward because axial length of a –20D eye will be 24 mm + 6.66 mm = 30.66 mm that will place the corneal vertex 6 mm forward than in emmetropia.

   b. The cornea is larger than in emmetropia. In absence of stretching of the anterior segment, it is not possible to explain this phenomenon.

   c. The angle kappa is negative.

   d. The anterior chamber is deeper than in emmetropia.

   e. Pupil is large and sluggish.

   f. The angle of anterior chamber is wide.

2. **Signs in posterior segment:** The posterior segment changes start early. It takes many years for them to develop fully to produce typical changes in retina and choroid. The posterior segment changes can be divided into following parts depending on the intraocular structure involved are as follows.

Optic nerve

a. The optic nerve looks larger than its actual size due to far placed nodal point and a large circle of blur as compared to emmetropia. The size of the disk looks normal when seen by direct ophthalmoscope through the correcting lens.

b. The disk is pale.

c. The cup looks proportionately large giving a false impression of the glaucoma.

d. The pallor may be mistaken as mild optic atrophy.

Peripapillary area:

a. Temporal crescent: The retina stops short of reaching the border of the disk and the choroid is visible in a crescent fashion with concavity toward the disk.

b. Annular crescent: The crescent may be seen all around. This is relatively rare.

c. Supertraction of retina: The retina in contrast to temporal crescent where it stops short is drawn over the nasal disk border, mostly due to oblique entrance of the optic nerve. This may also be found in emmetropic eye sometimes.

Choroid and retina:

a. The first visible change is appearance of tigroid fundus (tessellated fundus) where the large choroidal vessels become visible following atrophy of retinal pigment epithelium and choriocapillaries. This condition does not have any adverse effect on the vision and may be found even in emmetropic eyes with normal vision.

b. The next stage consists of disappearance of large part of choroidal tissue exposing sclera. The patches are similar to large patches of healed choroiditis. The patches may be confluent or scattered.

c. The choroidal atrophy is more pronounced around the posterior pole.

d. The most important and major cause of non-improvement of vision or sudden lowering of vision in progressive myopia is Foster-Fuchs spot (fleck).

Foster-Fuch spot: This is an oval red area surrounded by pale area. The red color is imparted by subretinal neovascularization and hemorrhage. The spot may be on the macula or be paramacular. The subretinal hemorrhage and neovascularization may be spontaneous or secondary to lacquer cracks.

Lacquer cracks: These cracks are breaks in Bruch's membrane and retinal pigment epithelium. About 4% of myopic eyes develop lacquer cracks in the early part of the progressive myopia. The lacquer cracks may be mistaken as angioid streak, which are independent of myopia, but they themselves are capable of developing subretinal neovascularization. The lacquer cracks are fine branching pale lines that may cross each other. Their presence is fraught with danger of loss of vision due to choroidal hemorrhage.

The peripheral changes are limited to retina. They consist of cystoid and lattice degeneration. Other peripheral degenerations are not common in progressive myopia. Peripheral retinal holes may develop with or without peripheral retinal degeneration that may lead to rhegmatogenous retinal detachment.

Vitreous:

a. Vitreous changes in progressive myopia are common. They start in young age producing vitreous opacities (muscae volitantes).

b. In late stages, the vitreous may completely liquefy.

c. Posterior vitreous detachment.

d. Vitreoretinal adhesions.

e. Traction detachment.

Sclera

Sclera in pathological myopia is thinner than in emmetropia. The sclera rigidity is low, the stretching of sclera is confined to posterior segment; in very high myopia posterior staphyloma may develop round or in the posterior pole. The posterior staphyloma is a bulge in the sclera lined by choroid and retina. The retinal blood vessels dip in the ectatic choroid. The staphyloma on retinoscopy is found to be more myopic than rest of the eye. It is best visualized by indirect ophthalmoscope and CT.

Complications of progressive myopia: Eyes with progressive myopia are prone for many complications spread over both anterior and posterior segments. The complications are more marked and vision-threatening in posterior segment.

The posterior segment complications are subretinal hemorrhage, subretinal neovascularization, vitreous liquefaction, posterior vitreous detachment and rhegmatogenous retinal detachment. It is presumed that myopic disk rarely develops papilledema.

The anterior segment complications consist of presenile development of age-related cataract in the form of posterior capsular opacity and central nuclear sclerosis. The eyes with vitreous degeneration and liquefaction are more prone for vitreous disturbance and nuclear drop during lens implantation. Pseudophakic retinal detachment is also more common in progressive myopia. Myopic eyes are more prone to develop chronic simple glaucoma and high degree of esotropia.

Management of progressive myopia: The optics involved in management of progressive myopia is same as in simple myopia that is bringing the posterior plane to the retina. This is obtained by minus lenses, the focal length of which should be equal to the far point of the myopic eye. This helps the rays to enter the eye as parallel rays. This is best obtained following retinoscopy under complete cycloplegia. It is better to under correct high myopia, no doubt this results in poor distant correction, but at the same time gives comfortable near vision and brings accommodation and convergence within physiological limits. A high myope in range 10–15 may be under corrected up to –3D depending upon near vision requirements. Another disadvantage of full spectacle correction is minification of image. The high minus lenses give considerable amount of peripheral restriction of field, hence they may be given myodisk that have power in the central 15 mm and the periphery is flat. Better results are obtained by contact lenses that have less peripheral distortion, absence of minification and a good cosmetic appearance. A high myope in presbyopic age may be given near correction in the form of spectacle over contact lens or a bifocal contact lens.

Surgical Treatment of Myopia in General

Surgical treatment for myopia is becoming more popular than about 2 decades ago. The main cause behind the popularity are safety of present day surgery, scope of resurgery, elimination of low myopia, reduction of high myopia to a lower level, elimination of peripheral distortion and minification and overall better cosmetic appearance.

The surgical treatment should be undertaken, only when the person is over 20 years of age, the power has been stable for at least 1 year. The patient if made aware of the fact that elimination of power in no way influences the changes in the posterior segment.

The surgical treatment is divided into two broad groups:

1. More popular and practiced surgery on the cornea.
2. Less common and less practiced are lens related surgeries.

The surgeries on the cornea can be:

1. Incisional.
2. Laser.
3. Incisional with laser application.

Lens related surgeries can be:

1. Clear lens extraction.
2. Clear lens extraction with posterior chamber intraocular lens (PCIOL).
3. Phakic IOL.

Surgeries on Cornea

Incisional corneal surgery (radial keratotomy): This was the most widely performed surgery for myopia about 2–3 decades ago. This has been given up in favor of better non-incisional surgeries. The radial keratotomy is a microsurgery that requires the use of special microinstrument. The surgery is done under local anesthesia. The actual procedure consists of giving partial thickness radial incisions beginning on the periphery and ending centrally, leaving a 4 mm clear central zone in front of the pupil. The number of incisions and depth of incision depends on extent of myopia.

Non-incision procedure (photorefractive keratectomy): In this, excimer laser with 193 nm wavelength is used to photoablate the central cornea. It gives very satisfactory result in moderate myopia. The laser breaks the intermolecular bonds in the cornea. This molds the cornea, changing the power of the cornea.

Incisional cum laser procedure: Presently, this is most widely practiced procedure for myopia. In this procedure, a circular flap of 130–160 μ thickness is fashioned and everted. This is followed by ablation of mid-stroma by excimer and repositing the flap back. This flattens the cornea, reducing the myopia.

Procedures on the Lens

Clear lens extraction: This is mostly indicated in unilateral high myopia, above 16, but can also be done in bilateral high myopias. Here, the lens is removed as small incision cataract surgery (SICS) or by phako and the eye is left aphakic to be corrected by contact lens.

Lens extraction with PCIOL: The lens is extracted by phaco and a suitable PCIOL is placed in the back as per biometric reading.

Secondary myopia

All secondary myopias are considered to be pathological. Some of them are progressive. Some may be transient. They can be curvature or index in nature. Examples of progressive secondary myopias are keratoconus and central nuclear sclerosis. Others are non-progressive and may be transient. The examples of transient myopia are hyperglycemia, spasm of accommodation and drug induced.

One of the common causes of secondary myopia is keratoconus.

Keratoconus

Keratoconus is the commonest cause of curvature myopia. It is non-inflammatory in nature and considered to be a dystrophy of all the layers of the cornea. The defect lies mostly in the corneal collagen. The condition is bilateral, almost symmetrical and progressive. Its presence is generally felt by the end of 1st decade of life when the parents report too frequent increment of myopia, which is invariably compound myopic astigmatism. Though the condition is progressive, it gets stabilized by the 4th decade. By the time, the vision is reduced to a level from where it cannot be salvaged by spectacle or contact lens. Some patients at puberty pass into hydrops of cornea, which is a painful condition with opaque cornea, lacrimation and excessive photophobia.

Diagnosis

Diagnosis of fully developed keratoconus is not difficult by history of frequent change in myopic change of compound myopic astigmatism that cannot be corrected by spectacle or contact lenses. The early signs are:

1. Non-improvement of vision by pinhole.
2. Scissor reflex on retinoscopy.
3. Oblique astigmatism on keratometry.
   Late signs are:
1. Black dot at the center of pink retinal glow due to opacity at the apex of cone.
2. Vogt's striae in the stroma on slit lamp.
3. Fleischer ring at the base of the cone.
4. Egg-shaped mire on keratometry.

Management is as follows:

1. Optical correction by spectacle.
2. Optical correction by rigid gas permeable contact lenses.
3. When vision no longer improves by optical devices, then there are two options:
   a. Penetrating keratoplasty: This gives very satisfactory results because the peripheral cornea is normal to which the donor material of normal thickness can be stitched.
   b. Corneal collagen cross-linking by riboflavin and ultraviolet A from a solid ultraviolet source.
4. Refractive surgeries are contraindicated in keratoconus due to its irregular thinness.

Lenticonus

Lenticonus is a rare congenital anomaly of lens. It can be anterior or posterior lenticonus. The latter is more common, is generally unilateral. In both the conditions, there is a bulge in the capsule that contains capsule and part of the cortex, in the central 2–5 mm of the axis of the lens. This results in axial index myopia. The patient has diminished distant central vision that becomes worse if the pupil constricts. There is an oil drop appearance in the lens when seen through a slit lamp with dilated pupil. On retinoscopy, the central reflex is myopic and peripheral, relatively hypermetropic. There is a scissor movement on retinoscopy. The posterior lenticonus has more tendencies to develop cortical cataract.

Management comprises of optical correction, as long as possible. In children and young adults, pupil may be kept dilated to give better vision from the periphery of the lens. Once a stage has been reached, when optical correction no more suffices, the only option left is to do a lensectomy by phako and implanting a PCIOL.

Forward displacement of the lens

Forward displacement of the lens is again a rare phenomenon that is mostly traumatic, but can happen in ectopia lentis as well. The patient has diminished distant vision that can be corrected optically. The patient should be under observation for possible subluxation, lenticular opacity, secondary narrow angle glaucoma and frank location.

Hyperglycemic myopia

Hyperglycemic myopia is a fairly common refractive change in diabetes due to hydration of the lens resulting in index myopia that follows abnormally high blood sugar. The patient with diabetes may consult an ophthalmologist for the first time with diminished distant vision and is found to have high blood sugar. Other possibility is that a diabetic presbyope may report that he/she no more requires near vision correction. The exact blood sugar level that can cause myopia is not clear. It varies from patient to patient. The condition passes off following lowering blood sugar. Diabetes is more often associated with central nuclear sclerosis that also causes index myopia, irrespective of blood sugar level. Central nuclear sclerosis can be managed optically for sometimes, but the eye will be ultimately operated for cataract with IOL implant.

Pseudomyopia

Pseudomyopia is an iatrogenic myopia due to miscalculation of power. It is seen in children, who are in fact hypermetropes reporting with asthenopia. Such children are misdiagnosed as myopes and prescribed minus glasses subjectively. The vision initially seems to improve. Addition of minus lenses increase his accommodation, enhancing shifting of the retinal image forward requiring increase in power at every visit till the condition becomes unbearable due to headache and blurring of vision. The best way to avoid and treat such cases is to ask the patient to refrain from using minus glasses for few days and doing refraction under complete cycloplegia, preferably atropine and prescribe glasses as per retinoscopy findings, which invariably turn out to be hypermetropic or astigmatic. This makes it mandatory to do the refraction in all children less than 10 years under complete cycloplegia, irrespective of initial vision.

Drug-induced myopia

Drug-induced myopia is also an iatrogenic myopia. The drugs that can induce myopia can either be systemic or local. The commonly used drug that causes myopia is acetazolamide taken orally. The locally acting drugs are strong miotics. In the first instance, the myopia is index myopia due to changes in the cortex. In the second case, instilled drugs cause ciliary spasm that in turn induces accommodation causing the image to move forwards, away from the retina. Both the conditions are treated by discontinuation of the medicine. Miotic-induced myopia may require instillation of cycloplegia for 2–3 days.

Cyclotonia-induced myopia

Cyclotonia-induced myopia can happen following:

1. Instillation of strong miotics in emmetropes and worsening of already existing myopia, reducing hypermetropia.
2. Blunt injury causing spasm of ciliary body.

Both are treated by instillation of cycloplegia.

Space myopia (empty space/field myopia)

Space myopia is a transient myopia experienced by jet-pilots at great heights, from where neither the landmarks on the earth or anything in the black space is visible. The normal human eyes require the outline of an object to stimulate the rays to travel from object of interest to the retina. In absence of this, the eyes accommodate at an intermediate distance producing myopia. The condition can be averted in absence of a fixing point in the space by fixing the tip of the wing on either side of the aircraft by the pilot.

Night myopia

Night myopia is an acquired myopia low presbyopes who try to read in dim light and are happy with induced myopia that neutralizes part of their near requirement. The condition passes off when the patient is counseled properly to read in suitably lit place.

Overcorrection myopia

Overcorrection myopia is yet another iatrogenic myopia produced either by overcorrection of hypermetropia by refractive surgeries, by spectacle or contact lens. The former requires resurgery for myopia and the second requires adjustment for the contact lens or spectacle as per retinoscopy.

Myopia of prematurity

Myopia of prematurity is a condition of ill-understood etiology. It is generally seen in children with birth weight of 1,250 g or less. It is more common in children with retinopathy of prematurity (ROP), but can be seen in premature children without ROP as well. Incidence in the second instance is less. The myopia, when diagnosed early, may be found to range between –10D and –20D. Fortunately, myopia gets reduced to 1D–2D by 1 year. In some cases, myopia may not regress and persist and diagnosed as congenital myopia. The cause of regression is not known.

HYPERMETROPIA (HYPEROPIA)

Hypermetropia is that ametropia where parallel rays are brought to focus behind the photosensitive layer of the retina when accommodation is at rest. Accommodation can partially or completely eliminate hypermetropia (Figs 6.10A to C).

Hypermetropia is distributed all over the world. Some races are more prone to be hypermetropic. It is generally bilateral and equal (isometropic). However, some cases may be unilateral with normal vision in the other eye (anisometropia). Unilateral hypermetropia is more common than unilateral myopia. Unilateral hypermetropia is more prone to develop anisometropic amblyopia and squint.

All children except congenital myopics are born hypermetropic by about 3.0D sphere. This is a paradox because the axial length of

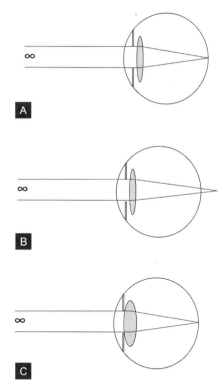

Figures 6.10A to C: Optics of hypermetropia. **A.** Emmetropia when accommodation is at rest, parallel rays are brought to focus on the retina; **B.** Hypermetropia when accommodation is at rest, parallel rays are brought to focus behind the retina; **C.** Hypermetropia when accommodation is active, the parallel rays are brought to focus on the retina (hypermetropia is corrected).

the newborn eye is 16.5–17.5 mm. To be ametropic, an eye should be about 24 mm. In the previous pages, we have seen that 1 mm of shortening of axial length from emmetropic eye results in hypermetropia of 3D. Thus, an eye 17 mm long should be 24–17 mm = 7 mm and be 21D hypermetropic.

The discrepancy is explained by two facts:

1. The lens of a newborn is more spherical than adult.
2. The cornea of newborn is steeper in relation to axial length. It has been pointed out earlier that 1 mm steeping of cornea causes 7D of myopia.

Thus, the two factors, i.e. lenticular steepening and corneal steepening added together neutralize the axial hypermetropia mostly, leaving only +3D of error of refraction.

As the child grows, the axial length increases rapidly and by 5–6 years, it reaches the emmetropic length. At this stage, 3 things can happen:

1. Eye fails to reach emmetropic length and the eye becomes hypermetropic.
2. The eye reaches the emmetropic length and becomes emmetropic.
3. The axial length overshoots emmetropic length and becomes myopic.

Though the axial length in adult hypermetropia is shorter, the refractive power of the cornea and the lens are within normal limits.

Classification of Hypermetropia

Like all errors of refraction, hypermetropia too has been classified in many ways. Unfortunately, none is sufficient enough to cover all types of hypermetropia (Figs 6.11 and 6.12).

Structural Hypermetropia

Structural hypermetropia can be caused due to following factors.

Axial length: A shortening of 1 mm of the axial length causes 3D of hypermetropia. Axial hypermetropia is rarely more than +6D except in congenital conditions like nanophthalmos. In microphthalmos, not only the axial length is short, but the cornea is also flatter, which added to short axial length makes hypermetropia worse.

Curvature: A flattening of 1 mm of the corneal or lenticular curvature causes 6D of hypermetropia.

Refractive index: If the refractive index is reduced to less than 1.37, the eye becomes hypermetropic. The exact relation between

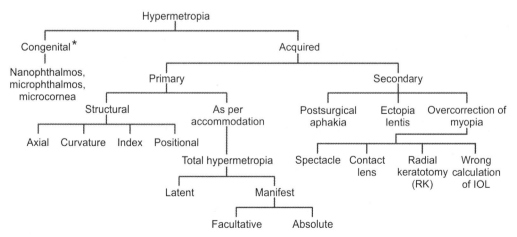

Figure 6.11: Mostly used classification of hypermetropia. *All congenital hypermetropias are pathological, present at birth and difficult to treat.

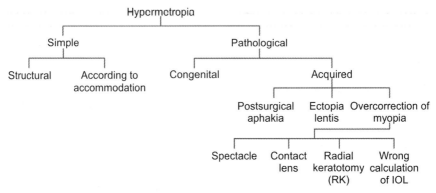

Figure 6.12: Another way of classifying hypermetropia

refractive index and hypermetropia is not well understood. The common causes of index hypermetropia are:

1. Age: As age advances, the cortex becomes less convergent and the lenticular curvature also flattens.

2. Hypoglycemia: Persons during initial stages of treatment for diabetes are prone to develop hypermetropia due to relative dehydration of the lens. Even those under treatment for diabetes for long time may become hypermetropic due to sudden increase in dose of antidiabetic, decreased calorie intake or enhanced physical activity.

Displacement: Backward shift of 1 mm the lens in optical axis causes 1.4D of hypermetropia. Total absence of lens as in aphakia of any etiology causes maximum hypermetropia, which is roughly +10D sphere.

Other causes of hypermetropia are mostly iatrogenic:

1. Pharmacological: Facultative hypermetropia may pass into absolute hypermetropia following ingestion of parasympatholytic drugs.

2. Hypermetropia can be unmasked by use of cycloplegic locally.

3. Optical: Overcorrection of myopia by contact lens or spectacle.

4. Surgical: Overcorrection of myopia by radial keratotomy (RK) or laser-assisted in situ keratomileusis (LASIK).

5. Residual hypermetropia following IOL implant.

Hypermetropia According to Available Accommodation

On the basis of accommodation, the hypermetropia can be latent and manifest. The manifest hypermetropia is again divided into facultative and absolute. The sum of all is called total hypermetropia (Fig. 6.13).

Total hypermetropia: This is the sum of all hypermetropias. It can only be fully elicited under complete cycloplegia by atropine. One example of total hypermetropia is aphakia where there is no lens; hence the eye is in the perpetual state of absence of accommodation. The other conditions that can precipitate absolute hypermetropia are internal and total III nerve palsy.

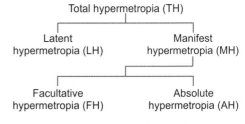

Figure 6.13: Classification of total hypermetropia

Latent hypermetropia: This is due to inherent tone of ciliary muscle and is present in all hypermetropic eyes without being felt by the person, because it is symptoms less. It can be unmasked by subtracting manifest hypermetropia from total hypermetropia. It varies between 0.5D and 1.0D sphere and gradually declines with age with little clinical significance.

Manifest hypermetropia: This represents total hypermetropia—latent hypermetropia and is sum of facultative hypermetropia and absolute hypermetropia. Thus,

$$AH + FH = MH = TH - LH$$

This can be elicited without cycloplegia provided the patient fixes a distant object. It is partly corrected by patient's available accommodation and the remaining correction is corrected by plus sphere. The strongest plus sphere with which the patient remains 6/6 denotes manifest hypermetropia. Thus, MH = Accommodation + Convex lens.

1. Facultative hypermetropia: This is that part of hypermetropia, which can be corrected by the effect of accommodation. The patient has 6/6 distant vision and remains 6/6 by adding plus lenses till a stage is reached when the vision starts declining. This power gives the amount of facultative hypermetropia. It is the difference between manifest and absolute hypermetropia.

2. Absolute hypermetropia: This is not corrected by the effort of accommodation the patient has diminished distant vision. All facultative hypermetropes are likely to be converted into absolute hypermetropia after 60 years of age. The following examples depict various components of hypermetropia:

    a. Suppose an eye has a total hypermetropia of +5D as arrived following retinoscopy under atropine and has a latent hypermetropia of 0.5D.

    b. The patient manifest hypermetropia is +5.0D – 0.5D = +4.5D, which can

be arrived by retinoscopy even without cycloplegia provided, the patient fixes a distant object, relaxing accommodation completely.

    c. Out of this, +4.5D manifest hypermetropia, +1.5D sphere is facultative. Hence, he/she is left with absolute hypermetropia of +3D sphere that require to be corrected by plus lenses because eyes with absolute hypermetropia are bound to have subnormal distant vision.

Same can be arrived in a different way:

1. Let us consider an eye with subnormal vision that subjectively shows to have hypermetropia of +5.0D. This is absolute hypermetropia.

2. The eye retains vision 6/6 till this power is increased to +7D showing that he/she has been corrected +7D – (+5D) = +2D by accommodation.

3. +7D is manifest hypermetropia.

4. Under full cycloplegia, refraction comes to +7.5D out of which, +0.5D is latent hypermetropia.

5. Thus, he/she has got a +7.5D of the total hypermetropia.

Clinical Pictures

Symptoms

The term farsightedness for hypermetropia is irrelevant. It gives an impression as if all hypermetropic eyes have good distant vision. In fact, 50% of eyes in adults and all secondary hypermetropias like aphakia, dislocated lens and nanophthalmos are bound to have subnormal distance vision.

The symptoms depend on available accommodation, which in turn depends on:

1. Age of the patient:

    a. Children are more likely to be symptoms free because of their ability to accommodate more.

b. The 75% of hypermetropes above 60 have diminished distant vision due to less availability of accommodation.

2. Near vision requirements: Adults who are engaged in prolonged near work are more likely to develop symptoms of asthenopia and blurred distant vision.

3. All aphakes are bound to have diminished distant as well as near vision.

4. Patient may report with esotropia and are found to have hypermetropia.

5. Asthenopia.

6. Difficulty in near work.

7. Diminished distant vision.

8. Recurrent blepharitis, stye chalazion, chronic conjunctivitis.

9. The symptoms may be any of the above or a combination of two or more.

Signs

In case of low hypermetropia, there may be no external signs that may point toward presence of hypermetropia even distant vision may be normal and the patient may be able to read small prints without glasses.

The signs become evident in moderate to high hypermetropia. They include:

1. Relatively narrow interpalpebral aperture due to small eyeball.

2. Eyeball is small in axial hypermetropia. It is normal in curvature and index hypermetropia. Obviously, it will be within normal limits in aphakia.

3. The cornea is smaller than in emmetropia.

4. Anterior chamber is shallow and prone to angle closure after 40 years of age.

5. Angle kappa is positive, giving an impression of divergent squint.

6. Exophoria.

7. Accommodative esotropia.

8. Small pupil that takes more time to dilate with weak cycloplegia.

9. Low accommodative convergence/accommodation (AC/A).

10. Sclera has sharp curve at the equator.

11. The ciliary muscles are well developed.

12. The circular fibers are hypertrophied (this is not visible externally).

13. The fundus is small. It has shot-silk appearance. The retinal vascular reflexes are accentuated, may be mistaken as sclerosed.

14. The disk is small, giving an appearance of pseudoneuritis.

15. Fovea is dull.

16. Vision may be normal or subnormal.

17. Anisometropia is more common.

18. Uncorrected eyes are likely to develop amblyopia.

19. Amblyopia is more common in unilateral hypermetropia.

20. Presbyopia sets in early than in emmetropia.

Management

1. This depends upon the available accommodation.

2. The effort should be to bring back the posterior focal plane that is situated behind the retina to the retina.

3. This is achieved by prescribing plus lenses.

4. The principle involved in prescription of glasses to hypermetropes is:

   a. Unlike myopia, all persons with hypermetropia need not be corrected.

   b. Only symptomatic patients should be corrected.

   c. Extent of hypermetropia in persons under 50 years should be determined under cycloplegia.

   d. All patients under 10 years should be refracted under atropine.

   e. Manifest hypermetropia below 1D can be ignored, unless the patient is symptomatic.

f. The first prescription should be lowest that gives 6/6 vision.

g. It is preferably increased over months till the manifest hypermetropia has been reached.

h. The best method is to add 1/4th of latent to the manifest (Donder).

i. Hypermetropia with accommodative squint should be given full correction.

   To see an object at 1 m, an emmetrope requires accommodation of 1D and convergence of 1 ma. A hypermetrope of 4D will require +4 + 1 = +5D of accommodation and 5 ma of convergence. This is the cause of esotropia in moderate to high hypermetropia.

j. Amblyopia should always be suspected in unilateral hypermetropia and when detected should be treated by antiamblyopia treatment.

k. In some children, hypermetropia gets neutralized as the child grows and the eyeball elongates. Hence, all the hypermetropic children during their growing age should be refracted yearly under cycloplegia.

l. Patients above 50 years who are prone to develop central nuclear sclerosis may discard their plus correction due to second sight.

m. Pre-presbyopic patients who complain of difficulty in near work should be given full distant correction. This generally eliminates additional near correction.

n. Astigmatism when present, should be fully corrected, it should neither be under or over corrected because astigmatism is independent of accommodation.

o. Contact lens power in hypermetropia is more than spectacle power.

p. Surgical treatment in hypermetropia is not as rewarding as in myopia and should be performed only after 20 years of age.

Complications of Hypermetropia

1. Hypermetropic eyes are more prone to develop amblyopia, especially in anisometropia and in presence of high astigmatism.

2. Accommodative esotropia is more common in children. This may be seen in children as young as 2–3 years. Conversely, all children with esotropia should be refracted under atropine and prescribed glasses as per retinoscopy, including bifocals if needed.

3. The following two are the acute complications that are seen after 40 years of age:
   a. Acute narrow angle glaucoma.
   b. Non-arteritic anterior ischemic optic neuropathy.

Secondary hypermetropia mainly includes postsurgical aphakia, ectopia lentis, overcorrection of myopia, etc. Among these aphakia is the most important and is detailed below (refer Fig. 6.11).

Aphakia

Aphakia is the absence of crystalline lens from the pupillary area. It is most important cause of index, total hypermetropia. The commonest cause of aphakia is surgical removal, either by intracapsular cataract extraction (ICCE) or extracapsular cataract extraction (ECCE). Spontaneous absorption of traumatic cataract also results in aphakia with clinical features indistinguishable from ECCE.

The other causes of aphakia are dislocation of the lens as in Marfan's syndrome, Marchesani syndrome, homocystinuria, blunt trauma and spontaneous dislocation, generally seen in long-standing anterior uveitis and buphthalmos. Congenital aphakia is extremely rare.

Optics of Aphakia

Aphakia is the extreme form of hypermetropia where in spite of the high error of refraction, the vision can be fully restored optically, provided to media and the fundus are normal. The normal phakic emmetropic eye has a dioptric power of roughly +60D when accommodation is at rest. This refractive power of +60D is divisible into two parts:

1. A large corneal, that accounts for +43D.

2. Remaining +17D is attributed to clear lens.

An aphakic eye is nearer to Donders/Listing's concept of reduced eye of a single refracting surface, i.e. the cornea. This brings about the fundamental change in image formation in aphakic eye. In reduced eye, the anterior focal plane is 17.2 mm in front of the cornea and the posterior focal point is 24.4 mm from the cornea. The two principle points are taken to be on the anterior surface of the cornea. The two nodal points are so close to each other that, they are also taken to be single for calculation. This point is taken to be 7.75 mm (8 mm) from the anterior corneal surface (Fig. 6.14).

In aphakia, absence of lens brings about drastic change in image formation:

1. The anterior focal plane shifts forwards to 23.3 mm from the anterior cornea surface.

2. The posterior focal plane is shifted back to 31 mm from anterior corneal surface, which is 7 mm behind the retina. Thus, theoretically, if an eye were 31 mm long, which is almost impossible in clinical practice, should behave like an emmetropic eye.

3. This can otherwise be corrected by a plus lens with enough converging power, to bring the posterior focal plane back to retina. This can happen if:

   a. An artificial lens put over the nodal point as happens more or less in pseudophakia (incidentally, the power of lens in the posterior chamber is +20D and not +17D, which it replaces).

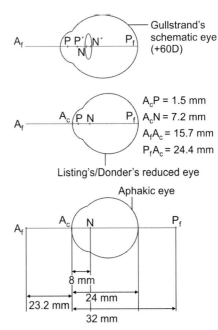

A$_c$P = 1.5 mm
A$_c$N = 7.2 mm
A$_f$A$_c$ = 15.7 mm
P$_f$A$_c$ = 24.4 mm

Listing's/Donder's reduced eye

Aphakic eye

8 mm

24 mm
23.2 mm
32 mm

A$_f$P$_f$ is the principal axis
A$_f$ is the anterior focal point
P$_f$ is the posterior focal point
P and P′ are the two principal points
N and N′ are two nodal points

Figure 6.14: Comparison between Gullstrand's schematic eye, Listing's/Donder's reduced eye and aphakic eye

   b. Putting a plus contact lens on cornea.

   c. Putting a +10D lens in a spectacle at the anterior focal plane. A +10D lens at anterior focal plane has an effective power of +17D lens in situ.

   d. Thus, if an eye was emmetropic before lens extraction, a plus +10D lens at anterior focal plane should correct the defect. An eye that was hypermetropic before lens extraction will require more than +10D sphere and a myopic will require less than +10D sphere in spectacles.

   e. The concept that addition of pre-existing power with +10D will determine the final power is not correct neither will a –5D preoperative will be corrected by +5D nor a plus +5D will require a +15D to be corrected. The best option is to do the refraction and prescribe according to the retinoscopy because aphakia following classical lens extraction is always associated with some degree of astigmatism against the rule. The astigmatism varies between 1 and 2 cylinders in horizontal axis. Preoperative astigmatism, unless very high cannot be correlated to postsurgical aphakia. It may be enhanced or decreased depending on its type, i.e. with the rule or against the rule.

The refraction in aphakia is static refraction because the eye has no accommodation hence there is no need of cycloplegia, the retinoscopy can be done under simple mydriatic, irrespective of age.

4. A commonly used formula to determine the power of the postsurgical aphakia in an ametropic eye is,

   A = +10D + ½a, where A stands for postoperative power and a stands for preoperative spectacle power. Example:

   a. A preoperative myopia of –5D will require a lens of +10D + (–5/2) = +10 – 2.5 = +7.5D sphere.

   b. In case of –20D, correcting required will be +10 + (–20/2) = +10 – 10 = 0D.

   c. A –10D will not be neutralized, but will require a corrective power of +5D.

   d. A +5D preoperative will not require +15D but +12.5D.

      Theoretically, an eye that is 31 mm long, i.e. 31 – 24 = 7 mm × 3 = –21D should require no glasses for distant vision, but this is not possible due to the fact that an eye with –21D has myopia too much of pathological changes in the posterior pole that does not permit the vision to improve beyond a certain limit.

5. As there is no accommodation, the distant vision must be supplemented with a +3D sphere. This near correction has a fixed focus, so a patient may require two separate near glasses, one for 25–30 cm for reading and another for intermediate distance of writing and eating. All aphakes do not tolerate bifocal, trifocal or progressive lenses unless the distant correction is low.

The greatest disadvantage of aphakic correction by spectacle glasses is 25%–33% magnification because an aphakic corrected by a plus power in spectacle acts as a Galilean telescope where the plus lens acts as a objective and a hypothetical minus lens in the eye as eyepiece. Magnification of 33% will make 1 m long object to look 1.33 m. This does not create much problem if:

1. Both eyes are aphakic and have almost equal power.

2. The other eye has very poor vision due to various reasons. The common causes of reduced vision in the other eye are advanced cataract, corneal opacity, fundus changes and divergent squint.

3. The problem arises in uniocular aphakia when the other eye has good vision and no magnification.

The difference in refractive power in two eyes is called anisometropia and the difference of size of the images in two eyes is called aniseikonia, both of which are accentuated in uniocular corrected aphakia. The normal eyes do not fuse with aniseikonia of more than 5%. This results in diplopia, which is the main cause of intolerance of glasses in uniocular aphakia. This can be mitigated by:

1. No power is given to the operated eye, which will ultimately get suppressed and diverge.

2. Occlude the normal eye, which the patient is unlikely to accept because the image seen through the operated eye corrected by glasses has many disadvantages. Moreover,

patching of one eye is not cosmetically accepted.

3. The diplopia can be avoided if the magnification could be brought down to 5%–7%. The two methods available to reduce the magnification and aniseikonia are:

    a. Contact lens.

    b. IOL.

Optical Correction of Aphakia

Optical correction of aphakia can be done by:

1. Spectacles.

2. Contact lens.

3. IOL.

Spectacle correction: Before the advent of IOL, spectacle correction of aphakia following traditional lens extraction was most popular and widely used method. It consists of:

a. Doing refraction under mydriasis.

b. Glasses for distance are prescribed as per retinoscopic finding that generally amounted to +9D sphere to +11D sphere with +1D to +2D cylinder at 180°. The spherical value in myopia was less than +10D and more than +10D in hypermetropia. The value of cylinder was not affected by preoperative spherical ametropia.

c. As there was no lens, there was no accommodation resulting in absence of near vision, which required supplementation of +2.5D to +3.5D on the distant correction.

Contact lens: These lenses are prescribed either as per keratometric finding or based on retinoscopic power. The power of the contact lens was more than +10D. It fails to correct astigmatism fully and near vision defect requires supplementation of +2.5D to +3D spectacle over the contact lens. The contact lens:

a. Is put on the cornea, nearer the nodal point than spectacle.

b. The power of the contact lens is more than the spectacle.

c. Contact lens gives a magnification of 8%–10%.

d. This is nearer to tolerable magnification of 5%.

e. The patient may tolerate up to 8% of magnification.

f. The contact lenses not only reduce the magnification, it also abolishes peripheral aberration and increases peripheral field of vision.

Intraocular lens (IOL): These are the most widely used methods of correction in aphakia. The IOL can be put either in the anterior chamber or posterior chamber. The anterior chamber lenses are no more in vogue as primary procedure. The posterior chamber intraocular lenses (PCIOLs) can be either in the sulcus or in the bag. The latter is most widely used primary procedure. Here, the power of the lens is calculated by biometer before the operation and the lens is implanted during lens extraction. The power of the IOL is more than spectacle or contact lens. As there is no astigmatism in pseudophakia, following phacoemulsification, there is no need of correction of astigmatism. If any astigmatism is left, it can be corrected either in the spectacle or by using a toric IOL as primary procedure. Theoretically there is no accommodation; however, some IOL's are available, which are capable of inducing accommodation. Otherwise, near vision is corrected by +2D to +2.5D sphere in the spectacle. The other method of avoiding spectacle correction for near is to make the eye slightly myopic with a vision 6/9 to 6/12 and fairly good near vision.

The posterior chamber IOL (PCIOL):

1. Is almost on the nodal point.

2. There is no magnification.

3. The power of IOL is more than +17D.

4. All the drawbacks of spectacle and contact lenses are absent in PCIOL.

Advantages and Disadvantages of Various Optical Devices in Aphakia

Drawbacks of spectacles in aphakia consists of:

1. Anisometropia.
2. Aniseikonia.
3. Magnification.
4. False sense of good vision—a corrected vision of 6/6 in aphakia is in fact equal to 6/9 to 6/12 of emmetropia.
5. Required separate addition of +3D sphere for near vision at 30 cm.
6. Spherical aberration leading to pincushion distortion (Figs 6.15A and B).
7. Prismatic effect.
8. Reduced peripheral field.
9. Ring scotoma (Fig. 6.16).
10. Jack in box phenomenon.
11. Cosmetic blemish (Fig. 6.17).

Advantages of contact lens over spectacle are:

1. Less magnification/aniseikonia.
2. Reduced chances of diplopia in uniocular aphakia.
3. Enlarged field.
4. Elimination of spherical and prismatic aberration.
5. Cosmetically better.

Disadvantages of contact lenses in aphakia:

1. Costly.
2. Requires separate near correction.
3. Difficulty in inserting and removing:

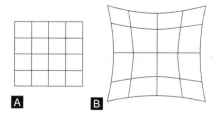

Figures 6.15A and B: Pincushion effect. **A.** A grill as seen through a plain sheet of glass; **B.** The same grill seen through an aphakic convex lens.

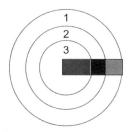

Figure 6.16: Ring scotoma. **1.** Is the incorrected field with blurred vision; **2.** Ring scotoma with no vision; **3.** Corrected central vision.

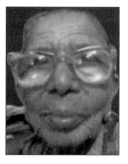

Figure 6.17: Cosmetic blemish in aphakia

a. Children may not be able to perform both.
b. Elderly may not be able to insert contact lens because:
   i. There is no near vision.
   ii. Diplopia, if the other eye has good vision.
   iii. Tremors in the hand.
   iv. Inability to flex the wrist due to arthritis.
4. Requires utmost cleanliness.
5. Lingering chances of contact lenses induced microbial keratitis.
6. Inability to locate the contact lens, if it is dislodged.

Advantages of PCIOL over spectacle and contact lenses correction:

1. All disadvantages/shortcomings of spectacles and contact lenses are absent in PCIOL.

2. Advent of IOL has completely eliminated all surgical procedures on cornea that were practiced once to correct high ametropia of aphakia.

ASTIGMATISM

Astigmatism is that error of refraction where all parallel rays are not brought to focus at a point may be in front or behind the photosensitive layer of the retina with or without accommodation. Accommodation even in hypermetropic astigmatism does not correct astigmatism. Some of the astigmatisms are worsened by accommodation. In hypermetropic astigmatism, the sign may change (Figs 6.18A to C).

It is difficult to find a real stigmatic eye. All eyes have some degree of astigmatism. All children at birth at astigmatic, which passes off within first few months, only in a few eyes it fails to resolve, these eyes remain astigmatic throughout the life. Unlike spherical errors, the value of the astigmatic correction rarely changes, especially in corneal astigmatism. Low degree of astigmatism is very common. It is generally associated with spherical ametropia, but only astigmatism without spherical error is no exception.

Astigmatism above 2D cylinder is considered to be high astigmatism. Primary astigmatism as high as 6D cylinders have been reported. Astigmatism has strong hereditary tendency. It is known to run in families. It is common to find astigmatism in siblings. There is no racial or sex difference in incidence of astigmatism.

Optics of Astigmatism

In astigmatism, all rays are not focused in a pinpoint. They are focused in two different planes in different meridians. These planes are called focal planes as opposed to focal points in stigmatic eyes. The eyes in astigmatism behave like a torus and the rays are focused in a manner similar to seen in Sturm's conoid.

The distance that separates the two principal planes is called Strum's interval or focal interval and represents the value of the cylinder that will counter the toracity. The circle of least confusion in Sturm's conoid denotes the spherical value of astigmatism. In simple astigmatism, the spherical value is nil. In compound and mixed astigmatisms, the spherical error is represented by a definite value. The aim of treatment of astigmatism is to abolish the Sturm's interval as far as possible.

Accommodation and Astigmatism

Accommodation does not correct astigmatism. The value of cylindric power remains the same with or without accommodation. By accommodating, the planes shift anteriorly. Thus, all types of astigmatism are converted into compound myopic astigmatism.

Types of Astigmatism

The types of astigmatism can be (Fig. 6.19):

1. Primary astigmatism: When no definite cause can be found.
2. Secondary astigmatism:
   • Trauma
   • Degeneration
   • Dystrophies.
3. Consecutive astigmatism:
   • Post-LASIK
   • Post-IOL.

Primary Astigmatism

The causes of primary astigmatism can be in the cornea, lens or retina. Corneal astigmatism is the commonest type of primary as well as secondary astigmatism. It accounts for about 90% of astigmatism.

Corneal Astigmatism

Corneal astigmatism can be:

1. Regular.
2. Irregular.

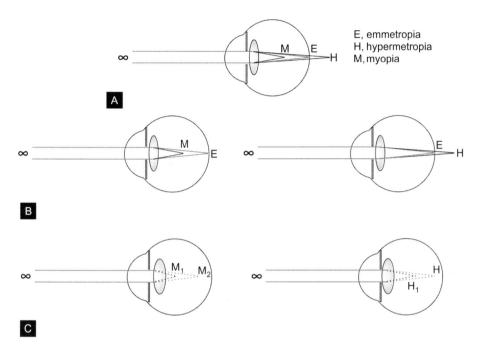

Figures 6.18A to C: Astigmatism and its types. **A.** Various types of stigmatic (spherial) error of refractions; **B.** Myopic and hypermetropic astigmatism when accommodation is at rest; **C.** Change in myopic and hypermetropic astigmatism when accommodation is active.

Regular astigmatism

Regular astigmatism is that astigmatism that has:

1. Two different meridians:
   • Vertical
   • Horizontal.
2. The axes are at right angles to each other, except in bi-oblique astigmatism where they are not at right angles:
   • One at 20°
   • The other at 120°.
3. The refraction in each meridian is uniform throughout.
4. The refraction changes gradually from one meridian to the other.
5. It is the commonest type of primary corneal astigmatism.

Types of regular astigmatism

1. According to the steepness of the vertical meridian:
   • With the rule
   • Against the rule.
2. According to relation of the two axes:
   • At right angles to each other
   • Not at right angles to each other.
3. According to the symmetry of the axes:
   • Symmetric—mirror image
   • Asymmetric.

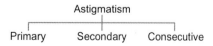

Figure 6.19: Various types of astigmatism

4. According to type of error of refraction:
   - Myopic
   - Hypermetropic
   - Combination.
5. According to position of image in relation to the retina:
   - Simple
   - Compound
   - Mixed.

Astigmatism with the rule

In almost all emmetropic eyes, the vertical meridian is more curved than the horizontal by 0.25D, hence it is little myopic than the horizontal. It is asymptomatic. The change in curvature is brought about by the pressure of the normal lid. It is so common that this is taken as physiological and called astigmatism with the rule, hence astigmatism with the rule is that error of refraction that requires minus cylinder in horizontal axis, i.e. 180° ± 20° or plus cylinder at 90° ± 20°. Children are more likely to have astigmatism with the rule.

Astigmatism against the rule

This type of regular astigmatism is less common than the former. In this type of astigmatism, the horizontal meridian is more curved than vertical meridian and requires a plus cylinder at horizontal axis or a minus cylinder in vertical axis to correct the astigmatism. The cause of this is not well understood. The persons above 50 years are more likely to have astigmatism against the rule.

In by gone days, lens extraction was done through an incision in the upper limbus between 3 and 9 O'clock. This resulted in development of astigmatism against the rule that was corrected by a cylinder ranging from +1D to +2D cylinder at 180° ± 20°.

Oblique astigmatism

Oblique astigmatism is a type of regular astigmatism where the two meridians are at right angles to each other, but instead of being at 180° and 90°, they are at 45° and 135°. They are generally mirror image of each other, i.e. if the axis in the right eye is at 45°, the axis in the left eye will be 135°. The sum total of the two axes will be 180°. They may be at other angles as will, i.e. +/– on either side of 45° and 135°, so long their sum of total remains 180°. The cylinders are generally nearer to 90° on each side.

Bi-oblique astigmatism

Bi-oblique astigmatism is also a regular astigmatism where the two principle meridians are not at right angles and their sum total is not 180°, i.e. one axis is at 100° and the other at 30°.

According to error of refraction

It can be purely myopic or hypermetropic or a combination of the two where sign of the sphere and cylinder are different.

According to position of the image

According to position of the image in relation to retina, i.e. position of the two focal lines (Fig. 6.20).

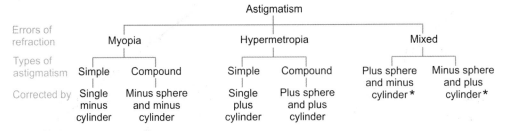

Figure 6.20: Classification of astigmatism. *The value of the cylinder will be more than the value of the sphere.

Simple myopic astigmatism: In this type error of refraction, one set of rays are brought to focus on the retina and the other in front (Fig. 6.21).

This is corrected by single minus cylinder. If the patient accommodates, the already myopic meridian moves forward making it more myopic and the emmetropic meridian follows it converting simple myopic astigmatism to compound myopic astigmatism.

Compound myopic astigmatism: Both the meridians are ametropic and the rays come to focus at two different focal planes in front of the retina (Fig. 6.22).

They require myopic sphere and myopic cylinder to correct. The value of the cylinder is the difference between the two meridians (focal planes). If the patient accommodates, the compound myopic astigmatism is enhanced as the two principal planes move farther away from the retina.

Simple hypermetropic astigmatism: In this one meridian is emmetropic and the other is hypermetropic (Fig. 6.23).

The condition is corrected by single plus cylinder. If the patient accommodates:

1. The emmetropic meridian becomes myopic.

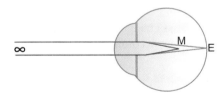

Figure 6.21: Simple myopic astigmatism

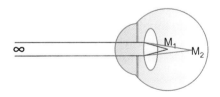

Figure 6.22: Compound myopic astigmatism

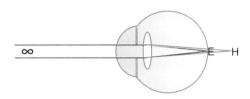

Figure 6.23: Simple hypermetropic astigmatism

2. Hypermetropic meridian becomes:
   a. Emmetropic and overall refraction is converted into simple myopic astigmatism.
   b. The hypermetropic plane fails to reach emmetropic status and the eye is converted into mixed astigmatism.
   c. If the accommodation overshoots emmetropic, it becomes myopic and the eye becomes compound myopic astigmatism.

Compound hypermetropic astigmatism: Here, both the planes are focused behind the retina and the condition is corrected by plus sphere and plus cylinder. By accommodation, following things can happen (Fig. 6.24):

1. If the spherical and the cylindrical values are so high that none of them can be brought to focus on the retina, the eye remains compound hypermetropic astigmatism.
2. The spherical and cylindrical values are small and both of them move forward in front of the retina; the condition is converted into compound myopic astigmatism.
3. One meridian comes to focus in front of the retina and other remains behind the retina, the eye is converted into mixed astigmatism.

   To overcome all this problems, there are two objective methods:

1. The best is to abolish accommodation with cycloplegia in all ages and prescribe glasses as per retinoscopy.
2. Fogging by putting plus lens in front of the eye under examination and converting all astigmatisms to a situation where

the eye behaves like a compound myopic astigmatism and then correct the error by subjective methods.

Mixed astigmatism

Mixed astigmatism is that astigmatism where some rays are focused in front of the retina and the others behind the retina; the condition becomes worse as accommodation converts both the types into compound myopic astigmatism. The condition is corrected by sphere and cylinder of opposite sign, i.e. plus sphere with minus cylinder or minus sphere with plus cylinder.

In mixed astigmatism, the value of the cylinder is always more than the sphere, the circle of least confusion falls either on the retina or near the retina. This makes the eye to have unexpected good vision.

Clinical features of regular astigmatism

Signs: As follows:

1. Externally, there may be no sign that may point toward presence of astigmatism.
2. Some children may tilt the head to compensate the axis of cylinder.
3. Astigmatic children may squeeze the eyes to overcome part of spherical error.
4. Cylindrical part of the error is not corrected by squeezing the lids.
5. The child may be brought with squint and found to have astigmatism.
6. Vision:
   a. Depends on degree of astigmatism. Low astigmatic may not complain of diminished distant vision.
   b. Vision with pinhole may not improve as much as in spherical error, e.g. an eye with 6/18 vision in a case of spherical error will improve to 6/6 with pinhole provided the media is clear, fundus is normal and there is no amblyopia. An astigmatic eye with 6/18 will hardly improve to 6/12 or 6/9 partial under the same conditions.

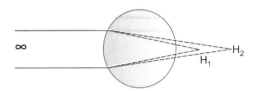

Figure 6.24: Compound hypermetropic astigmatism

   c. Power of cylinder in astigmatism may be unexpectedly high, i.e. spherical ametropic eye with 6/12 vision will improve to 6/6 or 6/5 with ±0.5D to ±0.75D sphere. But an astigmatic with the same vision may require as much as ±1.25D to ±1.75D cylinder to reach the same correction.
7. Retinoscopy will show different power at different meridians. There may be scissor movement in bi-oblique astigmatism.
8. Keratometry will have different readings in different meridians.
9. In high astigmatism, the circles of Placido's disk may be oval.
10. Fundus:
    a. The disk looks oval.
    b. Vertically oval disk is more common in astigmatism.
    c. The edges may be blurred.
    d. Oblique entry of nerve is more common.
    e. Usual changes of spherical ametropia always accompany astigmatic changes.

Symptoms:

1. The patient may be asymptomatic and found to be astigmatic on routine examination.
2. Diminished distant vision rarely exceeds 6/18 in simple astigmatism. Loss of vision is maximum in compound astigmatism; it is less in mixed astigmatism of same degree.
3. Diminished near vision in pre-presbyopic age.

4. Patient may hold the reading material near or move the head toward the table work to get magnification without accommodation.

5. Asthenopic symptoms: These are more in low and oblique astigmatism. They are more marked in hypermetropic astigmatism.

6. Non-visual symptoms of chronic infection like blepharitis, recurrent styes and chalazia are more common in astigmatism than in spherical ametropia.

Management: As follows:

1. All astigmatic eyes do not require treatment.

2. Astigmatism can be treated:
   a. Optically by:
      i. By spectacles.
      ii. By contact lens.
      iii. By combination.
   b. Surgically.

3. Points to remember:
   a. Power of cylinder rarely changes in regular astigmatism.
   b. The axis may change with age.
   c. Sign and axis, both change in simple and compound astigmatism if the power of addition is more than spherical ametropia in myopic astigmatism.
   d. Small astigmatism less than 0.5D should be corrected only if there are visual as well as asthenopic symptoms. This should be done following refraction under cycloplegia and glasses prescribed only after postcycloplegic period.
   e. In high astigmatism, cylindrical error should be corrected fully. There is no scope for over or under correction.
   f. Mixed astigmatism and bi-oblique astigmatisms are preferably corrected by contact lens and residual power given in spectacle.
   g. Low and moderate astigmatisms can be fully corrected by contact lens. Rigid gas permeable contact lenses are better suited. Soft contact lenses are not suitable to correct astigmatism. They will correct only the spherical part. Residual part is treated by spectacles.
   h. High astigmatism is treated by toric contact lenses.
   i. If the patient has diminished near vision in pre-presbyopic age, the patient is relieved by using distant astigmatic correction only.

Surgical correction: It is not as rewarding as in spherical ametropia.

Irregular astigmatism

Irregular astigmatism is always acquired and pathological. Instead of two principal meridians, there are multiple meridians, which are inclined to each other at various angles. The power may not only change in different meridians, but also in the same meridian. It can be unilateral or bilateral. The commonest cause of irregular astigmatism lies in the cornea and to less extent in the lens. The common causes are pterygium, limbal dermoid, keratoconus, iris prolapse, corneal opacities, keratectasia, descemetocele, corneal vascularization, multiple corneal foreign bodies and keratoplasty. The symptoms are diminished distant vision, near vision may also be affected by irregular astigmatism in any age. Scattering of light, glare, vision may improve with pinhole but not with spectacle. Placido's disk shows irregular rings.

Management: The best treatment for irregular astigmatism is by hard or rigid gas permeable contact lenses. The soft lenses get themselves molded according to the curvature of the cornea, hence fail to reduce astigmatism. The best treatment is by penetrating keratoplasty that leaves a clear cornea in front of the pupil. A contact lens may be required in postkeratoplasty status.

Lenticular Astigmatism

Lenticular astigmatism is less frequent than corneal astigmatism and is always pathological. It is not always possible to treat it with spectacle or contact lens. It is best treated by removal of the lens and replacing it by IOL. The lenticular astigmatism can be curvature, index or positional. The examples of curvature astigmatism are lenticonus, both anterior and posterior. The index astigmatism develops in cortical opacification. The positional lenticular astigmatism is caused by tilting of the lens. The commonest cause is blunt injury. A tilted IOL aggravates astigmatism in a pseudophakia.

Retinal Astigmatism

Retinal astigmatism is due to forward irregular bowing of the retina due to central serous retinopathy, cystoid macular edema or a growth pushing the globe from behind. The condition is not amenable to optical correction, but may improve with medical treatment.

ANISOMETROPIA

TYPES

Anisometropia is the binocular state where refractive power of the two eyes is not equal. This is in contrast to isometropia, where the refractive status is the same. Isometropia is physiological, but like all physiological conditions, a perfect isometropic person is rare.

Antimetropia

Antimetropia is a term that denotes refraction in two eyes of different types, i.e. one is myopic and the other is hypermetropic.

The word **monovision** denotes an abnormal binocular status where:

1. The patient habitually uses one eye and the other eye is either suppressed or is amblyopic.

2. Uses one eye for distance and the other eye for near.

Aniseikonia

Aniseikonia (anisokonia) is that binocular visual status where the retinal images of the two eyes are not of the same size.

Anisophoria/Anisotropia

Anisophoria/Anisotropia is a binocular condition of vision where angle of squint is different in two eyes in different gazes.

Consequences of Anisometropia

The most important consequence of anisometropia is its effect on retinal image sizes in two eyes. This becomes more evident following optical correction. The corrected image may be magnified or minified. The former happens following correction by convex lenses and latter by concave lenses:

1. A difference of 1D between the two uncorrected eyes brings about 2% changes in size of images.

2. For every diopter of correction, 1° of aniseikonia is introduced, which is roughly 1%.

3. To have a binocular single vision, both eyes should have isokonic images. The two eyes are able to fuse up to 2% of aniseikonia without effort. It can tolerate up to 5% change in two retinal images that is brought about by difference in anisometropia of 2.5D.

4. Some patients especially children can fuse two images, even with anisometropia of 4D, beyond, which it is not possible for anyone to fuse the two images.

5. Inability to fuse two images of different size results in,

    Diplopia → Suppression → Amblyopia → Squint

6. Children with hypermetropic anisometropia/aniseikonia are more likely to develop esotropia and adults exotropia.

7. Children may also be exotropic if the vision in one eye is very low.

Etiology of Anisometropia

Like all errors of refraction, anisometropia can be congenital or acquired. The congenital conditions may be considered to be primary and non-pathological. Acquired anisometropias are secondary to some obvious pathology like uniocular aphakia, keratoconus, postkeratoplasty and wrong calculated power of IOL. The congenital causes are mostly genetic. The genetics depend upon the genetics of prevailing axial error of refraction, i.e. myopia/hypermetropia. It is said that all newborn have detectable anisometropia that passes of in next few months and are not of clinical significance. Anisometropia can be axial or refractive. The latter is mostly corneal, hence astigmatic in nature. A combination of two is also possible. Axial anisometropia is more common.

A 3%–4% of populations have anisometropia of clinical significance. Many may not be aware of it. Undetected anisometropia is a major cause of amblyopia and squint in children. About 75% children with squint have hypermetropic anisometropia.

Clinical Anisometropia

Broadly anisometropia can be defined as given below (Fig. 6.25):

1. Myopic or hypermetropic.
2. Antimetropic.
3. Spherical or cylindrical.

Terminologies

1. Simple anisometropia: One eye is emmetropic and the other is either myopic or hypermetropic.
2. Compound anisometropia: Both eyes are ametropic of same sign, i.e. myopia or hypermetropia of different degrees.
3. Mixed anisometropia: Both eyes have ametropia of opposite signs.

4. Simple astigmatic anisometropia: One eye is emmetropic, the other eye has simple astigmatism, may be myopic or hypermetropic.
5. Compound astigmatic anisometropia: Both eyes have astigmatism. Both have astigmatism of same sign, but of different degrees.
6. Mixed anisometropia: Both eyes are astigmatic, one myope and other hypermetrope.

Clinical Features of Anisometropia

Signs

1. There may be no sign that may give away presence of anisometropia. Otherwise a child may be brought for esotropia and found to have hypermetropic anisometropia. Simple ametropic anisometropia is common cause of esotropia.
2. Presence of anisometropia is best elicited by retinoscopy under cycloplegia.
3. Suppression and amblyopia are common in anisometropia.
4. Suppression in anisometropia is elicited by FRIEND chart, worth four dot test or synoptophore. Synoptophore examination will reveal reduced stereoacuity as well. Stereoacuity is low in anisometropia, more than 1D.
5. Oblique illumination may reveal unilateral aphakia and unilateral keratoconus, which are two major causes of anisometropia.

Symptoms

1. The patient may be anisometropic and not aware of it.
2. The child is brought with uniocular diminished vision.
3. The child is brought with diminished vision in both eyes and found to be anisometropic—compound or mixed; stigmatic, astigmatic or antimetropic.

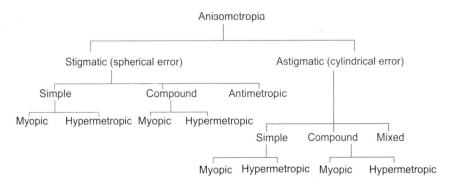

Figure 6.25: Classification of anisometropia

4. An antimetropic anisometropia may use myopic eye for near and hypermetropic eye for distance without requiring near correction in presbyopic age.

5. Variable squint.

6. Asthenopia.

Management

1. Children require management of anisometropia more urgently than adults because they are more likely to develop amblyopia than adults, except in antimetropic anisometropia.

2. Loss of binocular vision is proportionate to degree of anisometropia. More is anisometropia, less are the chances of retaining binocular vision.

3. In small degree of anisometropia, less than 2.5D, binocular vision may be present.

4. Anisometropia should be detected and diagnosed as soon as possible by routine vision test in schools.

5. Children under 6 years, which is most crucial age to manage amblyopia, may not cooperate for vision testing, but the parents or teachers may reveal, child sits too close to television or cannot see the writings on the blackboard. This happens in simple anisometropia and on retinoscopy, the difference in the two is revealed.

6. Presence of squint requires retinoscopy under atropine because the squinting eye may have greater degree of ametropia.

7. When amblyopia is found, it should be treated by usual antiamblyopic method, vigorously, even in the presence of anisometropia.

8. Correct error of refraction optically. The commonly followed guideline for optical correction consists of:

   a. Anisometropia more than 1D should be corrected. Least amblyopia develops.

   b. The first choice for correcting anisometropia up to 3D is spectacle.

   c. Decreasing the vertex distance of spectacle increases the image size in myopia and decreases image size in hypermetropia. Hence, myopic lenses should be snug with the face.

   d. Even when difference between the two eyes is 3D, the eye with higher power should be under corrected.

   e. Even in presence of diplopia, the eye with higher power should be given power equal to the eye with lower error.

   f. Children with anisometropia should be managed vigorously, from the earliest possible age.

   g. In children under 6 years, antiamblyopic treatment should get preference over cosmetic correction of squint.

h. Contact lenses are good for aniseikonia up to 6%–7%.

i. The best treatment for unilateral aphakia is to put an IOL in the posterior chamber as a primary procedure.

j. If the eye is already aphakic at the time of first presentation, the options open are:

    i. Correction by contact lens.

    ii. Secondary IOL.

k. High unilateral myopia may be treated by:

    i. Contact lens.

    ii. Refractive surgery.

    iii. Clear lens extraction.

    iv. Clear lens extraction with IOL.

However, it should be remembered that refractive corneal surgeries are contraindicated in children.

Treatment

Optical: Anisometropia can be managed to some extent optically either by spectacle or contact lenses. Spectacles are rarely tolerated if the difference in two eyes is more than 4D. In such cases, ametropia should be corrected optically to the extent that will not produce diplopia. Generally, the eye with lower power is corrected fully and the eye with higher power is given less number. An anisometropic person, who uses one eye for distance and one for near does not require any optical correction.

Contact lenses are preferred in high degree of anisometropia. They are widely used in uniocular aphakia with good vision in the other eye. Contact lenses are best answer to low degree of anisometropia due to less magnification as compared to spectacle.

Surgical: The most widely used surgical method is secondary IOL in already aphakic eye.

In case of unilateral high ametropia, the best alternative is to do refractive corneal surgery.

In case of unilateral myopia, clear lens extraction with or without IOL may give good vision.

7 Optical Devices Used to Examine the Eye

OPTICAL DEVICES

The devices used to examine the eye can be optical or non-optical. The optical devices are divided into two broad groups:

1. Magnifiers.
2. Non-magnifiers.

Commonly used magnifiers are:

a. Corneal loupes:
   i. Uniocular.
   ii. Binocular.
b. Lenses:
   i. Used with indirect ophthalmoscope; +15D, +20D and +30D.
   ii. Used with slit lamp; +76D and +90D.
c. Ophthalmoscopes:
   i. Distant direct ophthalmoscope.
   ii. Direct ophthalmoscope.
   iii. Indirect ophthalmoscope.
d. Slit lamp biomicroscope.
e. Operating telescope.
f. Operating microscope.

Commonly used non-magnifying optical devices are:

a. Hruby lens.
b. Gonioscope.
c. Applanation tonometer.
d. Pachymeter.

Non-optical devices used are:

1. Ultrasound; A and B.
2. Computed tomography (CT).
3. Magnetic resonance imaging (MRI).
4. Optical coherence tomography (OCT).
5. X-ray.

MAGNIFICATION

Magnification is an apparent enlargement of an object without real physical change in size of an object. It is the ratio between the object and its image. The two methods by which magnification can be achieved are as follows.

Moving the Object Nearer the Eye

Let E is the eye, R is the retina, N is the nodal point of E. BB' is the visual axis. AB is an object away from the eye subtending an angle B'NA' on the retina R, which is equal to angle ANB. Let's call it $\alpha°$. CD is the position of the same object when moved nearer the eye and it subtends an angle C'NB' on the retina R. This is equal to angle CND. Let us call it angle α_1. From the statement above, magnification in this particular situation is ratio between C'B' and A'B' (Fig. 7.1).

If this ratio is less than 1, it is called minification or demagnification and if more than 1, it is called magnification.

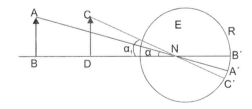

Figure 7.1: Change in size of the retinal image on moving the object toward the eye

Moving the object AB (O) from B to D increases the size of the image in a ratio of α_1/α where α is the angle subtended by AB at nodal point and α_1 is the angle subtended by the object at CD at the nodal point. This is inversely proportionate to first and second positions. Shorter the distance of the second position, larger will be the image (magnification). It is directly related to vergence of light from AB to CD.

If a magnifier is moved closer to the eye, there is no change in magnification; it only increases field of view.

More is the vergence, larger will be the magnification. Moving the object nearer the eye is not always possible, even when it is possible; it is restrained by accommodation, which is arbitrarily taken as 25 cm that results in magnification. A plus lens with focal length 25 cm, which has a power of +4D, will bring the object at anterior focal plane of the lens. The rays will become parallel and not require accommodation.

From Figure 7.1, it is obvious that ratio between B'A' and B'C' is also equal to ratio between α_1 and α.

Thus, magnification (M) is not only C'B'/A'B' but also α_1/α. The formula of magnification is given as $M = \alpha_1/\alpha$.

Magnifier as an Alternative

When it is not possible to move the object nearer the eye, the second alternative is a magnifier that will change the angle formed by the object on the retina. This is brought about by using either a single plus lens as in corneal loupe or combination of lenses as in telescopes and microscopes.

Types of Magnification

Various types of magnification met within ophthalmic practice are:

1. Angular magnification (seen in optical instruments with an eyepiece and an objective).
2. Linear (lateral/transverse) magnification. This is seen in real images. This is not used in ophthalmology.
3. Axial magnification. This is square of transverse magnification.

Various types of magnifiers used in ophthalmic practice are given in Table 7.1 and Box 7.1.

Table 7.1: Various types of magnifiers used in ophthalmology

Name of the magnifier	Example
Simple magnifier	Uniocular (corneal loupe) Binocular (Binomag)

Slit lamp biomicroscope	For examination of the anterior segment; no additional attachment required
	Examination of the posterior segment; special lenses are required
	    Direct method: Hruby lens
	    Indirect method: El Bayadi, Volk

Ophthalmoscope	Direct ophthalmoscope; simple magnifier
	Indirect ophthalmoscope; astronomical telescope
	    Uniocular
	    Binocular

Examining telescope	Galilean telescope; power variable
Operating microscope	Astronomical telescope where prisms are used to make the image upright

Box 7.1: Magnifiers in ophthalmology

The direct ophthalmoscope acts as a simple magnifier
Indirect ophthalmoscope acts as an astronomical telescope
The examining telescope acts as a Galilean telescope
Aphakic correction acts a Galilean telescope

In all magnifiers, there is an enhanced resolution of the image.

Resolution

Resolution is an optical property of an imaging system to resolve the details in the object seen by separating two points at a standard distance. Closer are the two points, better is the resolution; it depends on illumination and magnification. Bright illumination and low magnification give better resolution, thus, visualization depends more on resolution than magnification. However, an instrument with high resolution will give better magnification.

Angular Magnification

Angular magnification is applied to those devices that have an eyepiece and an objective. The image formed by the eyepiece is virtual image at infinity. It cannot be measured, hence, the size is taken as angle subtended by the object at the focal point. This is called angular size.

Magnification in Various Optical Devices

Magnification differs in construction of the magnifier that can have single lens or a combination of lenses.

Magnification by Single Lens Magnifier (Simple Magnifier)

Magnification by single lens magnifier is a linear magnification that is given as:

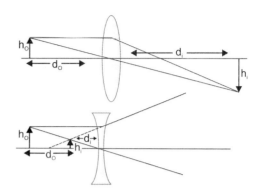

Figure 7.2: Linear magnification

$$M = \frac{f}{f-d_0}$$

or

$$M = \frac{d_i}{d_0} = \frac{h_i}{h_0} = \frac{v}{u}$$

where, f is the focal length and d_0 is the distance of the object from the lens, d_i is the distance of the image from the lens, h_i is the height of the image, h_0 is the height of the object, v is the distance between the object and the lens, u is the distance between image and the lens (Fig. 7.2).

Note: Real v is taken as positive and virtual v is taken as negative.

Magnification by Combination of Lenses (Compound Magnifier)

Commonly used compound magnifiers in ophthalmology are:

• Operating telescopes
• Operating microscopes
• Spectacles.

OPERATING TELESCOPES

Operating telescopes are nothing, but miniature telescopes mounted on a spectacle frame. Their optics is similar to any commonly used telescopes (Figs 7.3 and 7.4).

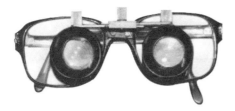

Figure 7.3: Operating telescope (frontal view)

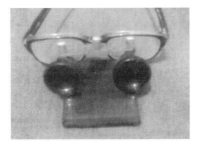

Figure 7.4: An operating telescope

Telescopes are generally meant to see objects far away, which are not seen by naked or spectacled eyes. They are used as operating loupes in ophthalmology to see minute structures in working distance with a magnified image that is not laterally reversed.

Principle

Operating telescopes are made on the principle of Galilean telescopes in contrast to astronomical telescopes, which gives an inverted image, not suitable for examination of anterior segment.

The telescope has an objective and an ocular (eyepiece). The objective is directed toward the object and the eyepiece is toward the eye of the observer. The objective is a plus lens and eyepiece, a minus lens. The objective of the operating loupe forms a real image of the object at its far point. The eyepiece is so located that its focal plane is at the focus only to reach the eye as parallel rays.

Comparative Features

In contrast to this, in an astronomical telescope, both the objective and the eyepiece are convex. In Galilean telescopes, the image formed by the objective is virtual and becomes object for the eyepiece. The objective in Galilean telescope is weak plus lens and the eyepiece is strong negative lens. These are separated by the algebraic sum of their focal lengths (Fig. 7.5).

Magnification

The magnification of Galilean telescope is:

$$M = \frac{\text{Power of ocular}}{\text{Power of the objective}}$$

The final image of a Galilean telescope is magnified and erect.

The objective has got a focal length of f_o, which is longer than the focal length of the eyepiece, which is f_e because the eyepiece is stronger than the objective.

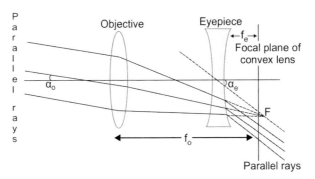

Figure 7.5: Optics of Galilean telescope, magnification = power of the oculus/power of the objective

MICROSCOPE

Microscopes are generally used to see minute things at a close range. The commonly used microscope is a clinical microscope where transparent slides are illuminated by a separate light coming from behind the slide. In ophthalmology, the microscope is used as slit lamp and surgical microscope (Fig. 7.6). The optics of microscope and astronomical telescope are same (Fig. 7.7).

The only difference is that the two focal points of telescope coincide, while in microscope they are separated by the distance called tube distance. The disadvantage of a clinical microscope is that this gives an inverted image, which is not suitable for microsurgery of the eye. To avoid this, the image formed is rotated by a prism in the microscope to give an erect, magnified image that is not laterally reversed at a comfortable working distance. The object (the eye being operated) is kept very near the objective that has a short focal length. The eye must be at a focal plane of the

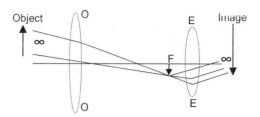

Figure 7.7: Optics of astronomical telescope. OO is the oculus, EE is the eyepiece, F is the common focal point and image is formed at infinity (∞), highly magnified and inverted.

objective. The objective gives a linear magnification. The eyepiece acts as a simple magnifier and allows parallel rays to reach the observer's eye.

The total magnification is product of linear magnification of the objective and angular magnification of the eyepiece, i.e. M = $M_o \times M_e$ where M is the total magnification, M_o is the magnification of the objective and M_e is the magnification of the eyepiece (refer Chapter 10 Low Vision Aids).

SPECTACLE MAGNIFICATION

Spectacle magnification is a common knowledge that when looking through a plus lens, put at close quarter, the object looks large. While looking through a minus lens kept at any distance from the eyes, the object looks small, but always erect.

Emmetropic Eye

To be emmetrope, the eye must have a refractive power of +60D.

Hypermetropic Eye

The hypermetropic eye is supposed to have a hypothetical minus lens in it. This needs to be corrected by putting a plus lens in front of the eye at anterior focal plane to bring to an emmetropic state. In contrast to this, a myopic eye has a hypothetical plus lens in it that

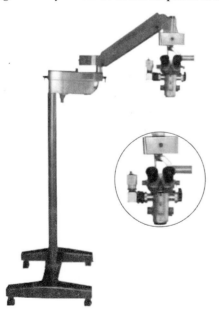

Figure 7.6: An operating microscope
[*Courtesy:* Appasamy Associates (with permission)]

needs to be neutralized by putting a minus lens at anterior focal plane.

Aphakic Eye

An aphakic eye has all the properties of hypermetropic eye minus the accommodation. An aphakic eye is considered to have an imaginary –10D to –12D lens in it. This creates a Galilean telescope like situation when a plus lens is put at its anterior focal plane, giving a 25% magnification that is reduced to 5%–7%, when a contact lens is put on the cornea, which is nearer to the nodal point. The magnification is totally abolished when a posterior chamber lens is used. The posterior chamber lens is almost on the nodal point of the eye.

To correct ametropia, the lens used should have focal point equal to far point of the eye under consideration. The far point of a myopic eye is in front of the eye and far point of hypermetropic eye is a hypothetical point behind the eye. The hypermetropic eye acts as a Galilean telescope, while myopic eye acts as a reversed Galilean telescope. When fundus of a myopic eye is seen through a direct ophthalmoscope, the disk looks large because the hypothetical plus lens in the eye and minus lens in the ophthalmoscope put together give a Galilean telescope effect. In contrast to this, hypothetical minus lens in the hypermetropic eye and plus lens of the direct ophthalmoscope give a reverse Galilean telescope effect causing minification of the image.

OPTICS OF OPHTHALMOSCOPES

Ophthalmoscopes are illuminated optical devices to see interior of the globe. The illumination can be inbuilt or may be reflected. The reflected illumination is no more used except for examination of ocular media, which can also be done by inbuilt illumination of ophthalmoscope. The process of examination by ophthalmoscope is called ophthalmoscopy or fundoscopy. The term fundus is loosely used to denote the spherical inner side of the globe from ora serrata to optic disk.

Distant Direct Ophthalmoscopy

Distant direct ophthalmoscopy is a confusing term in which the optics of the ophthalmoscopy is not utilized. This process gives only an idea about presence of opacity in the cornea, lens and vitreous. In fact, this examination denotes not only presence but also location, size and movement of the opacities in the media. The similarity between the two terms ophthalmoscopy and distant direct ophthalmoscopy is limited to use of reflected light in both the procedures.

Method of Examination

1. The patient sits comfortably at a distance of half a meter from the observer with fully dilated pupil. Simple mydriatics are sufficient to dilate the pupil. No cycloplegic is required.

2. A source of light is kept about 25 cm behind the head and slightly laterally from the head of the patient. This keeps the face and eyes in dark.

3. A plane mirror is used to reflect the light in the dilated pupil in the manner it is done, while doing retinoscopy.

4. A concave mirror can also be used, but the reflected ray is very bright and sharp causing inconvenience to the patient.

5. In an eye with clear media, the pupillary area lightens up with a pink retinal glow without any black spot (Fig. 7.8A).

   Presence of black spot in the pink glow indicates presence of opacity in the media (Figs 7.8B to D).

6. The relative position of the opacities can be determined by parallax. The parallax is elicited in relation to the pupillary plane, which roughly corresponds to the anterior lens capsule.

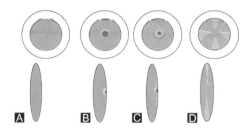

Figures 7.8A to D: Appearance of opacities in the media in distant direct ophthalmology. **A.** Transparent lens in emmetropia; **B.** Posterior polar opacity; **C.** Posterior capsular opacity; **D.** Peripheral cortical opacity.

7. The patient is asked to move the eye in different meridians. If the black spot is stationary, the opacity is in the lens. If the black spot moves with the movement of the eye, it is in the cornea. If the opacity moves against the movement of the eye, it is most probably in the vitreous.

A gray reflex during distant direct ophthalmoscopy in the pupillary area instead of a pink glow means shallow retinal detachment, growth in the posterior pole, large atrophic choroidal patch, coloboma of the choroids and large opaque nerve fibers (Fig. 7.9).

Dull reflex is seen in hazy vitreous, dense posterior capsular opacity in posterior chamber intraocular lens (PCIOL) and thin after cataract (Fig. 7.10).

Total absence of pupillary glow means mature cataract, large vitreous hemorrhage, endophthalmitis or total retinal detachment (Fig. 7.11).

Note: This procedure is no more used in routine practice because all the information

can be gathered during plane mirror retinoscopy, direct ophthalmoscopy and examination by slit lamp.

Direct Ophthalmoscopy

Direct ophthalmoscopy is done by an instrument called direct ophthalmoscope. This is the most commonly used optical device to examine the fundus and opacities in the media. It gives accurate subjective information not only of the fundus background but also about transparency of media and rough estimation of error of refraction.

It gives an image of the retina, which is erect, virtual and magnified.

Principle
The principle of ophthalmoscopy is based on:
1. Light enters the eye through the pupil.
2. The light illuminates the retina.
3. Some of the light is reflected back through the pupil in the same direction.
4. It forms an image on the retina.
5. It can be visible to an observer, if his/her pupil is in the same path of the reflected light.

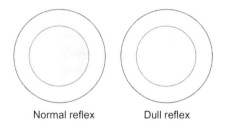

Normal reflex   Dull reflex

Figure 7.10: Normal and dull reflexes

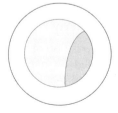

Figure 7.9: Gray reflex in the pupillary area

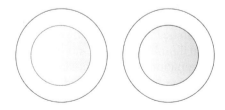

Figure 7.11: Absence of glow

6. If a light is placed in front of the unaccommodated observed eye and the observer brings his/her pupil behind the light, the reflected light from the illuminated spot on the retina is visible to the observer.

Direct Ophthalmoscope

The present-day direct ophthalmoscope is a compact, handheld, self-illuminated optical device, which works either on dry battery or through a step-down transformer. The direct ophthalmoscope has two main parts:

1. The body, which is hollow and houses the battery or a step-down transformer, switch and a rheostat.
2. The head forms the main part of the device. It contains:
   a. An illumination system.
   b. An optical system.

Illumination system: It comprises of a low-voltage bulb that throws parallel rays, which are reflected by either a plane mirror or a suitable prism placed in the path of the rays above the bulb. The rays from the bulb are deviated at 90° to the reach the pupil. Behind and little above the mirror is a peephole for the observer to see the illuminated area.

Still behind the peephole is a wheel that contains the optical part.

Optical system: It consists of a wheel that can be rotated around a central axis. The wheel has small apertures that contain a series of plus and minus lenses. The range is generally between –30D and +30D in gradually increasing and decreasing strength. These lenses are meant to correct the refractive error of observer's eye and observed eye. Between the bulb and the reflecting mirror is a disk with apertures of various sizes and shapes. The apertures can be small, intermediate or large. The small aperture is used to see the fundus with undilated pupil and the largest with widely dilated pupil. Some direct ophthalmoscopes have small slit and a graticule also. The slit is meant to give a rough optical section of the cornea and the lens, and diagnose macular edema and hole. The graticule is meant to measure size of the lesion on the fundus, size of the disk and cup-disk ratio. The swelling of the disk is measured by adding plus lenses and depth of the cup is measured by adding minus lenses. Elevation of 1 mm needs +3D and 1 mm of excavation needs –3D.

All direct ophthalmoscopes have built-in rheostat to control illumination and of course a switch to put the illumination on or off. Some ophthalmoscopes have cobalt blue and red-free green filters incorporated. The filters are placed between the bulb and reflecting mirror.

Optics of Direct Ophthalmoscope

Optics of the direct ophthalmoscope lies in the eye observed. The instrument acts only as a viewing and illuminating system.

The basic optical principles involved in direct ophthalmoscopy are (Figs 7.12 and 7.13):

1. A source of light is reflected by a plane or mildly concave mirror into the observed eye or traced to observer's eye from the handheld instrument.
2. This illuminates an area of the fundus.

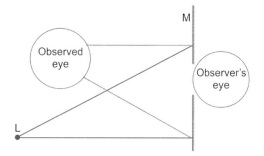

Figure 7.12: Path of light rays in direct ophthalmoscope. Path of rays of light from the source of light (L) to the mirror (M) reflected into the observed eye and traced to observer's eye. In case of handheld direct ophthalmoscope, the mirror can be replaced by a suitable reflecting prism.

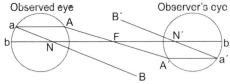

Figure 7.13: Principle of direct ophthalmoscopy. bNFN'b' is the principle axis of the two eyes; F is the point where the focus of both the eyes coincide; N and N' are the two nodal points. A ray AFA' is refracted to reach the observer's eye at a' forming an image a'b' of ab, of the same size as ab. aA is a ray parallel to optical axis bNFN'b'. A is the point where aA meets the observer's eye and refracted as A'a'. B'N'a' passes through the nodal point N' undeviated and meet the observer's eye at a'. a'b' is the image of ab on the observer's eye.

3. The light from the illuminated area is again reflected back along the optical axis to reach the eye of the observer.

4. The illuminated area is the object for the optical device.

5. To see the illuminated area, the observer's eye should be in the line of the rays reflected from the illuminated fundus.

6. The eye of the observer should be very near the observed eye, i.e. anterior focal plane (15.7 mm) in front of the cornea of the observed eye.

7. The emerging rays from the observed eye behave differently depending upon refractive status of the observed eye:

   a. Emmetropia: The rays emerging from the observed eye are parallel and are brought to focus on the retina of the observer (Fig. 7.14).

   b. Hypermteropia: The emerging rays are divergent and do not reach the retina of the observer. They meet behind the eye of the observer unless the observer's eye either accommodates or a plus lens is kept in front of the eye (Figs 7.15A to C).

   c. Myopia: The emerging rays are converging and come to focus in front of

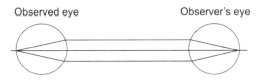

Figure 7.14: Path of rays in an emmetropic eye. Rays coming out of the observed eye are parallel to reach the observer's eye.

the retina and can be focused only if they are made parallel by interposing minus lens in front of the observer's eye (Figs 7.16A to C).

8. The above statements are true, if the observer is emmetrope and has a relaxed accommodation. Otherwise, the observer can have his/her error corrected by spectacle or put required lens against the peephole of the direct ophthalmoscope.

9. The area of the fundus illuminated is largest in myopia and smallest in hypermetropia.

Magnification by Direct Ophthalmoscope

The image formed during direct ophthalmoscope is magnified, erect and virtual, situated behind the observed eye. The image formation depends upon the dioptric power of the observed eye. The ophthalmoscope acts only as a source of illumination. The area of the fundus illuminated acts as the object. The dioptric power of the eye acts as a strong convex sphere of +60D with short focal length. The magnification is similar to simple magnifier/corneal loupe where the power of the uniocular corneal loupe is +40D (Figs 7.17 and 7.18).

It can be calculated by the formula:

$$M = \frac{D}{4} = \frac{60}{4} = 15$$

where, M stands for magnification and D for dioptric power of an emmetropic eye.

In case of myopia of 5D, this will be:

$$M = \frac{65}{4} = 16.25$$

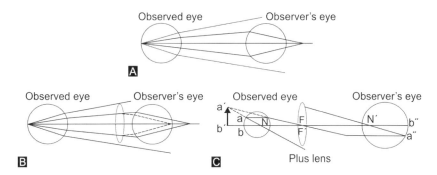

Figures 7.15A to C: Path of light rays in hypermetropia as seen with direct ophthalmoscope. **A.** Diverging rays emerging from the hypermetropic observed eye form an image behind the observer's eye; **B.** When a suitable plus lens is put in front of the observer's eye, the diverging rays are brought to focus on the retina making the fundus of the observed eye clear; **C.** a′b′ is the erect virtual image of ab.

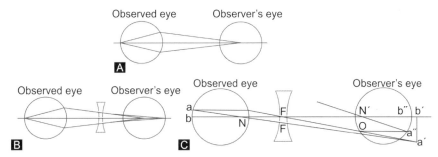

Figures 7.16A to C: Path of light rays in myopia as seen with direct ophthalmoscope. **A.** Converging rays from the observed eye are brought to focus in front of the observer's eye; **B.** Converging rays from the observed eye are brought to focus on the retina with a concave lens of suitable focal length placed at the anterior focal length of the observed eye; **C.** A suitable concave lens placed at the anterior focal plane of the observed eye produces a virtual and enlarged image behind the observer's eyes.

In case of hypermtropia of 5D, this will be:

$$M = \frac{55}{4} = 13.15$$

Note: The above equations explain why a myopic disk looks larger than a hypermetropic disk.

Method of Doing Direct Ophthalmoscopy

The best results are obtained by fully dilated pupil because it circumviates any central opacity in the cornea or in the lens. However, fundus can be seen with undilated pupil, if the patient looks at a distant object. To see with undilated pupil, a smaller aperture in the ophthalmoscope may be used. The small aperture reduces the field of vision. It is good only for examination of the disk. In an attempt to see the macula, the pupil instantaneously constricts obliterating the fundus.

To operate the ophthalmoscope, the examiner holds the instruments on the right hand, stands on the right side of the patient facing the patient and examines the right eye. The reverse is done to examine the left eye. The pupil of the patient is well dilated.

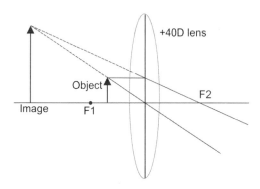

Figure 7.17: Principle of a simple corneal loupe

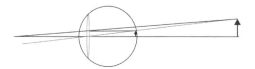

Figure 7.18: Magnification by a direct ophthalmoscope

The patient fixes a distant object. This dilates the pupil more and abolishes the accommodation further. The observer should develop skill to examine the fundus with both eyes open.

Indirect Ophthalmoscope

Indirect ophthalmoscope is one of the most widely used optical devices to examine the fundus and perform retinal surgery. It is unavoidable tool in retinal surgery. It was invented almost at the same time in 1851 as direct ophthalmoscope. It did not become popular due to its inherent property of producing an inverted image, which required long orientation, time and both the hands remain engaged during indirect ophthalmoscopy. Though the concept of binocular indirect ophthalmoscope was known since 1851, it was only when binocular indirect ophthalmoscope was developed by Schepen (1947), to whom the present day popularity of this versatile instrument goes.

Types

There are two types of indirect ophthalmoscopes:

1. Original type of uniocular indirect ophthalmoscope that is no more in use.
2. Modern binocular indirect ophthalmoscope, which can either be attached to a headband or spectacle mounted. The former is more popular than latter.

Optics of Indirect Ophthalmoscope

The optics of all the indirect ophthalmoscopes is the same (Fig. 7.19). They all consist of:

1. An illumination system.
2. Magnifying cum observation system.

The optics of indirect ophthalmoscope is better comprehended in uniocular indirect ophthalmoscope. Once it has been understood, it may be translated to principle of binocular indirect ophthalmoscope.

Principle of Indirect Ophthalmoscope

Indirect ophthalmoscope makes the eye more myopic by putting a high plus lens in front of the eye under examination. The high convex lens is referred to as condensing lens. The purposes of the condensing lens are:

1. To condense rays coming out of the eye under examination between the condensing lens and the observer.
2. To magnify the image.

Thus, a condensing lens in indirect ophthalmoscope is not only a simple condenser but also a magnifier. The magnification is little influenced by the refractive power of the eye under examination, but directly related to the diopter of the condensing lens. More is the diopter of condensing lens; less is the magnification and depth of focus. The illumination is less in condensing lens with low diopters. The condensing lens produces an inverted, real and magnified image of the fundus in the

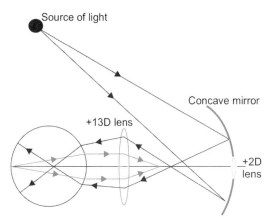

Figure 7.19: Optics of indirect ophthalmoscope

air between the lens and the observer, close to the focal length of the condensing lens. The power of the condensing lens decides the distance at which it should be held in front of the eye being examined. Higher the power of the condensing lens, lesser will be the distance. In the bygone days, +13D lens was the only lens used in indirect ophthalmoscope. It gave a magnification of 5X with very limited field. Nowadays, it has been abandoned in favor of +15D, +20D and +30D. Out of these, +20D is most popular to use as a tool of preliminary survey of the overall features, the +15D is used for detailed examination of macula and disk. However, there are better methods to examine these structures, using either –55D Hruby lens or +76D to +90D lens with slit lamp. The +30D is more useful to examine the retinal periphery, which is again better visualized when a scleral depressor is used along with. The features of condensing lens of various diopters are given in Table 7.2.

From Table 7.2, theoretically, a +60D condensing lens does not give any magnification. There is no stereopsis. The field is large. The +60D lens is not used with binocular indirect ophthalmoscope. It is used in slit lamp examination as El Bayadi lens where the image is formed 16 mm toward the observer. The magnification is given by the slit lamp; hence an El Bayadi lens of +60D will have a magnification of 10X or 15X depending on the power of the eyepiece.

Optics of Monocular Indirect Ophthalmoscope

The behavior of the rays, position and size of the image and area visible by indirect ophthalmoscope depend on power of the lens used. The behavior of the rays is different in eyes with different refractive status (Figs 7.19 to 7.22).

In emmetropic eye, the rays coming out of the fundus are parallel. They are brought to focus by the condensing lens and the image is formed at the principle focus of the condensing lens (Fig. 7.20).

In a hypermetropic eye (Fig. 7.21), the rays leave the eye as diverging; hence will seem to come from hypothetical point behind the eye. This image is enlarged and upright. The condensing lens uses this hypothetical image as object and forms an inverted image in front of the principal focus of the condensing lens, which is magnified. The image is farthest from the eye and nearer to the observer when compared to emmetropic or myopic eye.

Table 7.2: Features of condensing lens of various diopters

Diopter (D)	Distance from patient's eye	Magnification	Field	Stereopsis
+15D	6.6 cm = 3″	4X	30°	Normal
+20D	5.0 cm = 2″	3X	51°	¾ normal
+30D	3.3 cm = 1.5″	2X	60°	½ normal

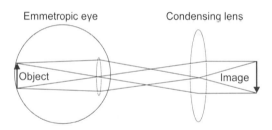

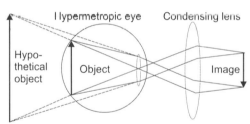

Figure 7.20: Image formation by indirect ophthalmoscope in an emmetropic eye. The rays emerging from the emmetropic eye are brought to focus at the principle focus of the condensing lens forming a real, inverted and magnified image.

Figure 7.21: Image formation by an indirect ophthalmoscope in a hypermetropic eye. The rays emerging from a hypermetropic eye are divergent and seem to originate from a plane behind the eye. The condensing lens takes this image as the object and forms real, inverted and magnified image between the condensing lens and its focus.

In myopic eye (Fig. 7.22), the rays emerging from the eye under examination are convergent; hence an inverted, enlarged image is formed in front of the eye. The condensing lens uses this as second object to form a second image in the focal length of the condensing lens.

Thus, we have seen that:

1. In emmetropia, the image is formed at focus of the condensing lens (Fig. 7.23A).
2. In hypermetropia, farthest from the eye and nearest to the observer (Fig. 7.23B).
3. In myopia, at a distance less than the focal length of the condensing lens, i.e. nearest to the eye (Fig. 7.23C).

The size of the image depends upon the position of the focus of the condensing lens in relation to anterior focal plane of the eye:

1. If the anterior focus of the eye and the principal focus of the condensing lens correspond, all the images irrespective of power of the eye will be of the same size (Fig. 7.24A).
2. If the condensing lens is moved toward the eye and the distance of its principal focus is less than the anterior focus of the eye under examination, the image will be larger in a hypermetropic eye and smaller in myopic eye (Fig. 7.24B).

3. If the condensing lens is moved away from the eye and its principal focus is beyond the anterior focus of the eye under examination, the myopic image will be largest and hypermetropic image will be smallest (Fig. 7.24C).

The magnification in indirect ophthalmoscope is refractive power of the eye under examination ÷ power of the condensing lens. Thus, a +15D will give a magnification of 60/15 = 4X, +20D will give 3X and +30D will give 2X magnification.

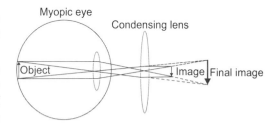

Figure 7.22: Image formation by indirect ophthalmoscope in myopic eye. The emergent rays are convergent and focused nearer to the lens than the principal focus and form an inverted image in front of the eye. The condensing lens forms the final image that is real, magnified and inverted at its own focal length.

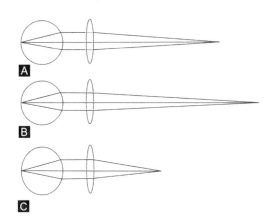

Figures 7.23A to C: Summary of image formation by condensing lens kept at same distance from the eye and position of the image formed by it in various types of errors of refraction. **A.** Emmetropia; **B.** Hypermetropia; **C.** Myopia.

Technique of Unilateral Indirect Ophthalmoscopy with +13D

1. Patient sits in front of the observer at 1 m distance with widely dilated pupil.

2. A source of light is kept behind and slightly lateral to the head of the patient. This keeps the face of the patient in the dark, but throws light on the face of the observer.

3. The patient fixes a distant point.

4. The observer uses a concave mirror to reflect the light from the source into the dilated pupil.

5. The concave mirror used has following properties:
   a. The focal length of 25 cm, which:
      i. Converges the parallel rays at 25 cm in front of it.
      ii. After this, these rays diverge to reach the pupil as divergent rays.
   b. A +2D lens is incorporated in the peephole of the concave mirror to relax the accommodation of the observer (this is optional).

6. A self-illuminated retinoscope with divergent rays can also be used. This will eliminate the use of a source of light mentioned above.

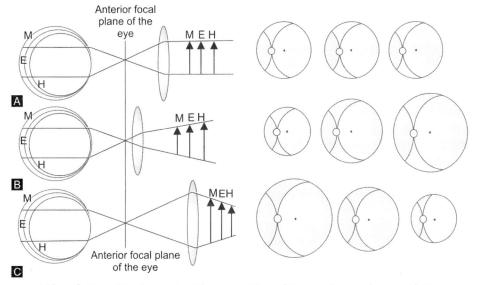

Figures 7.24A to C: Size of the image in different position of the condensing lens in relation to anterior focal plane of the eye. **A.** Principal focus of the condensing lens and the anterior focus of the eye are same; **B.** Principal focus of the condensing lens is less than anterior focus of the eye; **C.** Principal focus of condensing lens is more than anterior focus of the eye (E, emmetrope; H, hypermetrope; M, myope).

7. A pink glow is seen in the pupillary area, which may move with or against as per error of refraction of the observed eye. This movement is in no way related to indirect ophthalmoscope.

8. The observer places a +13D biconvex condensing lens in front of the eye, very near the eye and gradually moves the lens away from the eye.

9. At a certain distance, the whole of the pupillary area lights up with a pink glow.

10. The lens is moved farther from the eye till an inverted, real, magnified image of the fundus becomes visible.

11. The image is formed between the condensing lens and the observer near the focal plane of the condensing lens.

12. The observer should now ignore the pupillary glow and pay attention to the inverted image between the lens and the observer. This is the stage when the +2D incorporated in the peephole comes handy in a presbyopic observer.

13. The whole procedure requires patience and practice to study the fundus; it is better to focus the optic disk first. To see the optic nerve of the right eye, the patient is asked to look either at the right ear of the observer or tip of the right extended index finger of the observer. To see the left disk, the patient is asked to look at the left ear.

14. A difficulty that arises at this stage is unwanted, troublesome light reflex from the two surfaces of the condensing lens and the anterior surface of the cornea. The light reflexes are similar to Purkinje images. They are formed by the two surfaces of the condensing lens and anterior surface of the cornea. They have nothing to do with the image formation by the condensing lens, which in turn depends on the refracting power of the condensing lens. The troublesome reflex can be eliminated by holding the condensing lens at a distance of 9 cm, which is equal to the focal length of the condensing lens from the anterior focal plane of the eye. The other method is to tilt the lens. This separates the two images formed by the two surfaces of the condensing lens and looking between the two light reflexes.

15. The observer should put on his/her distant correction throughout the procedure and keep self 1 m from the patient. If observer moves nearer the patient, he/she requires additional accommodation to see the image clearly.

Binocular Indirect Ophthalmoscope

The principle and optics of binocular indirect ophthalmoscope (Fig. 7.25) is basically the same as in uniocular indirect ophthalmoscope. In binocular indirect ophthalmoscope, both the eyes of the examiner are used simultaneously. This gives much needed stereopsis. The other advantage is built-in illumination, which is far brighter than best illumination, any direct ophthalmoscope or uniocular indirect ophthalmoscope can give. It leaves one hand free to use a scleral depressor and draw the fundus picture.

Parts or features of the binocular indirect ophthalmoscope consist of:

1. Headband with built-in illumination system.
2. The interpupillary distance reducing mechanism.
3. A condensing lens to give a real, inverted, magnified aerial image near the focal point of the condensing lens toward the observer.

Headband: This is adjustable band with two adjustments, one horizontal for circumference of the head of the observer and the other at right angles to it to adjust vertically.

This mechanism prevents the whole of the illuminating system from sagging down.

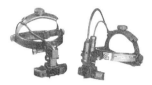

Figure 7.25: Binocular indirect ophthalmoscope [*Courtesy:* Appasamy Associates (with permission)]

Illumination system: It consists of:

1. Interpupillary distance adjustment.
2. Adjustment for the angulation of mirrors.
3. Adjustment for the size of the spot.
4. Two eyepieces.
5. Filters.
6. A side-view mirror.

The above adjustments are housed in a simple complex that is hinged at the front surface of the headband. The hinge permits the whole complex to move forward and backward (Fig. 7.26).

The illumination is given by an 18-watt halogen lamp. This gives very bright illumination. Bright illumination with low magnification gives better resolution and greater depth of focus. The lamp gets its electric supply from a step-down transformer, which has a rheostat, which controls the brightness of the illumination there are some models, which operate on rechargeable dry cells.

The angulation of the mirror is done through a screw at one side of a mirror. On the opposite side is an adjustment for the size of the spot and arrangement to interpose either a cobalt blue or a red-free filter.

Interpupillary distance reducing mechanism: To have binocular view, one eye of the patient is seen at a time. The eyes of the examiner and the light from the illumination source should be imaged by the condensing lens within the pupil of the patient. The distance between the pupil of an average observer ranges between 55 and 75 mm with an average of 60 mm. With 60 mm of interpupillary distance, the two eyes of the

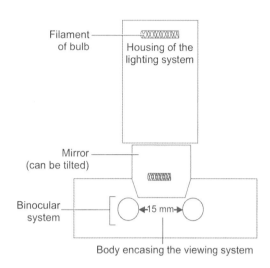

Figure 7.26: Front view of the illumination and viewing system of indirect ophthalmoscope

observer are imaged too far apart. Thus, they cannot be imaged in the pupil of the patient after passing through the condensing lens.

The ideal interpupillary distance should be 15 mm to have a binocular view. This has been made possible through two plane mirrors, kept parallel to each other and reflecting surfaces facing each other (Fig. 7.27). The light from the illumination system comes few millimeters above the line of vision. The light from the illumination and the observer's eye are imaged on the pupil of the observed eye forming a triangle after being reflected through the mirror in the headband. There is arrangement to change the interpupillary distance to suit the observer's eyes. To examine the other eye, the observer has just to move the head to focus the eye.

While doing indirect binocular fundus examination of one eye, the patient should be asked to keep the other eye open. If the patient keeps the other eye closed, the eye under examination will roll up.

Condensing lens: These are high-powered plus lenses with short focal length. They are used to concentrate parallel as well as diverging rays to

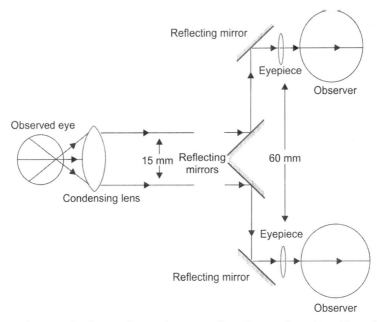

Figure 7.27: Mechanism of reducing observer's interpupillary distance from 60 to 15 mm by reflecting plane mirrors (or prisms)

a pinpoint focus or form an image at a given point. The lenses can be biconvex or plano-convex. They may be spheric or aspheric.

The condensing lens as a whole acts as a convex lens, but one of its surfaces acts as a convex mirror and the opposite surface acts as either concave mirror or a plane mirror, both forming unwanted and uncomfortable reflections. To avoid these uncomfortable reflections from the surface, they are generally coated with antireflecting chemicals. The other method to avoid these reflections is to tilt the lens, which moves the two reflections in opposite direction leaving a clear reflection-free area in between, through which the area of interest can be seen.

In the past, +13D lens was the only lens available. It was also used to concentrate light for examination by corneal loupe. This was cumbersome and required practice. The condensing lens used in the past with corneal loupe has been replaced by more sophisticated bright, halogen pen torches that can give both diffuse and pinpoint illumination. The second use in examination of fundus by indirect binocular ophthalmoscope or slit lamp biomicroscope, where it enhances the myopic value of the eye under examination by +13D, i.e. an emmetropic eye is converted to −13D myope, a −5D of myopia is converted to −18D and a +5D hypermetropic eye becomes −8D. Nowadays, +13D condensing lens has became obsolete and has been replaced by a battery of lenses ranging from +15D to +90D.

A condensing lens forms a real, inverted, magnified image in the space (refer Optics of Indirect Ophthalmoscope). Commonly used lenses are +20D and +30D for indirect ophthalmoscopy. Lesser is the power of the condensing lens, more is the magnification and larger is the working distance, but smaller is the field of vision. Thus, a +15D condensing lens will have a magnification of 4X, working distance 75 mm and field of vision 40°. A +30D condensing lens will have a magnification of 2X, working distance of 30 mm, but the field will be increased to 60°. Comparison between properties of condensing lens of various diopters is shown in Table 7.3.

The condensing lenses used in slit lamp biomicroscopy differ from those used in indirect ophthalmoscopy. They range between +78D and +90D. A +78D gives a magnification of 0.93X and field between 80° and 90°, while a +90D will give a magnification of 0.66X and field 75°–85°. Thus, it will be observed that when a condensing lens of power more than the total dioptric power of the eye, i.e. +60D is used, there is infact minification. But in reality, the magnification by slit lamp can be deduced by multiplying this figure by the magnification of the slit lamp. For example, the actual magnification with a +60D will be 10X; +78D will be 0.93 × 10 = 9.3 and by +90D will be 0.66 × 10 = 6.66.

The comparison of the direct and indirect ophthalmoscopes is given in detail in Table 7.4.

EXAMINATION OF FUNDUS BY SLIT LAMP

There are various methods of examining fundus (Fig. 7.28). They are:

1. Direct.
2. Indirect.

Direct methods comprise of direct ophthalmoscope, Goldmann and Koeppe's modified lens, and Hruby lens. The indirect methods consist of indirect ophthalmoscope using +15D to +30D condensing lens and slit lamp biomicroscope using +60D to +90D convex lenses.

The easiest way of examining the fundus is by direct ophthalmoscope. The advantages are that it gives an erect image. The magnification is maximum, i.e. 15 times and the learning curve is very short. It can be used with dilated or normal pupil. It is very handy instrument. The only drawback is that only a small area of fundus, i.e. less than 10° is seen at a time and the periphery is not visible, which is the seat of many retinal lesions.

Next best is by indirect ophthalmoscope that requires practice to reorient inverted image. The most difficult is examination of fundus by slit lamp.

Optics

The optics involved in examination by slit lamp depends upon the following points:

1. The standard slit lamp can focus up to 4 inches from the oculus, i.e. 4 × 2.5 = 10 cm = 100 mm.
2. For all practical purposes, this distance is taken as 9.5 cm.
3. Plane focused by the slit lamp is 11 inches from the eye of the examiner, i.e. 11 inches = 11 × 2.5 cm = 27.5 cm, which is taken as 180 mm.
4. This is too far from the retina, hence, retina cannot be focused by a standard slit lamp.
5. Hence, this requires modification in the optical system of the slit lamp.
6. The modifications can be brought about by two methods:
   a. Neutralizing the refracting power of emmetropic eye from +60D to 0 by:

Table 7.3: Comparison of various diopters of condensing lens

Diopters	Working distance	Magnification	Field	Stereopsis	Illumination
+15D	75 mm	4X	30°	Normal	Low
+20D	50 mm	3X	50°	¾ normal	Medium
+30D	38 mm	2X	60°	½ normal	Bright

Table 7.4: Comparison of direct and indirect ophthalmoscopes

Features	Direct	Indirect
Handheld	Always	Handheld indirect ophthalmoscope is monocular and is no more in clinical use
Laterality	Always uniocular	May be uniocular or binocular; latter is more convenient, hence more popular
Attachment to head-band	Not possible and not required	Preferred mode of attachment; however, may be spectacle mounted
Condensing lens	Not required	Must

Image
  Location
  Orientation
  Type
  Magnification
  Factor deciding magnification
  Telescopic effect
	Behind the observed eye
	Erect
	Virtual
	15X
	
	Dioptric power of the eye
	Galilean
		In front of the eye
		Inverted
		Real
		3X–5X
		
		Dioptric power of the condensing lens
		Astronomical

Brightness	Not very bright (10 watt) so details in hazy media are not visible	Very bright (18 watt); details are visible even in hazy media
Visibility	Poor in high errors of refraction	Error of refraction does not interfere with visibility

Field
  Area
 	
  Size
	From disk to a little behind ora serrata
	2 × disk size, i.e. 7°
		From disk to ora serrata
		
		8 × disk size, i.e. 25°–30°

Stereopsis	Nil	Good
Working distance	Very short	Arms length
Scleral depressor	Cannot be used	Is a standard procedure

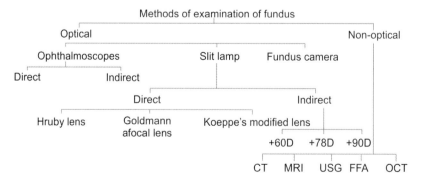

Figure 7.28: Various methods of examining the fundus (CT, computed tomography; FFA, fundus fluorescein angiography; MRI, magnetic resonance imaging; OCT, optical coherence tomography; USG, ultrasonography).

i. Neutralizing +45D of the cornea by an afocal flat contact lens as in Goldmann three-mirror gonioscope (Fig. 7.29).

ii. Koeppe's modified lens: The Goldmann and Koeppe's modified lenses (Fig. 7.30) form virtual, erect image on the retina in the vitreous, 18 mm in front of the retina.

iii. Neutralizing +60D, i.e. total refracting power of the eye by inserting a –60D (in fact it is a –58.6D planoconcave Hruby lens) lens between the slit lamp and the cornea. This is not a contact lens. It is fitted on a standard slit lamp at 10–15 mm in front of the patient's cornea. It gives a virtual, erect and minified image of the retina, which is enhanced by magnification of slit lamp (Fig. 7.31).

b. By indirect method that follows the optics of usual binocular indirect ophthalmoscope gives a real, inverted image minus magnification. There are two commonly used condensing lenses:

i. El Bayadi lens +60D: This forms an image of the same size, i.e. 1X between the lens and the observer. The image is formed 17 mm

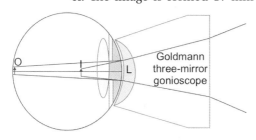

Figure 7.29: Optics of Goldmann three-mirror gonioscope used to examine the posterior pole. O is the retinal image; L is a thick contact lens of Goldmann three-mirror gonioscope, which forms virtual, erect and diminished image of I at O in the vitreous, just behind the lens.

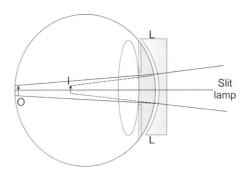

Figure 7.30: Optics of Koeppe's modified lens. O is the retinal image; LL is a thin planoconcave contact lens that forms virtual, erect image of O at I in the mid-vitreous.

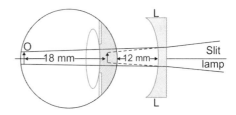

Figure 7.31: Optics of Hruby lens. O is the retinal image; LL is the –58D non-contact Hruby lens kept at 12 mm in front of the eye under observation, I is the virtual, erect and diminished image of O, 18 mm from the O in the anterior chamber (AC).

from the condensing lens toward the observer (Fig. 7.32).

ii. Lens +90D: This also gives an inverted, real, demagnified (minified), i.e. 0.75X image in the air between the lens and the observer.

iii. Most widely used lens is a +78D that has all the properties of +60D and +90D. The magnification and the field being in between.

Non-optical Methods of Examining Fundus

The non-optical devices are considered as ancillary devices. The fundus fluorescein angiography (FFA) and OCT are effective only in clear media, while X-ray, CT, MRI and ultrasonography (USG) have advantage of being useful even in the presence of opaque media.

Slit Lamp Biomicroscope

Slit lamp biomicroscope is a versatile optical instrument, which is commonly referred as slit lamp only. Basically it is nothing, but a sort of oblique illumination system that gives excellent illumination and magnification. The instrument is used to examine the outer structure from skin of the lid to inner structures like optic nerve and macula. The instrument has two parts:

1. An illumination system with a slit and other accessories like filters, etc.
2. A compound microscope.

Both the parts are incorporated in a single mechanical supporting system (Figs 7.33A and B).

Most of the instruments work on step-down transformer for electric supply. A small version, which is handheld, works on dry battery.

The modern slit lamp consists of:

1. An illumination system.
2. A microscope.

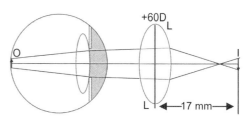

Figure 7.32: Optics of El Bayadi lens. O is the retinal image; LL is the +60D El Bayadi lens; I is the real, inverted same size image of O at 17 mm from the +60D lens toward the observer.

3. A coupling system.
4. A mechanical support.
5. An adjustable table.

The light can be projected from above or below.

Illumination system: The illumination system (Figs 7.34 and 7.35) consists of:

1. A halogen bulb of $2 \times 10^5 - 4 \times 10^5$ lux kept in upright position.
2. Condensing lens system: Light from the bulb is first concentrated by a pair of condensing planoconvex lenses kept with their parallel surfaces facing each other with a gap in between.

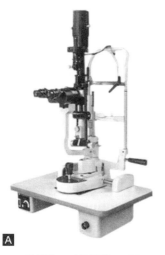

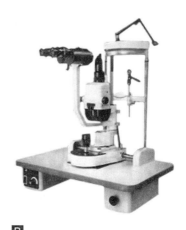

A   **B**

Figures 7.33A and B: Different types of slit lamp. **A.** Illumination system above the microscope; **B.** Illumination system below the microscope [*Courtesy:* Appasamy Associates (with permission)].

3. The filament of the bulb is first imaged on the objective after going through the condensing lens and mechanical slit. The slit is imaged on the patient's eye.

4. Slit aperture: There are two slit apertures, one controlling width and the other height. The former is vertical and the latter is horizontal. The width can be changed by narrowing the vertical slit as and when required. This is achieved by knob incorporated in the body. The width can be changed by a horizontally-placed disk with circular holes of various sizes; this narrows both vertical and horizontal apertures. The slit can be converted in circles of various sizes, ranging from pinpoint upwards. The axis of the slit can be changed by a separate milled knob.

5. Filters: Various types of filters can be incorporated between the bulb and the slit. The two common filters used are cobalt blue and red free.

6. Reflecting mirror/prism: It is placed at the top of illumination system, when the light comes from below and at the bottom when light comes from above. The purpose is to change the direction of the beam from vertical to horizontal to reach the eye of the patient (refer Figs 7.34 and 7.35).

Microscope: It is a binocular compound microscope that produces an enlarged, real inverted image that is made upright by a prism. Each arm of the binocular consists of an eyepiece and an objective (Fig. 7.36 and also refer Fig. 7.6).

1. Eyepiece: The power of the eyepiece is variable, gives a magnification of 10X and 15X. The power of eyepiece is +10D sphere. The power of the eyepiece can be changed by 8D on each side, i.e. minus or plus by rotating the eyepiece. Generally, the commonly used magnification is 10X. This can be changed by replacing 10X lens by 15X lens. The other arrangement that enhances magnification is a flip

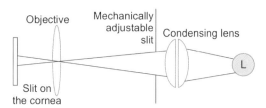

Figure 7.34: Optics of the illumination system in a slit lamp biomicroscope

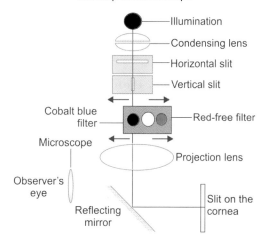

Figure 7.35: Basic attachments in the illumination system of a slit lamp

lever that changes the magnification to a higher level without changing the power of the eyepiece. The binocular tubes are not parallel to each other. They are inclined to each other by 10°–15°. This gives a single vision. The working distance of microscope is 100 mm.

2. Objective: It consists of two planoconvex lenses with their plane surfaces parallel to each other separated by a thin gap. The total power of the objective is +22D. The eyepiece and the objective are not homoaxial. Objective is at a higher level. Rays from the eyepiece is replaced by a suitable prism that rotates the ray by 90°. This ray is picked up by a prism little above the first prism. This again changes the direction of the ray by 90°. Thus, the rays emerging from the objective is at a higher level, but parallel to the first ray.

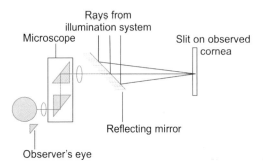

Figure 7.36: Composite picture of illumination system of microscope

Coupling mechanism: The microscope and illuminating mechanism constitute two different systems that are coupled round a common pivot, so that both can be moved separately in a horizontal plane. The reflecting mirror is at a lower level than the horizontal axis of microscope, but the two are parfocal, i.e. they are focused at the same point. Both the arms can be locked at desired angle separately.

Mechanical support: It can be divided into two parts as given below:

1. The base: This anchors the illumination system and the microscope to a common platform allowing them to move together in a horizontal frame both anteroposterior and side-to-side. There is a device called joystick to adjust the vertical height of both the system. The whole of the base can be locked at a desired distance and angle from the eye of the patient.

2. The frame: This has two vertical pillars joined by a sturdy, horizontally-placed curved headband and chin rest, 9–10 inches from the headband. The height of the chin rest can be adjusted vertically. There is an adjustable fixation light for the patient to fix when the eye is being examined.

Adjustable table: Whole of the slit lamp microscope is anchored on a smooth top table. The height of the table top is adjustable.

Under the table top is a drawer that houses the step-down transformer, which supplies power to the illumination system. The step-down transformer is provided with a rheostat to control the illumination. The power supplied can be put off by a separate switch.

Accessories: Commonly supplied accessories, which are supplied with a standard slit lamp are:

1. An applanation tonometer.
2. A Hruby lens.
3. The other options are photographic attachment for anterior segment photography, side tube for teaching, gonioscope, keratometer, pachymeter, laser delivery system.

Handheld slit lamp: A miniature version of a slit lamp, complete with a microscope and illumination system is available to use in non-ambulatory patients and for use in camps and mass survey. It works on dry battery. It does not have the usual accessory attachments that are available with table-top slit lamps.

Other processes: Those used in slit lamp biomicroscopy can be divided into two groups:

1. Examination of anterior segment.
2. Examination of posterior segment.

The examinations of the anterior segment that requires slit lamp are given below:

1. Gonioscopy.
2. Applanation tonometry.
3. Contact lens fitting.
4. Tear meniscus examination.
5. Laser iridotomy.
6. Laser capsulotomy.
7. Optical pachymetry.
8. Photography of the anterior segment.

GONIOSCOPY

The examination of angle of anterior segment is called gonioscopy and the instrument used is called gonioscope.

Optics of Gonioscope

The angle is situated in such a place that it is obscured by overhanging scleral ledge and is not visible by any form of oblique illumination.

The rays arising from the angle strike the posterior surface of the cornea and are reflected back to the opposite angle. This happens because of total internal reflection (Fig. 7.37). The angle formed by the rays arising from the angle of the anterior chamber (AC) at the air-cornea interface is more than 45°, which is higher than the critical angle, hence is reflected to the other angle without going out. The solution to overcome this problem is by eliminating the cornea from the air-cornea interface and replace it by a glass-air interface by putting a contact lens with refractive index equal to the refractive index of cornea. When a contact lens is put over the cornea, the cornea tear film coupling solution and the contact lens form a composite refractive medium. The ray from the angle passes through the cornea without deviation, then passes through the contact lens of gonioscope. This is either reflected by the mirror/prism of the gonioscope to be picked up by slit lamp or an operating microscope. Operating microscope is used with direct gonioscope and slit lamp with indirect gonioscope.

The gonioscope is not capable of any magnification. The magnification is provided by the slit lamp.

Types

On the basis of principle of refraction and reflection, the gonioscopes are divided into two classes. These are:

1. Reflecting gonioscope (indirect gonioscope).
2. Refracting gonioscope (direct gonioscope).

Indirect Gonioscope

The indirect gonioscope consists of a conical body; the wider part is away from the cornea. The conical lens has a contact lens in it. The curvature of the contact lens is steeper than the cornea and the diameter is more than the cornea (Fig. 7.38).

There are plane mirrors on the wall of the body of gonioscope inclined on the inner surface of the cone. One end of the mirror on the contact lens and the other, away from it. The number of mirrors varies between one and four each with a different purpose.

The cornea, the tear film coupling solution and the contact lens form a composite refracting medium.

The gonioscope may require a viscous solution to be put on the cornea to keep the lens in place. If the diameter of the contact lenses as in Goldmann and Allen-Thorpe gonioscopes is larger than the cornea, a viscous substance is required to couple the lens to the cornea. The viscous substance generally used is methyl cellulose. The Zeiss four-mirror

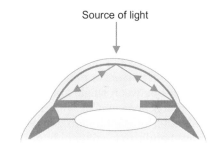

Figure 7.37: Total internal reflection of rays in the anterior chamber

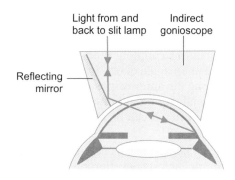

Figure 7.38: Optics of indirect gonioscope

gonioscope that has a diameter less than cornea does not require viscous solution to couple. If the gonio lenses are flatter than the cornea and require viscous fluid to couple are also called suction lenses. The contact lenses that do not require viscous fluid are called non-suction lenses. The images formed by non-suction gonioscopes are not of very good quality. They require longer learning curve. The advantages are that they can be used for indentation gonioscopy and rapid evaluation.

The commonest indirect gonioscope is Goldmann three-mirror gonioscope. It is one of the largest and heaviest gonioscope and can be used to see not only the angle of the AC but also up to periphery of the fundus. The gonioscope produces an image of the opposite angle. The image is virtual, erect and of the same size. Thus, when the gonio mirror is positioned at upper pole, it shows the image of the angle at the lower pole. The center part of the gonioscope can be used for slit lamp examination of the optic nerve head and the posterior pole without much magnification.

Indirect gonioscopes are also classified as per number of mirrors or prisms used. The number varies between single and four mirrors. The gonioscopes may be with handle or without handle. The Goldmann gonioscopes do not have handle to keep them in position. The Goldmann gonioscopes are kept in place by the capillary action supported by the lids and the fingers of the examiner.

One-mirror gonioscope: This is smallest gonioscope used. It only visualizes the angle of AC at the site opposite the position of the mirror. It requires coupling fluid. The mirror is inclined at an angle of 62°. It needs to be rotated along the anterior-posterior axis to see the angle all around. It is most convenient to use and master. It can be used to indent the angle (Fig. 7.39).

Two-mirror gonioscope: Its function is same as one-mirror gonioscopes. The only difference is that it has two identical mirrors inclined at an angle of 62°. Its main advantage is that it needs

to be rotated half the circle. It visualizes the angle only. It requires viscous coupling and can be used for indentation gonioscopy. The two-mirror gonioscopes gives best in situ view of the angle.

Goldmann three-mirror gonioscope: It is not only a gonioscope but also a device to examine the fundus from disk to the ora. It is a large and heavy device. It has three plane mirrors inclined at different angles (Figs 7.40A to C). The smallest mirror has a dome-shaped top and is inclined at 60°; it is used to examine the angle of AC. The second is larger, inclined at 67° used to see the pars plana. The third mirror is inclined at 73° and is used to see the fundus from ora serrata to the edge of the posterior pole. The images are mirror images without change in size and are not laterally reversed. The three-mirror gonioscopes require coupling substance. It has a minus contact lens that neutralizes the +45D of cornea when placed over the cornea with viscous substance. The commonly-used viscous substance is methyl cellulose. The overall diameter of the base of the gonioscope is 12 mm, which is larger than the diameter of the cornea. As the edge of the base extend up to sclera, it is also referred to as scleral lens in contrast to Zeiss and Posner four-mirror gonioscopes that have diameters of 9 mm that is smaller than cornea and rests solely on cornea, hence called corneal gonio lenses. The four-mirror gonioscopes do not require any coupling fluid.

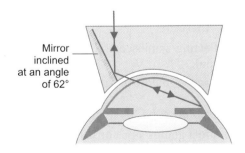

Figure 7.39: Optics of one-mirror gonioscope

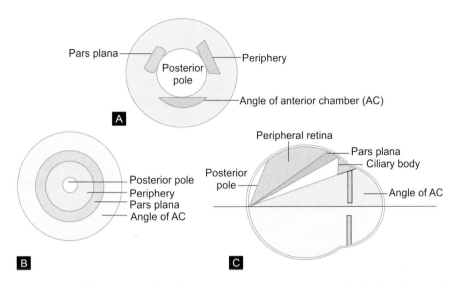

Figures 7.40A to C: Different parts of Goldmann three-mirror gonioscope. **A.** Various shapes of prisms/mirrors used in three-mirror gonioscopes; **B.** Areas visible by prisms/mirrors by three-mirror gonioscopes (front view); **C.** Areas visible by prisms/mirrors by three-mirror gonioscopes (side view).

Central part is used to see the optic nerve and posterior pole by slit lamp. To see the posterior pole, the light is directed on the circular contact lens; while seeing the other parts, the light is directed on the mirror concerned.

Methods of gonioscopy

There are three methods of gonioscopy. They are:

1. Gonioscopy in situ.
2. Manipulative gonioscopy.
3. Indentation gonioscopy.

Gonioscopy in situ: It is best performed by Goldmann two-mirror gonioscopes. The three-mirror gonioscope is not suitable for this purpose. Gonioscopy in situ is the routine way of examination by keeping the long axis up the gonioscope at right angles to the vertex of the cornea. The patient is asked to look straight ahead. The lights of the room and the illumination of the slit lamp are dimmed. The height of the slit lamp is used just up to the pupillary border. This prevents constriction of the pupil. A pinpoint constricted pupil may change the width of the angle so does a dilated pupil.

The angle is examined without pressing a gonioscope or moving on the surface of the cornea. The angle is examined for visibility of all the structures. Non-visibility of structures raises suspicion of occlusion of the angle that can be appositional or synechial. This brings the second step, i.e. manipulative gonioscopy.

Manipulative gonioscopy: It is a technique to look over the hump of the steep iris. This is achieved by asking the patient to move the eye toward the angle being examined.

Indentation gonioscopy: This is best done by four-mirror handheld gonioscope. The test consists of keeping the lens constantly on the cornea without pressure indentation opens appositional closure of the angle.

Advantages of indirect gonioscopy

1. It can be performed as office procedure in a limited space with a minimum instrument, i.e. gonioscope and standard slit lamp, which gives variable illumination, magnification and slit size.
2. Learning curve is short.

3. The duration of procedure is short. The patient may not be aware of the procedure being done, hence cooperative.

4. Image is sharp and bright.

5. Indentation gonioscope is possible by indirect gonioscope only.

6. The posterior pole view is stereoscopic.

Disadvantages of indirect gonioscopy

1. The mirror image requires practice to master.

2. The two eyes cannot be examined simultaneously; hence, the angles on two sides cannot be compared at the same time. Surgery cannot be performed.

3. The non-ambulatory patient cannot be examined.

4. Infants and non-cooperative children cannot be examined.

Direct Gonioscopes

Direct gonioscopes (Fig. 7.41) are less frequently used in diagnosis of adult glaucoma, but are essential tools for diagnosis and surgery of glaucoma in children. They come in various shapes and sizes, put directly on the cornea after a coupling fluid has been put over the cornea. The rays arising from the angle, after traversing the aqueous and cornea, enter the gonio lens and are refracted directly, almost at right angles to the lens-air interface. These are picked up either by a handheld microscope, operating microscope or handheld slit lamp. Standard table-modeled slit lamp is of no use as the patients have to be supine and being children, are examined under general anesthesia.

The most widely used direct gonioscope is a solid dome-shaped gonioscope that is available in various sizes for neonates, infants and children. The diameter of the corneal end ranges between 16 and 22 mm. The curvature of the corneal end is steeper than cornea.

The gonioscope itself gives a magnification of 1.5X, which is enhanced to 10X, 12X, 15X by the operating microscope. The image given is erect, but not mirror image. The lens gives a panoramic view of the angle all around, hence, need not be rotated. Using two gonioscopes, one for each eye, the two eyes can be examined simultaneously and compared. The direct gonioscopes are the only gonioscopes for the surgery at the angle. The direct gonioscopes, other than Koeppe's, have handles to manipulate.

Advantages

1. The image formed is straight and not mirror image, hence orientation is easy.

2. It gives a panoramic view of the angle all around at the same time, hence need not be rotated.

3. The angle becomes deep as the lens-iris diaphragm goes back in supine position.

4. It can be used in anesthetized child.

5. The angle of the two eyes can be examined and compared simultaneously.

6. It is the most suitable diagnostic gonioscope for infants and children.

7. Only gonioscope employed for goniosurgery.

Disadvantages

1. Cannot be used as office procedure.

2. The patient has to be supine.

3. Posterior segment cannot be visualized.

4. Magnification with handheld microscope is not very good.

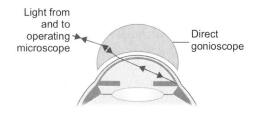

Figure 7.41: Optics of direct gonioscope

APPLANATION TONOMETRY

In applanation tonometry, slit lamp is used to illuminate the tonometer tip and fluorescein-stained cornea (Fig. 7.42). Magnification has very little importance in this procedure.

The applanation tonometry is the best available procedure to record intraocular tension. It is least affected by scleral rigidity, which is an inherent deterrent of indentation tonometry.

Principle

The principle of applanation tonometry is based on principle of Imbert-Fick, which states that the pressure inside a thin-walled dry sphere is equal to the force needed to flatten a known surface area divided by area flattened. Let P be the pressure inside, F be the force to flatten the surface and A be the area flattened. Then we have, P = F/A (Fig. 7.43).

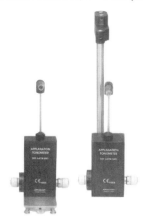

Figure 7.42: Obasic parts of applanation tonometer [*Courtesy:* Appasamy Associates (with permission)]

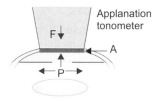

Figure 7.43: Principle of applanation tonometer. F is the force applied, A is the area of the cornea flattened and P is the pressure inside AC.

Optics

The principle of applanation tonometry sounds good for an experimental model. The human eye has few lacunae to fulfill all these criteria, but it is nearest to it in natural setting. The other factors that hamper the working of tonometer are that the cornea resists flattening. The tear in between the tonometer and the cornea, drags the tonometer toward the cornea. However, in practice these factors are negated by applanating a small, circular area of 3 mm in diameter at center of the cornea, causing negligible displacement of the fluid. There are various applanation tonometers available that work on Imbert-Fick principle. Out of which, the Goldmann applanation tonometer is the most popular applanation tonometer, requiring use of slit lamp. The applanation tonometer has an optical part that consists of a conical barrel, whose narrow end faces the cornea. The narrow end contains two prisms, the area that comes in contact with the cornea has a diameter of 3.06 mm. The wider end faces the observer.

Though the law is eponymed as Imbert-Fick law, it was indeed postulated by Goldmann. It does not fit in any principle of physics, may it be hydrolics or mechanics. This law has been challenged for its correctness because, as per the law, the structure has to be a perfect sphere, which the eye is not. The cornea is not equally curved although; it is steeped in the center. The sphere should be filled with liquid again. This is contradicted by the fact that all the contents in the eyeball are not homogeneous fluid. The outer cover of the sphere should be infinitely thin membrane, without rigidity. The cornea and sclera have definite thickness with variable rigidity and resists flattening. The outer surface of the sphere should be dry. The cornea on which the tonometer is applied is not dry; it is always covered with tear film, which due to its surface tension, drags the tonometer prism toward the cornea. Taking all this in consideration, the law has been modified as:

$$W + S = Pt \times A_1 + B \text{ or } Pt = (W + B)/(A_1 + B)$$

where, Pt is the intraocular pressure, A_1 is the internal area flattened, W is the weight required to flatten the known area, B is the pressure in the AC and S is the surface tension (Fig. 7.44).

However, these corrections have so far not been taken into account in all models available. The argument in favor of Goldmann tonometer are; only a small area is applanated, hence fluid displaced is negligible and asphericity of cornea and capillary pull of the tear meniscus negate each other.

Types

The applanation tonometers are available in two models:

1. Slit lamp mounted.
2. Handheld.

The slit lamp-mounted tonometer is more widely used as office procedure, while the handheld model is used in mass survey and in operation theater. The former can only be used in erect position. The latter has the advantage of being used both in supine as well as sitting position. The handheld models work on dry batteries. Both the types basically use Goldmann's principle of applanation. The handheld model can be optical or computerized.

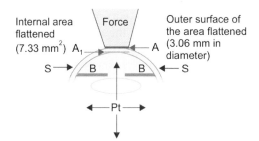

Figure 7.44: Modified principle of applanation tonometer. S is the surface tension, Pt is the intraocular pressure and B is the pressure inside AC [*Courtesy:* Dr Manav Deep Singh (with permission)].

Slit Lamp-mounted Applanation Tonometer

The slit lamp-mounted applanation tonometer has following parts:

1. An optical part—biprism.
2. Mechanical part:
   a. A housing contains a knob that controls the pressure applied to the biprism.
   b. An arm that joins the biprism to the housing. This also transmits the force to the biprism.

The tonometer can be plate/pivot mounted or overhanging.

Biprism: A plastic conical cylinder, the narrow end of which faces the cornea under examination is attached to a wider part. The wide part faces the observer (Fig. 7.45). The diameter of the end facing the cornea under examination is 3.06 mm. The cornea can be visualized through the cone by a slit lamp. The purpose of the two prisms is to split the light beam to convert the circular area on the cornea into two semicircles on each side of a line. In non-astigmatic eyes, this line is horizontal, i.e. 0° and 180°. In astigmatism, this becomes oblique and semicircles become oblong, which can be corrected by rotating the prism. The long axis of the biprism complex is parallel to the table top of the slit lamp. The biprism is attached to the housing below in a plate of pivot-mounted tonometer and above in overhanging housing by the arm.

The Goldmann applanation tonometer is a variable-force tonometer.

The housing contains a coil spring and an assortment of levers that adjust the force applied to the biprism. The observer looks through the broader end of the biprism through the oculus of the silt lamp. The illumination of the slit lamp is direct on the translucent end of the biprism and the stained cornea.

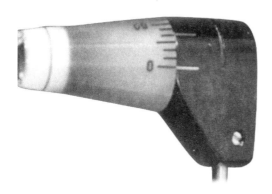

Figure 7.45: Biprism of an applanation tonometer
[*Courtesy:* Dr Lalit Verma (with permission)]

Technique of tonometry: It involves:

1. The patient is explained that it is a painless procedure, but an essential part of ocular examination.

2. The eyes are anesthetized by 4% xylocaine or 0.5% Paracaine (proparacaine hydrochloride).

3. The lower lid is pulled down and a sterile fluorescein strip is left in the lower fornix for few seconds.

4. The patient is asked to blink few times to spread the stain uniformly over the cornea.

5. Patient is asked to sit comfortably on a slit lamp with a tonometer attached to it.

6. The patient puts chin on the chin rest and the forehead comfortably against the headband and keeps the head steady.

7. The viewing system of the slit lamp is aligned in such a way that the oculus of the slit lamp, the biprisms and the center of the cornea are in one line.

8. The angle between the viewing system and the illumination is locked at 60°.

9. The illumination is put at maximum to illuminate the stained area.

10. The magnification is kept at lowest.

11. The illumination in the room is dimmed.

12. Only one eyepiece of the binocular is used to see the applanated area. To examine the right eye of the patient, the observer uses his/her right eye and the left eyepiece of the binocular (different clinicians practice different methods to have a uniocular view of the eye under examination).

13. The knob that controls the pressure exerted on the cornea is set at 1 and not at 0. If the knob is set at 0, the prism head oscillates over the corneal surface that may injure the corneal epithelium.

14. When the knob is set at 1, it transmits a pressure of 10 g and at 2, the pressure is raised to 20 g.

15. The light from the illumination is directed to the tip of the biprism. The color of the light is changed to cobalt blue, by interposing a cobalt blue filter. Under cobalt blue light, the fluorescein, which otherwise looks green in white light, turns yellow.

16. Whole of the applanation housing is moved slowly toward the cornea till it just touches the vertex of the cornea and gives an appearance of solid yellow circle. With little more movement, the solid circle is converted into an empty circle surrounded by a yellow circle (Figs 7.46A to F).

17. With further movement, the circle breaks into two semicircles:
    a. Remaining above.
    b. Drifting below the horizontal line.

    The ends of each circle are apart from each other.

    Moving the biprism still toward the cornea, the semicircles move toward each other.

18. When the outer edge of the two semicircles just touches each other, the end point has been reached.

19. The amount of pressure applied is read on the control knob and multiplied by a

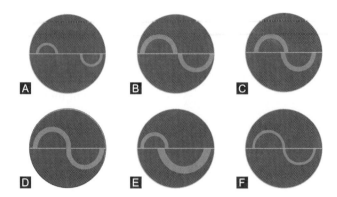

Figures 7.46A to F: Fluorescein pattern in applanation tonometry as seen through cobalt blue filter. **A.** Tonometer touching the film; **B.** Tonometer touching the corneal epithelium; **C.** Proper position of the circles to measure intraocular pressure; **D.** End point; **E.** Too much of fluorescein; **F.** Too less fluorescein (E and F indicate unsatisfactory fluorescein rings).

factor 10 to give intraocular pressure in mm Hg.

20. The intraocular tension in the other eye is measured in the same way, by just moving the housing horizontal.

Handheld Applanation Tonometer

The handheld applanation tonometers use the Goldmann principle of applanation. There are many models available. The commonly used are:

1. Contact applanation tonometers.

2. Non-contact applanation tonometers.

Contact tonometers: The commonly used handheld contact tonometers are:

1. Perkins handheld tonometer.

2. Draeger handheld tonometer.

Perkins tonometer: It is a handheld, portable tonometer that has biprism like Goldmann tonometer and a cobalt blue filter (Fig. 7.47). It generally works on dry battery, which is encased in its body. The body also acts as handle of the tonometer. It does not require slit lamp like other slit lamp-based tonometers. The applanation pressure can be changed by a rotator dial.

The patient can be examined either in sitting or supine position. The latter feature makes it useful in examining children under general anesthesia.

Draeger tonometer: This is less popular than Perkins tonometer. It uses a biprism of different kind. The applanation weight is supplied by an electrically operated motor.

Non-contact tonometers: These are so called air-puff tonometers, which differ from pneumotonometer, which is a modified contact tonometer. The non-contact tonometers are also based on applanation principle of Goldmann except, they do not require a biprism like contact tonometer and slit lamp. These tonometers generate a jet of air that applanate the cornea. The applanation is enhanced linearly over a given time. It also directs collimated beam of light on the corneal vertex and a receiver that detects parallel reflected rays from the applanated cornea and notes down the time required to reach the instrument, which is digitally converted into mm Hg.

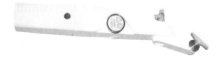

Figure 7.47: Perkins handheld tonometer
[*Courtesy:* Dr Lalit Verma (with permission)]

UNIOCULAR/BINOCULAR LOUPES

Uniocular Corneal Loupe

Uniocular corneal loupe is one of the most handy and cheap magnifiers used in ophthalmology (Figs 7.48A and B). It gives a good magnification of 10X and the image is erect. It requires little practice to master. The device consists of two planoconvex lenses of +20D each, which when put together make a total power of +40D (Fig. 7.49).

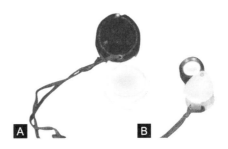

Figures 7.48A and B: **A.** Condensing lens; **B.** Uniocular corneal loupe.

Optics

The lenses are encased in a sturdy body. The lenses are placed in such a way that the plane surfaces are parallel and face each other. Lenses are separated by a clear gap of 2–3 mm in between. This reduces peripheral and prismatic aberration. The focal length of the combined lenses is 100/40 = 2.5 and the magnification is 40/4, i.e. 10. The object of interest must be kept at a distance less than the focal length of the device, i.e. 2.5 cm and illuminated by an external source of light. The instrument forms an erect, virtual, 10 times magnified image on the same side of the object. The optics involved is explained in the Figure 7.50.

The image is not laterally reversed. The uniocular corneal loupe is good for examination of the cornea, aqueous, lens, posterior opacification and anterior vitreous. In the past, a condensing lens of +13D was used to concentrate light on the object to illuminate it. The condensing lens has been replaced by pen torch.

Disadvantages

The disadvantages of uniocular corneal loupe are as follows:

1. The examiner has to move too close to the eye under examination that is less than 2.5 cm, to keep the area of interest within focal length of the loupe.

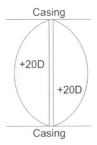

Figure 7.49: Construction of a corneal loupe

2. Both the hands of the examiner are engaged, one holding the loupe and other, the light. Hence, this device cannot be used to perform surgeries on the anterior segment.

3. There is no stereopsis.

4. The loupe has to be moved to and fro to keep the plane of interest in focus.

These difficulties are avoided by binocular corneal loupes.

Binocular Loupes

The binocular loupes are popularly known as Binomags.

Optics

Binocular loupes consist of two +6D spheres mounted in a frame that is hinged to a headband in such a way that the distance between the eye of the observer and the lens

Table 7.5: Comparison of uniocular and binocular corneal loupes

Features	Uniocular	Binocular
Lens	+40D	+6D
Incorporated prism	Nil	4Δ base in
Magnification	10X	1.5X
Stereopsis	Nil	Fairly good
Working distance	Less than 2.5 cm	12–20 cm
Hands engaged	Both	One (to hold the source of illumination)
Utility in surgery	Nil	Can be used to do surgeries on anterior segment

assembly can be adjusted (Fig. 7.51). Generally two prisms of 4Δ (Δ = prism diopter) with base in are added to spherical lenses to ease the convergence of the observers. As the power of the spherical lenses in the loupe is only +6D, the magnification is very less in comparison to uniocular loupe. The binocular loupes give a magnification of 6/4 = 1.5X only. The incorporated prism has no role in magnification. The binocular loupe has longer working distance. Increasing the power of the spherical lens in the binocular loupes increases the magnification, but reduces the working distance.

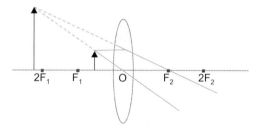

Figure 7.50: Optics of uniocular corneal loupe

Advantages

The two advantages of the binocular loupes are:

1. Good stereopsis.
2. These leave both the hands free that is helpful in manipulation of the eye under examination.

A source of light can be incorporated in the headband above the frame of the lenses. In absence of such an arrangement, a separate source of handheld light is required. The binocular loupe can be used not only to see the anterior segment but also to produce sufficient magnification to do surgeries ranging

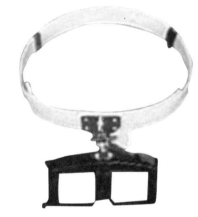

Figure 7.51: Binocular corneal loupe

from removing foreign bodies to intracapsular or extracapsular lens extraction.

The comparison of uniocular and binocular corneal loupes is given in Table 7.5.

8 Clinical Methods in Error of Refraction

CLINICAL METHODS

Clinical methods in error of refraction consist of:

1. History related to errors of refraction.
2. External examination.
3. Recording of vision:
   a. Distant vision:
      i. Without correction.
      ii. With correction.
   b. Near vision:
      i. Without correction.
      ii. With correction.
4. Determination of power of correction for distance and near.
5. Scope of further improvement:
   a. Subjective method of improvement of vision.
   b. Objective methods of improvement of vision.
6. Eliciting causes of non-improvement of vision: Examination of posterior segment by direct ophthalmoscope, indirect ophthalmoscope, fundus fluorescein angiography, ultrasonography and optical coherence tomography (OCT).
7. Prescription of glasses.

HISTORY RELATED TO ERRORS OF REFRACTION

History related to errors of refraction consists of:

1. Onset.
2. Progress.
3. Bilaterality.
4. Association of non-refractive ocular condition.
5. Association of non-ocular discomfort.

Complaints can be ocular or non-ocular (Fig. 8.1).

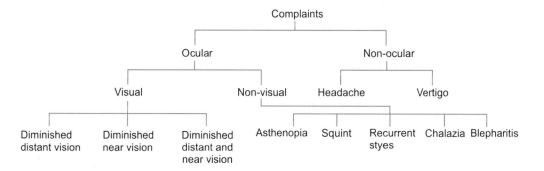

Figure 8.1: Visual complaints in error of refraction

The ocular complaints in relation to error of refraction can be visual or non-visual.

Diminished Vision

Diminished distant vision in errors of refraction is generally gradual, bilateral, painless and equal. But can occasionally be unequal or even unilateral or sudden.

Causes

Causes of bilateral sudden diminished vision due to error of refraction are:

1. Hyperglycemia: Rise of blood sugar causes index myopia.
2. Hypoglycemia: Causes index hypermetropia.
3. Drug induced: Many drugs, especially sulfa drugs in general and acetazolamide in particular are known to produce transient myopia that disappears with stoppage of medicine. Parasympatholytic drugs taken orally or locally precipitate and unmask hypermetropia. Similarly, instillation of strong miotics causes cyclotonia resulting in myopia (Box 8.1).

The commonest cause of diminished near vision is presbyopia, which is generally gradual, progressive, painless, bilateral and almost equal in both eyes, setting in about 40 years of age.

Box 8.1: Myopia

Myopia of childhood progresses relentlessly even with best correction and subsides after few years
Use of glasses has no effect on progression
Myopia is never cured spontaneously; however, small degree of hypermetropia in children may be neutralized by increase in axial length in teens
This is generally attributed to use of indigenous medicine, diet rich in vitamins, yoga, exercise, etc.

True unilateral presbyopia does not occur. If the patient in presbyopic age can read without presbyopic glasses, overwhelming chances are that he/she is myopic only in one eye and the other eye is either emmetropic or hypermetropic. Patient uses myopic eye for near and the other for distant vision, hence does not uses glasses for near or distance vision.

Causes of bilateral diminished near vision: These are the following:

1. Presbyopia.
2. Decompensated hypermetropia in prepresbyopic age.
3. Uncorrected high astigmatism.
4. Bilateral aphakia.
5. Bilateral pseudophakia.
6. Minus contact lenses in near presbyopic age.

Causes of unilateral diminished near vision: These are as follows:

1. Instillation of cycloplegic in one eye.
2. Unilateral traumatic cycloplegia.
3. Traumatic shift of lens backwards.
4. Subluxation of lens.
5. Posterior dislocation of lens.
6. Unilateral aphakia/pseudophakia.
7. Unilateral high hypermetropia.
8. Forward movement of the central retina:
   a. Central serous retinopathy.
   b. Macular detachment.
   c. Retrobulbar mass pushing the central retina forward.
9. Overcorrection of unilateral myopia by radial keratotomy (RK) or laser-assisted in situ keratomileusis (LASIK).

Diminished vision with usual glasses: The causes can be for distance/near/both.

Diminished distant vision with usual glasses: Features are detailed below:

1. In myopia:
   a. Increase in power is generally seen in children with progressive myopia. They require enhancement of power of glasses almost every year that gets stabilized in late teens.

b. Onset of central nuclear sclerosis in elderly.

c. Onset of keratoconus at puberty.

d. Overcorrection of hypermetropia by LASIK.

e. Hyperglycemia.

f. Instillation of strong miotics.

2. In hypermetropia:

   a. Reduction of hypermetropia in children at the onset of puberty.

   b. Increase in hypermetropia with advancing age.

   c. Use of parasympatholytic drugs orally or locally.

   d. Onset of central serous retinopathy.

   e. Hypoglycemia.

Diminished near vision with usual glasses: Following are the characteristics:

1. Diminished accommodation with age will require addition of plus power to the present power. A patient at 40, requires an addition of +1D to distant correction, +2D to +2.5D at 50 and +3D at 60. After that, the progression will stop.

2. Onset of central nuclear sclerosis will require reduction in plus power. A person who had been using addition of +2D at 50 years may not require near correction due to onset of myopia, secondary to central nuclear sclerosis.

3. Consumption or instillation of drugs that cause cycloplegia will require addition of plus lenses.

4. Hypoglycemia will require addition of plus lenses. Typical example is an untreated diabetic who is put on antidiabetic for first time suddenly realizes that he/she is unable to see with near glasses since he/she started antidiabetic treatment.

5. Central serous retinopathy.

Non-visual Symptoms of Error of Refraction

The common non-visual symptoms of error of refraction are:

1. Asthenopia.

2. Recurrent external infection.

3. Squint.

Asthenopia

Asthenopia is feeling of ocular tiredness. It manifests variously with non-specific symptoms:

1. Unexplained pain in and around the eyeball.

2. Heaviness in the eyeballs.

3. Headache, which is generally aggravated by prolong near work, prolong distant vision or intermediate vision like seeing a movie, television, long drive or working on a computer.

4. It is generally associated with chronic redness of the eyes due to recurrent subclinical infection of the lid margin and conjunctivitis. The patient may have normal or subnormal vision.

5. On careful examination, the patient may have hypermetropia, hypermetropic astigmatism or mixed astigmatism:

   a. Hypermetropia causes more asthenopia than myopia.

   b. Astigmatism and uncorrected presbyopia causes more discomfort.

6. It is bilateral, slow progressive and may be associated with muscle imbalance, with or without diplopia.

7. Children rarely complain of asthenopia.

8. All the cases with asthenopia should have refraction under cycloplegia and orthoptic evaluation.

9. It is treated by full correction with special reference to astigmatism and presbyopia. Prescription of proper glasses and orthoptic exercises promptly relieve asthenopia.

Recurrent External Infections

Recurrent external infections consists of recurrent stye, chalazia, blepharitis and chronic conjunctivitis. The infection is generally transferred by fingers. An asthenopic patient has tendency to touch and rub the eyes with fingers. In spite of all efforts, the fingers cannot be fully disinfected and the chance of infection lingers. Proper personal hygiene can reduce recurrent external infections. Conversely, all cases of recurrent stye, chalazia and blepharitis should be refracted under cycloplegia and prescribed glasses accordingly. This will relieve asthenopia as well.

Squint

Squint may be the main complaint to bring a child for ophthalmic consultation. The child on examination is found to have error of refraction with or without anomaly of accommodation. Such children are generally esotropic and corrected by plus lenses. A presbyopic adult may present with exotropia, myopes may present with both types of horizontal tropias, while anisometropia is commonly associated with exotropia. A child with high degree of astigmatism may tilt the head to overcome squint.

EXTERNAL EXAMINATIONS

External examinations in errors of refraction consist of detailed examinations of lids, cornea, pupil and lens.

Signs of Errors of Refraction

1. There may be no sign to betray errors of refraction.
2. The child may squeeze the lids to get a pinhole effect and the parents may think that either the child has squint or this is a part of mischief.
3. The high myopic eyes are larger than emmetropic or hypermetropic eyes because of increased axial length. All large eyes need not have error of refraction. The myopic eyes have large cornea and pupil. The pupil in myopia dilates faster than emmetropia or hypermetropia.

4. High hypermetropes have smaller cornea, small pupil and shallow anterior chamber. The pupils in hypermetropes take more time to dilate.
5. Myopes have negative angle kappa.
6. Hypermetropes have positive angle kappa.
7. Pseudosquint is more common in errors of refraction.
8. The patients with errors of refraction are more likely to have true squint in the form of phorias breaking into tropias or frank tropias.

Assessment in Case of Error of Refraction

1. The first and foremost test to be done in error of refraction is to note distant vision. Generally, near vision is tested only in presbyopic age. Sometimes, a pre-presbyopic may also complain of diminished near vision that is mostly due to uncorrected high hypermetropia or instillation of cycloplegia.
2. The next step is to find out if the diminished distant vision is due to error of refraction or organic disease.
3. This is found out by a simple test commonly called pinhole test. This test is also known as Scheiner's test (original Scheiner's test was done by two pinholes, which is no more used).

   Original Scheiner's test: This test was originally done to diagnose the type of error of refraction roughly. The original Scheiner's device had two pinholes set apart on each side of the pupil. Only one eye was examined, the other eye was occluded and the patient was asked to look at the Snellen's chart or equivalent. The device produced two parallel pencils of rays, which entered the eye. In case of myopia, they crossed each other in front of the retina. In case of hypermetropia, they crossed each other behind the retina and formed two small circles on the retina. The two points of light were brought to a single point by moving the Scheiner's disk to the far point of the eye and the error of refraction was determined from the far point. The whole test was cumbersome and is no more in clinical use. The double pinhole test or Scheiner's test has been replaced by a single pinhole test. The pinhole put in front of the eye under examination improves the vision in ametropia (Fig. 8.2).

Once it has been confirmed that the diminished vision is due to error of refraction, the next step is to find out the type and extent of error of refraction.

4. This can be done in two ways:
   a. Subjective test—this is less reliable.
   b. Objective test —this is accurate.

Subjective Test

Subjective test comprises of putting spherical lenses in front of the eye and noticing if the vision improves. If the vision improves with lens of either sign, i.e. plus or minus, the power of the lens of the same sign is gradually increased by adding lenses of the same sign in steps of 0.5D sphere till best vision is reached.

For example, a patient has distant vision of 6/18 that improves with pinhole has obviously an error of refraction. Now, +1D sphere is put in front of the eye and the result noted. If the vision improves, the power of the plus sphere is gradually increased till the best vision is attained. If the vision deteriorates from 6/18 with +1D; the power of the sphere is gradually reduced till 0 power is reached. Now the sign of addition is changed to minus and the power that gives best vision is minus power for that particular eye.

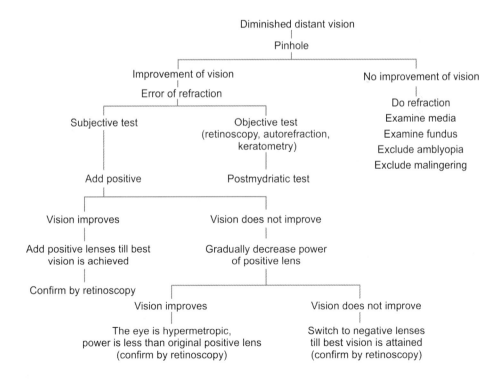

Figure 8.2: Approach to diminished distant vision

Fogging Method

Fogging is very useful method in abolishing accommodation, thus eliminating facultative hypermetropia in turn. This is very effective, non-cycloplegic abolition of accommodation. It is used in assessing acceptance under cycloplegia as well. In this method, plus lenses stronger than maximum correction of one of the hypermetropic meridians or minus lens weaker than myopic error is applied in front of the eye under examination. The power of the lenses is increased till the vision becomes clear by putting plus lenses in front of the eye. Accommodation is artificially abolished producing myopia. This can also be used in finding out the correct power of astigmatism.

Subjective test should be avoided in children.

Single Pinhole Test or Modified Scheiner's Test

Single pinhole test is very easy inexpensive useful test to differentiate between errors of refraction and organic causes responsible for diminished vision. The device used is called pinhole (PH) supplied with every trial set. It is a circular opaque disk, size of which is almost that of any other lens in the trial set. It has a central hole. The ideal diameter of a pinhole is 1.2 mm. If a regular pinhole is not available, it can be fashioned by making a 1.2 mm hole in an opaque cardboard. Sometimes, handheld pinholes with handle are also available (Figs 8.3A and B).

A pinhole 1.2 mm in diameter neutralizes up to 3D of error of refraction. Holes larger than 1.25 mm do not neutralize errors of refraction well. To have best result, the pinhole should be kept at the anterior focal plane (the usual distance for spectacle lens). Logically, a constricted pupil should also improve vision in errors of refraction. The constricted pupil being nearer the nodal point fails to neutralize

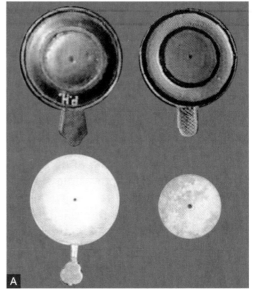

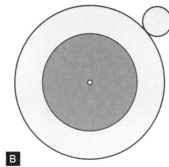

Figures 8.3A and B: Pinhole. **A.** Photograph of various types of pinholes; **B.** Pinhole.

error of refraction effectively. A pinhole does not correct high errors of refraction fully. A patient with 6/18 and a spherical error may get 6/6 or better vision with pinhole, but a person with 6/60 will improve to 6/18 or at the most 6/12. A pinhole does not effectively neutralize all astigmatism as well.

An effective improvement with spectacle lenses should not always be expected in all the cases with improved vision with pinhole. The best example is irregular astigmatism where vision does improve with pinhole, but not with lenses.

The optics involved in improvement of vision by a pinhole is increase in depth of focus. The other causes that contribute less are:

1. Narrow beam entering the eye through nodal point.
2. Cutting peripheral aberrations.

Depth of Focus

Depth of focus is defined as the range of movement of object in relation to retina that keeps an image clear. This denotes the distance through which when an object moved, forms a clear image on the given screen. In case of photography, the screen represents the film and the aperture of the shutter represents the pupil. In the eye, it is the retina that acts as the screen. The depth of focus depends both on the distance of the object from the film as well as size of the aperture. The size of aperture of photographic camera is counter part of the pupil of the eye.

Other subjective methods (Box 8.2) are fogging by sphere, stenopaic slit, astigmatic fan, cross cylinder and duochrome test. Duochrome test is precise for spherical values, while the other two give correct cylindrical value.

Box 8.2: Subjective assessment

The subjective methods are pinhole test, stenopaic slit test, adding lenses empirically to get the best vision, fogging by sphere, fogging by cylinder, cross cylinder, astigmatic fan, astigmatic dial and duochrome.

RECORDING OF VISION

Recording of vision is subjective. It involves response of the patient that depends on mental status, age and cooperation of the patient.

Before we pass on the subjective assessment of vision, we must discuss few terms used in relation to vision or visual acuity. They are:

1. Visibility: This is the ability of a person to discern presence of an object or objects in the field of vision.

2. Field of vision: It is all the area that has visibility when a person fixes an object of interest.
3. Resolution: It is the ability to discriminate two points in space (field).
4. Vision: It is absolute limit of visibility. It depends on:
   a. Distance of the object.
   b. Size of the object.
   c. Color of the object.
   d. Brightness of the object.
   e. Contrast.
   f. Background.
   g. Ambient light.

These are applicable to a normal eye, an eye with poor focusing and subnormal neural path will obviously result in diminished visibility. There are two components that involve near and distant vision:

1. Optical (refractive status).
2. Neural.

In clinical practice, vision comprises of:

1. Distant vision.
2. Near vision.
3. Color vision.
4. Field of vision.
5. Contrast.

NEAR AND DISTANT VISION

Near and distant vision depends on:

1. Proper focus:
   a. Normal refractive status.
   b. Available accommodation.
2. Structurally intact healthy eye and intact neurological path.

Visual Acuity

Visual acuity (VA) is measured in two sets of number, one denoting the distance between the patient and the object, and the other denotes smallest letter visible clearly from testing distance. It is expressed in fraction:

$$VA = \frac{d}{D}$$

where, the numerator d represents the distance between the optotypes (Snellen's chart) and the patient and the denominator D represents the distance at which the numerator should be read by an emmetropic, structurally normal eye with normal neurovisual path.

The visual acuity is expressed as reciprocal of minimum separable visual angle that can be recognized.

$$VA = \frac{1}{\text{Minimum separable visual angle}}$$
(measured as minutes of an arc)

A patient who recognizes a letter with minimum separable visual angle of 1 minute has VA = 1/1 = 20/20 = 6/6.

One minute arc is equal to (1/60th) of an angle, which in turn is (1/360th) of a circle.

In case of 6/60 the top letter, which should be read at 60 m by a normal eye is being read at 6 m.

The vulgar fraction VA = d/D is called Snellen's factor.

Optotypes are the variable sized figures commonly alphabets, but can be figures of diagrams to test vision (Figs 8.4 to 8.10).

The quantitative estimation of visual acuity is minimal resolvable visual angle measured in minutes.

Visual Angle

Visual angle is an angle subtended by an object in the visual field at the nodal point.

N is the nodal point of the eye. OO' is the visual axis. AB is a linear object. B_1A_1 is the image formed on the retina. ANB is the visual angle at nodal point N (Fig. 8.11).

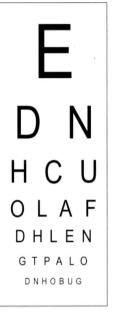

Figure 8.4: Snellen's chart (alphabets)

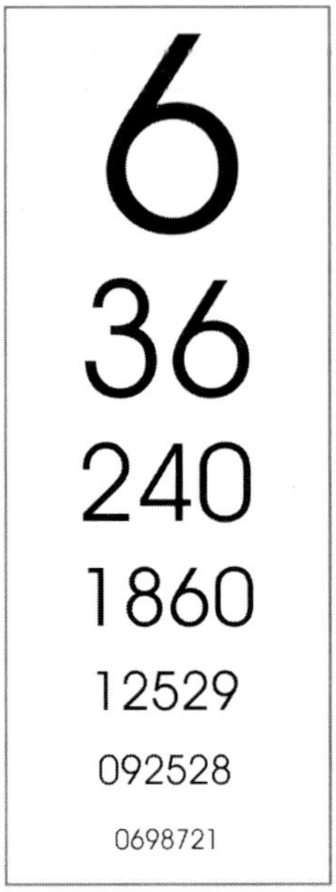

Figure 8.5: Snellen's chart (numbers)

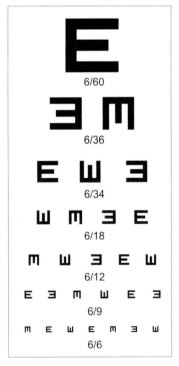

Figure 8.6: E-chart

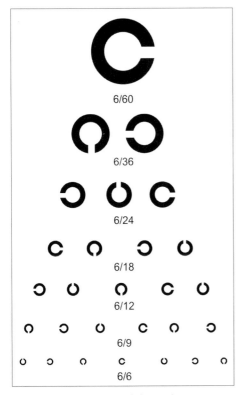

Figure 8.7: Landolt's C-chart

Visual acuity measures the smallest retinal image appreciated. In case of Figure 8.11, it is $A_1O'B_1$.

The size of the retinal image depends on the size of the object and the distance of the object from the retina.

AB is an object that forms image B'A' on the retina. When the same object is moved nearer the eye, it forms a larger image B'A" (Fig. 8.12A). This property is clinically used in patients who have vision less than 6/60. They are moved near the optotype till the top letter is visible. Say at 5 m. The Snellen's factor at this distance will become 5/60. Similarly, if the image of the object is at the same distance, this will also enlarge the retinal image and make it visible. This phenomenon is utilized by projecting proportionally large image

by a digital projector without moving the patient. Conversely, smaller objects put nearer the eye will form a same size of the image (Figs 8.12B and 8.13).

The magnification of retinal image besides distance of the object from the eye also depends on axial length and the nature of the dioptric power of the eye (Fig. 8.14).

The latter may be modified by adding correcting lenses at anterior focal plane, i.e.

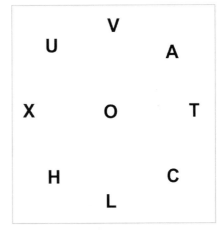

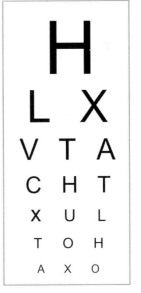

Figure 8.8: Snellen's test for young children and retarded (STYCAR)

15 mm in front of the cornea or a contact lens on the cornea or an intraocular lens (IOL) in the eye. Image is smaller in uncorrected hypermetropia and larger in uncorrected myopia than in emmetropia.

The vision corrected by lenses is also called absolute acuity of vision.

Assessment of Visual Acuity and its Grading

For clinical purposes, visual acuity is measurement of smallest object that is clearly seen at a certain distance. The patient should be able to appreciate the finest details of the object.

The neurophysiology involved in it is stimulation of two cones separated by an unstimulated cone in the macula. The average diameter of a macular cone is said to be 0.004 mm. Thus an average normal eye with normal dioptric power and neurosensory path should be able to appreciate a retinal image as small

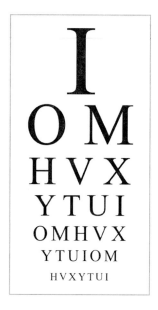

Figure 8.9: Reversible Snellen's chart. The letters look similar in the chart as well as in the mirror used at 3 m.

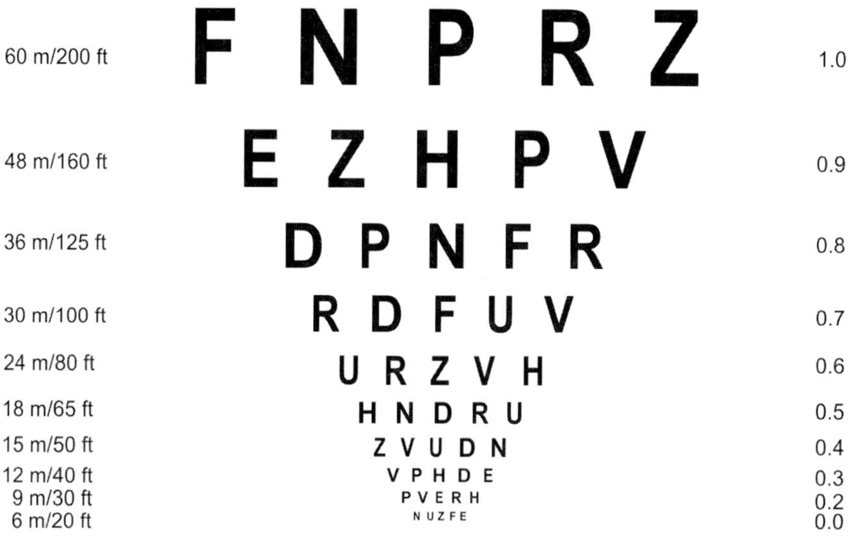

60 m/200 ft	F N P R Z	1.0
48 m/160 ft	E Z H P V	0.9
36 m/125 ft	D P N F R	0.8
30 m/100 ft	R D F U V	0.7
24 m/80 ft	U R Z V H	0.6
18 m/65 ft	H N D R U	0.5
15 m/50 ft	Z V U D N	0.4
12 m/40 ft	V P H D E	0.3
9 m/30 ft	P V E R H	0.2
6 m/20 ft	N U Z F E	0.0

Figure 8.10: Bailey-Lovie logMAR distance acuity and reading chart

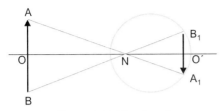

Figure 8.11: Visual angle

as 0.44 mm. This represents 1 minute arc of visual angle. This forms the basis of construction of all optotypes used in assessment of visual acuity. It has been discussed earlier, the visual angle depends not only on the height of the optotype but also distance of the optotype from the patient.

The commonly used formula to estimate the distance at which an optotype should be visible is given as follows:

$$= \frac{H}{88} \times \frac{6}{1} = D$$

where, D is the distance, H is the height of the optotype, 88 represents the height of the top letter in millimeter. For all practical purposes, it is taken as 90 mm or 9 cm. Thus, an optotype 9 cm should be visible at 6 m.

Vision Drums and Vision Charts

Vision charts can either be incorporated in the vision drum (Figs 8.15 and 8.16) or may be hung in frame individually. Each vision drum can accommodate four panels, one in English, one in vernacular language, one E chart and one C chart. They may also have,

Worth four-dot test, duochrome test and astigmatic fan along with the optotypes. The vision drums revolve along a long-axis and are self-illuminated. The illumination should be uniform. The drum can be rotated round the vertical axis, manually or electrically. Commonly four incandescent bulbs of 40 watts each are used, along the long-axis at equal distance from each other.

The figures are generally black on white background. They can also be white on black. The former gives better visibility as black on white gives better contrast than white on black. The panels in the vision drum are made of self-illuminated white materials that may be glass or plastic. The illumination is from behind the panel. In case of individual opaque panels, the source of illumination is in front of the panel.

The panels are available in two sizes, one for examination at 6 m and other for examination at 3 m.

The optotypes of the latter are half the size of the former.

Commonly used optotypes are alphabets, tumbling E, Landolt C, Sjogren's hands, numbers, pictures and dots (refer Figs 8.4 to 8.10).

Generally the optotypes are kept 6 m in front of the patient. In case of shortage of space, a plane mirror is kept at 3 m in front of the patient and a reversed vision chart is kept little above and behind the head of the patient. The image formed by the plane mirror is 3 m behind the mirror, erect, virtual and laterally reversed. To the patient, the image

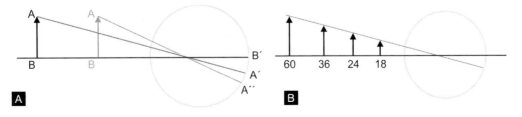

Figures 8.12A and B: Change in the size of retinal image on moving the object toward the eye

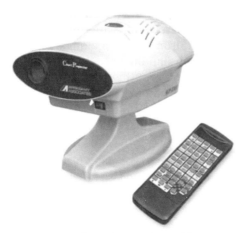

Figure 8.13: Auto chart projector [*Courtesy:* Appasamy Associates (with permission)]

seems to be situated at 6 m. And the reverse chart looks like a normal chart.

The following letters need not be reversed when using a mirror because they look same from both sides. They are—A H I M O T U V W X Y. For obvious reasons, E and C charts too need not be reversed.

The smaller vision charts are kept at 3 m in front of the patient; they too can either be self-illuminated or illuminated externally. Smaller charts can be projected via a projector on the screen. The vision charts used for preschool children entirely differ from Snellen's chart and its variation. Some of them are not even based on Snellen's fraction.

Construction of Figures on Snellen's Chart

Previously we have seen that measurement of vision is measurement of retinal image formed by the angle subtended at nodal point. It is defined as reciprocal of minimum resolvable visual angle measured in minutes. A minute is 1/60th of 1°. In fact, it is 0.017° of an arc. The 1° is (1/360) of a circle. 1 minute represents the distance between two cones separated by one normal cone.

Typical Snellen's chart comprises of seven lines of alphabets. The number of letter in each line increases as the size diminishes. The distance between the two lines is equal all through. The top line has largest single letter, which measures 88 mm that is rounded to 90 mm or 9 cm. The size of the letters decrease in a proportion of 60:36:24:18:12:9:6. This means that a smallest letter is 1/10th of top letter. As the numbers of the letters in each line increases, the size of the letters decreases by half octave after 6/36 and the vision is noted as 6/60, 6/36. Thus the distance between the second line is longer than the letters in last line. This is in contrast to logMAR chart of Bailey and Lovie where each line has five letters, irrespective of size and space between the two letters is equal to the size of the letter in that particular line.

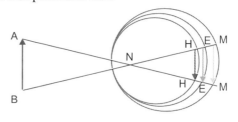

Figure 8.14: Relative size of the retinal image on different dimensions of the eye. MM is the image on a myopic eye, which is longer than emmetropic EE and hypermetropic HH. The hypermetropic eye has the shortest axial length.

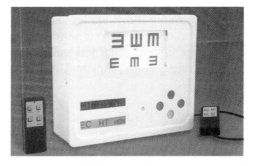

Figure 8.15: Self-illuminated, multipurpose with remote control to be used at 3 m along with refraction unit [*Courtesy:* Appasamy Associates (with permission)].

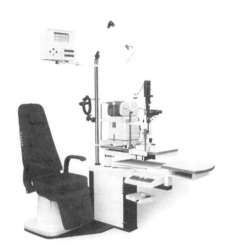

Figure 8.16: A refraction unit [*Courtesy:* Appasamy Associates (with permission)]

Each optotype (tumbling E, etc.) is so constructed that the top letter, i.e. 6/60 or 20/20 fits in a 9 cm × 9 cm square, which forms an angle of 5 minutes on the nodal point at 6 m (Figs 8.17A and B to 8.19).

The square is divided in 25 squares of equal size and each square forms angle of 1 minute of an arc. The distance between each arm is equal to thickness of each arm. The letters in 6/36 will have the same effect at 36 m as the last letter in 6/6 will have at 6 m. The letters in 6/6 will also form an angle of 5 minutes at the nodal point at 6 meters.

Optotypes of a particular type when moved nearer the eye will form angle larger than 5 minutes. Conversely, when moved away will form smaller angle and will be less visible.

The other charts based on Snellen's fraction are:

1. Snellen's test for young children and retarded (refer Fig. 8.8).
2. Allen's pictures.

The STYCAR comprises of two charts, one to be kept at 6 m and a smaller chart (that the child holds). The examiner points to a letter on the larger chart and ask the child to identify and point the same letter in the chart in their hand.

LogMAR Chart

Acronym logMAR stands for logarithm of the minimum angle of resolution. The chart is also known as Bailey-Lovie vision chart. The logMAR chart is little more complicated vision chart to understand (refer Figure 8.10). It has less clinical application and more prognostic value; it is good for mathematical calculation and statistical evaluation. It is most commonly used in noting progression in diabetic retinopathy as per early treatment of diabetic retinopathy study (ETDRS). It is also used in recording vision in low vision.

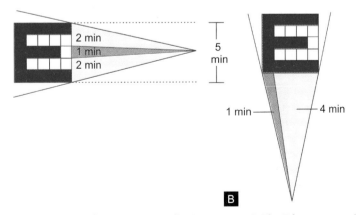

Figures 8.17A and B: Construction of optotype 'E' Snellen's optotype. **A.** The E forms an angle of 5 minutes (ash blue); **B.** Each arm of E forms an angle of 1 minute at the same distance (angle in cyan color).

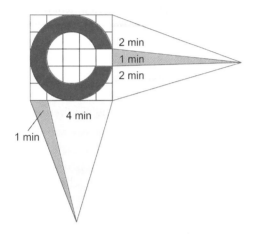

Figure 8.18: Construction of Landolt's C. The principle is same as in E-chart.

Each line has five optotypes of equal size, with equal distance between them. Total number of lines in a logMAR chart is 14 as compared to 7 lines of standard Snellen's chart. The 11th line of logMAR chart corresponds to 6/6 of Snellen's chart. In contrast to standard Snellen's chart, which is read at 6 m the logMAR chart is read at 4 m. To evaluate low vision, it is read at 3, 2 or 1 m as and when required. There is a geometric progression of height of letter from one line to the next.

The chart expresses decadic logMAR. The logMAR scale converts the geometric sequence of traditional Snellen's chart to linear scale. Each letter has a score value of 0.02 log unit. Thus, total score per line is 0.02 × 5 (number of letters) = 0.1 log unit.

The formula used to calculate the score of logMAR visual acuity = 0.1 + logMAR value of the best line read − 0.25 × number of letters read.

The chart measures visual acuity loss. Positive values indicate loss of vision. Negative values mean normal or better vision. They are written as lines lost or lines gained.

The optotypes of logMAR chart can be letters, tumbling E, Landolts broken C or geometric figures. Customized, portable charts are available for mass screen. Three different, but comparable charts are available, one for right eye and the other for left eye and third for refraction.

Advantages of logMAR over other charts: The followings are advantages of logMAR chart:

1. Equal number of letters per line (five).
2. Regular spacing between lines and letters.
3. Size of letters progress uniformly.
4. Final score of total letters read is precise.
5. Final score is based on total of all letters read.

Disadvantages of Snellen's chart as compared to logMAR: The disadvantages are as follows:

1. Number of letters in each line differs. The top line 6/60 has single letter, while the seventh line has seven letters.

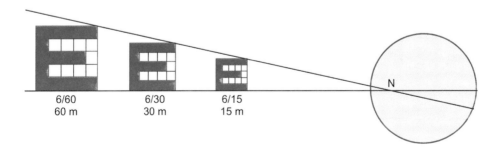

6/60	6/30	6/15
60 m	30 m	15 m

Figure 8.19: Relation between the size of the optotype and distance from the eye. The height of the optotype should be reduced to half if the distance is halved to form the same size of retinal image.

2. One mistake per line has different interpretation.
3. Progression in size of letters is irregular.

How to interpret visual acuity on a standard Snellen's chart read at 6 m?

If the person reads the top letter only, it is written as 6/60, which means that the top letter, which should be read at 60 m is being read at 6 m and the vision is 1/10th of normal. It may be written as 0.1 on decimal fraction and 20/200 as per American standard. 6/60 equals to +1.00 on logMAR scale (Table 8.1).

Similarly, if the second line that should be read at 36 m is being read at 6 m should be written as 6/36 and represents 1/6th of normal vision. This progression can go up to seventh line and that should be written as 6/6 on Snellen's chart or 1.0 on decimal scale. This is equivalent to +0.00 on logMAR and the patient reads the smallest letter at 6 m.

When a Snellen's chart, half the size of a standard chart is used, it is kept at 3 m, but it follows Snellen's fraction and is written as 6/60, 6/36, etc. depending on the line read (Table 8.2).

A person who can read the seventh line at 6 m can read the top letter at 60 m.

Table 8.2: Summary of comparison between Snellen's and American optotype

Snellen's (m)	American (ft)
20/200	6/60
20/80	6/24
20/40	6/12
20/20	6/6
20/10	6/3

Recording of Vision on Snellen's Chart

Recording of Distant Vision

Recording of distant vision is divided into two groups (Table 8.3):

Table 8.1: Comparison between the values of logMAR and other optotypes

SI No	LogMAR	Decimal	Snellen's (m)	American (ft)
1.	+1.00	0.100	6/60	20/200
2.	+0.90	0.125	6/48	20/160
3.	+0.80	0.160	6/38	20/125
4.	+0.70	0.200	6/30	20/100
5.	+0.60	0.250	6/24	20/80
6.	+0.50	0.320	6/19	20/63
7.	+0.40	0.400	6/15	20/50
8.	+0.30	0.500	6/12	20/40
9.	+0.20	0.630	6/9.5	20/32
10.	+0.10	0.800	6/7.5	20/25
11.	+0.00	1.000	6/6	20/20
12.	−0.10	1.250	6/4.8	20/16
13.	−0.20	1.600	6/3.8	20/12.5
14.	−0.30	2.000	6/3	20/10

Table 8.3: Recording of vision on Snellen's charts

Sl No	Line read	Number of letters in the line	Example of the alphabets	Vision
1.	First	1	E	6/60
2.	Second	2	DN	6/36
3.	Third	3	HCU	6/24
4.	Fourth	4	OLAF	6/18
5.	Fifth	5	DHLEN	6/12
6.	Sixth	6	CTPOLO	6/9
7.	Seventh	7	DNHOBUC	6/6
8.	Eighth	8	POTABLED	6/3

1. Those who can read the top letter (6/60) on the Snellen's chart or its equivalent at 6 m.
2. Those who cannot read the top letter, i.e. 6/60 at 6 m on Snellen's chart or its equivalent.

Steps in Testing Visual Acuity

For both the above groups, the following steps are taken:

1. The patient is seated at a distance of 6 m from the optotypes facing the optotypes.
2. The vision drum is illuminated, generally internally where electricity is available, otherwise it is illuminated externally.
3. The patient is asked to read the chart without squeezing the lids. Squeezing the lids produces pinhole effect that improves vision to a level more than actual vision. For example, a person can read only the top letter without squeezing; he/she will most probably be able to read third or even fourth line (Fig. 8.20).
4. Reading with both eyes is an optional step. It induces confidence in the patient and sooths apprehension in children.
5. It should be remembered that binocular vision is always better than uniocular vision when both eyes have vision.

6. Next step is to record vision in two eyes separately. For this, following steps are taken:
   a. By convention, the right eye is examined first.
   b. The other eye is occluded.
   c. The occlusion should be complete, obstructing all the rays without pressing the globe.
   d. This can be done by (Figs 8.21A to C):
      i. Palm of the patient.
      ii. Palm of the examiner.
      iii. Handheld occluder.
      iv. Trial frame mounted occlude.

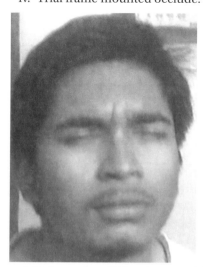

Figure 8.20: Squeezing of lids to improve vision

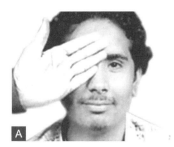
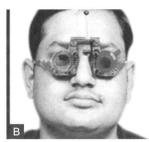
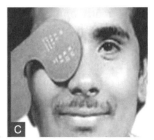

Figures 8.21A to C: Correct method for occluding the eye

Trial Frames

Trial frames are adjustable spectacle like frames (Fig. 8.22).

They have two rims, one for each eye. The rims are joined by a horizontal nose bridge, the length of which is adjustable that can be slide to adjust the interpupillary distance. Some of them have scales edged on it to measure the interpupillary distance in millimeters. Each rim has multiple slots on the front surface, which may be as many as 5 to accommodate optical devices like spherical lens, cylindrical lens, occluder, pinhole, stenopaic slit, prism, Maddox rod or red-green glasses. These devices can be put singly or in combination. The front most slots have degrees etched on the surface. They indicate axis of the cylinder put behind. The numbering of the degrees is done on the basis of an international convention. The numbering is generally at the lower half of the rim, but may be all around or may be placed obliquely. The numbering of the axis follows a definite rule, which means for the right eye, the zero is on the temporal side and 180° is on the nasal side. For the left eye, the zero is on the nasal side and the 180° is on the temporal side. In other words, 90° on both the eyes is vertically down in the middle. The axis is marked at difference of 5°, which is sufficient for clinical work. The cylindrical lenses are manually rotated to change the axis. Some sophisticated have milled screw to change the axis. The trial frames can be incorporated in the refraction unit also.

Recording of Vision of Person who can Read the Largest Letter or More on the Snellen's Chart

1. By convention, the vision in right eye is noted first, followed by left and then in both eyes.
2. Close the left eye and ask the patient to read, beginning from the top, if he/she reads the seventh line on a standard Snellen's chart in 6 m, the vision is noted as 6/6 or 20/20.

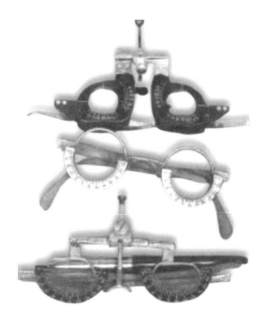

Figure 8.22: Commonly used trial frames

If the reads one line less, the vision is recorded as 6/9. Similarly, vision can be 6/12, 6/18, 6/24, 6/36 or 6/60.

While recording the vision, the lowest vision (Snellen's fraction) is recorded.

Close the right eye and record the vision as above.

3. Open both the eyes and note the vision in both eyes together.

Binocular vision is generally better than uniocular vision. It can never be less.

4. If the binocular vision is not more than uniocular vision separately, the cause should be sought in the eye with poor vision.

Causes of non-increment of vision: when both eyes are open:

1. There is no perception of light in one eye.
2. Vision in one eye is very poor as compared to the other eye.
3. One of the eyes has deep amblyopia.
4. One of the eyes has large angle of squint.
5. The patient turns his/her head in such a way that both the eyes do not fix simultaneously.
6. Malinger.

Recording of Vision in Person who Cannot See 6/60

There are four ways of making the person read the top letter:

1. In case of fixed vision drum, the patient is moved gradually toward the drum from seat 1 m at a time till the top letter becomes visible.
2. In case of handheld charts, the patient remains seated in the original position, the vision chart is moved gradually toward him/her till the top letter becomes visible.
3. Increase the size of the letter and note the size that is visible. The Snellen's factor is written on the computerized digital

meter. These devices are available with costly refraction units.

If the patient can read the top letter at 5 m, the vision is noted as 5/60. At 4 m 4/60, at 3 m 3/60 and so on up to at 1 m 1/60.

4. Counting finger at gradually decreasing distance.

This is alternative to 1, 2 and 3 mentioned above.

If the patient cannot read the top letter at 6 m, he/she is asked to count fingers at 5, 4, 3, 2 and 1 m till can count the fingers correctly. The rationale behind making the patient count the fingers are that the width of adult finger is almost equal to arms of the letter E of Snellen's chart. Thus, a patient who can accurately count fingers at given fixed distance has following acuity (Table 8.4).

Table 8.4: Acuity of vision in relation to the counting of fingers at different positions

Distance of CF*	Snellen's equivalent
5 m	5/60
4 m	4/60
3 m	3/60
2 m	2/60
1 m	1/60

*CF, counting finger

Precautions taken: while noting visual acuity by counting finger:

1. Light should fall on the palm of the examiner.
2. Keep the finger separated.
3. Ask the patient to count the number of fingers of the examiner.
4. Change the number of fingers at the same distance and ask the patient to count the number of fingers every time. Check the counting at least 3 times.
5. Never ask the patient to count his/her own fingers because even a person with no vision can tell the number of fingers at the end of his/her out stretched hand.

Recording of Vision in Person with Less Than 1/60

Error of refraction is rarely the sole cause of diminished vision in a person with less than 1/60 except in aphakia.

The examiner gradually moves toward the patient 1 m at a time and asks the patient to count as soon as the fingers are visible and is able to count. The vision is now written as CF 1/2 m, CF 1/3 m and CF 1/4 m.

OBJECTIVE METHODS OF ASSESSING REFRACTIVE STATUS

The objective methods employed in assessment of refractive status of the eye are more accurate than subjective method because subjective methods most of the time do not eliminate accommodation except in fogging. The subjective methods fail to unmask hypermetropia. The children may be prescribed minus glasses, while the child actually requires plus lenses. This happens due to strong accommodation in children. The subjective test also fails to estimate astigmatism precisely. The other source of error is patient's involvement especially children who may not cooperate or may not understand the instructions.

The various objective methods are:

1. Retinoscopy (skiascopy or shadow test).
2. Autorefraction.
3. Keratometry (for astigmatism and contact lens fitting).
4. Ultrasonography/especially for axial ametropia in presence of opacity in the media.

The first two methods are more commonly used in clinical practice in assessing types of errors in clear media.

Retinoscopy/Determination of Power of Correction

The method of retinoscopy is also called doing refraction. The word refraction encompasses steps performed to find out power of the optical device that may be spectacle or contact lens to give best vision. In other words, it denotes the objective method to find out the lens that when kept in front of eye, very near the eye between the retinoscope and the eye will cause the refracted rays emerging from the eye to come to focus in the plane of the eye piece of the retinoscope.

The retinoscopy indirectly finds out far point of the eye.

The retinoscopy indicates the total objective refractive power of the eye under examination. It is most suitable procedure to determine error of refraction in infants, nonverbal children, illiterate, deaf and mute and mentally retarded persons. The retinoscopy can detect difference as small as 0.25D. Retinoscope also picks up opacities in the media. The device by which retinoscopy is done is called retinoscope or skiascope. The basic function of which is to illuminate the retina through the pupil. The principle of retinoscopy is explained in Figure 8.23.

Types of Retinoscopes

There are two basic types of retinoscope, both of which follow the same rules of optics, i.e. the image moves opposite the movement of the object. The object in case of retinoscopy is the source of light that may be reflected by a mirror or it may be self-illuminated.

The two types of retinoscope are:

1. Reflecting (mirror):
   a. Plane mirror.
   b. Concave mirror.
2. Self-illuminated:
   a. Spot retinoscope.
   b. Streak retinoscope.

Mirror Retinoscopes

The mirror retinoscopes (Figs 8.24A and B) can either be single mirror or double mirror.

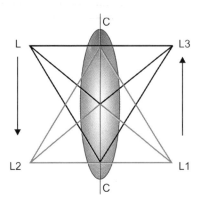

Figure 8.23: Principle of retinoscopy. CC is a convex lens; L is the source of light and L1 is its image on the opposite side and is away from it if L is moved to L2, the image L1 will move to L3 (the image in convex lens moves opposite the movement of the object). The lens CC may be considered as dioptric equivalent of eye of any refractive status, i.e. emmetropia, hypermetropia or myopia.

The optics involved in both the types of mirror is the same. The only difference is movement of the retinal glow in each type.

In the single mirror retinoscope, the device has only one type of mirror that can be either plane or concave (refer Fig. 8.24B). The difficulty with these types is that the examiner requires two retinoscopes in the working place. To overcome this difficulty, double mirror retinoscopes came into use.

Double mirror retinoscope is a small, handy, dumbbell-shaped device. That has two circular mirrors embedded on its body on either end. One of them is plane and the other concave. Both the mirrors have peepholes in the center through which the retinal glow and its movements can be observed by the examiner. In fact, the plane mirror is not absolutely plane. It is slightly curved, but not as much as the concave mirror on the other side. An ivory dot on the handle under the plane mirror makes it easy to identify the plane mirror in the dark room.

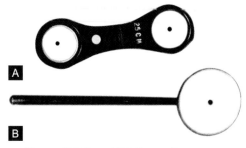

Figures 8.24A and B: Mirror retinoscopes.
A. Double mirror; **B.** Single mirror.

The concave mirror has curvature of 25 cm. The word 25 cm is engraved at the bottom of the concave mirror on the handle. The peephole in the plane mirror does not have any lens in it.

The peephole in the concave mirror has a +2D sphere lens incorporated in it. This is meant to relax the accommodation of the observer. This +2D lens is optional. The power of the lens is etched on the back surface of the retinoscope under the peephole.

The mirror retinoscope projects a conical beam of light on the retina, which is responsible for the circular shape of the retinal glow in spherical ametropia and oval in astigmatism.

Performing retinoscopy: To perform mirror retinoscopy, the requirements are:

1. An immediate source of light (ISL).
2. A retinoscope.
3. An eye with dilated pupil.

The immediate source of light is kept 25 cm behind the eye, slightly above and lateral to the eye. This reflects the light toward the observer, keeping the face of the patient dark. In plane mirror, the image of the ISL may be formed either between the patient and the observer or outside this zone, i.e. behind patient's eye or behind the observer's eye depending on type of ametropia. In clinical practice, the optometrist sits 1 m away, in front of the patient, thus the image of ISL formed is 1.25 m behind the observer and 2.50 m from the ISL (Fig. 8.25).

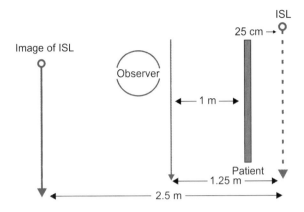

Figure 8.25: Relative position of ISL, patient and observer

To perform mirror retinoscopy, the light from the ISL is reflected through the pupil to the retina, which in turn sends it back as a retinal glow in the pupillary plane. This retinal glow shows movement in relation to the movement of the mirror, as follows:

1. It may move with the movement of the mirror.
2. It may not move.
3. It may move against the movement of the mirror.

The first condition is met with when the image formed is either behind the image of eye of the patient or the observer. In the second case, the error of refraction has been neutralized. In the third case, the images formed between the patient and the observer. These three observations constitute the basis of retinoscopy.

Streak Retinoscope

Streak retinoscope is a handheld device that looks similar to a direct ophthalmoscope in its outward appearance.

The streak retinoscope (Fig. 8.26) consists of a body that houses either dry batteries or a step-down transformer that illuminates the bulb. A bulb to illuminate. An array of plus

lenses above the bulb, a reflecting device that may be a plane mirror, a prism or a plano cylinder; a peephole to observe the outgoing beam of light, which is generally a streak. The light acts as immediate source of illumination. It consists of a bulb, the emerging rays of which can be converted into parallel or

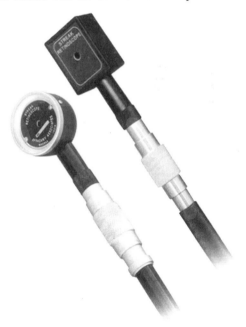

Figure 8.26: Streak retinoscope [*Courtesy:* Appasamy Associates (with permission)]

divergent rays, giving the effect of plane mirror or concave mirror by moving a plus planoconvex lens away or nearer the source of illumination (Fig. 8.27).

The emerging light can be circular spot when it is reflected by a plane mirror or a prism incorporated in it. It is a streak when a plano-cylindrical mirror is used to reflect light. The beam of light thrown by the streak retinoscope is called intercept.

Principle of Retinoscopy

Besides retinoscope, the phenomenon of retinoscopy requires:

1. Source of illumination: In mirror retinoscopy, it is 25 cm behind and slightly lateral to the eye of the patient (refer Fig. 8.26). It is an incandescent bulb of 40–60 watts, the light from which is reflected towards the observer. It keeps the face of the patient in shadow. In case of self-illuminated retinoscope (streak or spot), the source of illumination is inbuilt.

2. In both the cases, the observer generally sits at an arm's length (2/3–1 m) away and in front of the patient. However, this distance may vary between 1/2 and 2 m, requiring different adjustments, while calculating the power. Distance of 2 m gives more accurate findings, but is practically difficult because the observer need not only to see the retinal glow, but he/she is required to neutralize the movement of the globe by adding various types of lenses in front of the observed eye, which is best done at an arm's length.

3. Retinoscopy can be done under cycloplegia or without cycloplegia. The former is called static retinoscopy and the latter dynamic retinoscopy. Cycloplegic not only abolish accommodation but also causes mydriasis, which gives a better view of the retinal glow. A large circular glow circumvents central opacities in the cornea and lens. A small pupil may be obscured by opacities in the media.

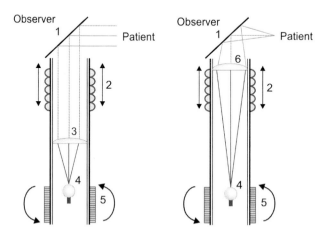

Figure 8.27: Outline of construction of streak retinoscope. **1.** Plane mirror; **2.** Arrangement to move the lens up and down; **3.** Convex lens near the bulb giving parallel ray effect (plane mirror effect); **4.** Bulb; **5.** Arrangement for changing the axis of the streak; **6.** Convex lens away from the bulb giving converging rays (concave mirror effect).

4. Static retinoscopy is done under complete cycloplegia (Table 8.5):
   a. Refraction in children under 10 should be done under long-acting cycloplegia like atropine 1% ointment applied 2 times a day for 3 consecutive days.
   b. Between 10 and 40 years, retinoscopy is done under short-acting cycloplegics like homatropine 2%, cyclopentolate 1% or tropicamide 1%. Addition of phenylephrine to any of the above cycloplegics enhances mydriasis without effecting cycloplegia.
   c. After 40 years, only short-acting cycloplegic is preferred.
   d. Simple mydriatic like phenylephrine 10% can be used after 60. Theoretically, dynamic retinoscopy, i.e. without cycloplegia should suffice at this age because there is hardly any accommodation left, but the practical problem is that by this age, most of the eyes would have developed lenticular opacities that hinder the retinal glow. Thus, a dilated pupil is preferred.
   e. The glasses are not prescribed immediately after retinoscopy. The practice is to allow the pupil to come to its normal size that takes few hours in tropicamide with 24 h in homatropine and cyclopentolate. It requires 10–15 days to abolish the effect of atropine.
      Any amount of miotics in any strength will not abolish drug-induced cycloplegia.
   f. The glasses are prescribed after 24–48 h of the refraction. This is commonly known as PMT, which stands for postmydriatic test. The better term should be postcycloplegic test.
5. Dynamic retinoscopy is that retinoscopy, which is done without cycloplegic. Refraction under simple mydriatic like phenylephrine is also dynamic retinoscopy,

while retinoscopy in aphakia and pseudophakia are static retinoscopy. In practice, the patient is asked to fix a distant object. This moderately dilates the pupil sufficient to do retinoscopy in absence of opacities in media. The light in the electric retinoscope can be reduced to prevent light-induced miosis. Dynamic retinoscopy measures refractive status both for distance and near. It does not require postcycloplegic test. The glasses for distance and near can be prescribed at the end of the retinoscopy.

Points to Remember

1. Miotics will not abolish mydriasis caused by phenylephrine.
2. It will cause cyclotonia that results in discomfort to the patient.
3. No miotics are recommended in both the forms of retinoscopy, i.e. static or dynamic.

Use of Atropine for Refraction in Children

Children under 10 must always be refracted under complete cycloplegia, which has accompanied benefit of widely dilated pupil. This is best achieved by instilling atropine. Atropine for ocular use is available as Atropine

Table 8.5: Regime of use of cycloplegic/mydriatic in various ages

Age	Cycloplegic/Mydriatic
Newborn	0.8% tropicamide with 2.5% phenylephrine every 5 min × 3 time
1–10 year	Atropine 0.5%–1% 2 time a day × 3
10–40 year	Homatropine 2% every 5 min × 3 Cyclopentolate 1% every 5 min × 3 Tropicacyil 0.8% every 5 min × 3
40 year and above	Tropicamide 0.8% 2 time every 5 min phenylephrine every 5 min × 3

sulfate in the form of drop or ointment. The strength of that ranges between 0.5% and 2%. The latter is used only in very resistant miosis mostly in chronic iridocyclitis in adults. The commonly used atropine is 1% aqueous solution. Each drop of 1% atropine contains 1/100th of a grain, which is equal to 0.6 mg. Thus, when one drop is put in each eye, the total quantity of atropine becomes 1/100th + 1/100th equivalent to 1/50th of a grain or 1.2 mg of atropine. Usual dose of atropine is 1/120th to 1/60th of a grain, which is equivalent to 0.5-1 mg. Thus, if both drops are absorbed, the child gets atropine in a dose more than within therapeutic limit. If the drop is by chance repeated within 12 h, the child gets a dose of 1/25th grain, which is equivalent to 2.5 mg that can cause severe toxicity. Atropine when instilled in eye is absorbed in two ways:

1. Partly through the conjunctiva and cornea.
2. Partly through systemic absorption following passage of atropine through puncta, canaliculus, sac, nasolacrimal duct in the throat. The absorption of atropine drops can be minimized by obliteration of the two puncta by index finger of the parents for a minute or so by which time, most of the atropine drop would have spilled over the lid. It is better to avoid atropine as drop below 10 years and if at all it has to be used, it should be diluted to 0.5% and instilled with a gap of at least 12 h. The better alternative is to use atropine ointment 2 times a day with a gap of 12 h. The amount of ointment should not exceed more than 2 mm in length. The advantage of ointment is that it is absorbed slowly and passes through the puncta in less quantity, reducing the chances of toxicity. Iris and ciliary body in children are more resistant to cycloplegics than in adults. Hence single application of cycloplegic, which is sufficient in adults, may not suffice in children.

The usual practice followed for children is to instill Atropine sulfate 1% ointment 2 times a day for 3 consecutive days in both eyes. This point should be impressed upon the parents. Otherwise, they may instill atropine only in eye with diminished vision/squint.

If pupil is still not sufficiently dilated, other cycloplegic like tropicamide is instilled in both the eyes 3 times a day, in each eye with a gap of 5 minutes between two drops. This is best done in the office of the optometrist.

The parents should be informed about possible side effects of atropine, both local and systemic.

Side Effects of Local Instillation of Atropine

1. Ocular: Glare, absent near vision, diminished distant vision, unmasking of tropia and increase in angle of squint.
2. Systemic: Flushing of face, dryness of mouth thirst and fever.

The parents are advised to inform the teacher about the temporary visual handicap due to cycloplegia in the child.

Postmydriatic (cycloplegic) test in children is done 15 days after the refraction.

In the meantime, the parents should be assured that loss of vision is temporary and will return to prerefraction level after the effect of atropine has passed off. The parents may be demonstrated this by putting plus lenses with improvement of vision.

The objective of retinoscopy is to find out the lens that will bring the far point of the observed eye in the plane of observer's eye.

The various components involved in retinoscopy are:

1. Dioptric status of the eye (error of refraction).
2. Illuminated object (retina).
3. Source of light (mirror).

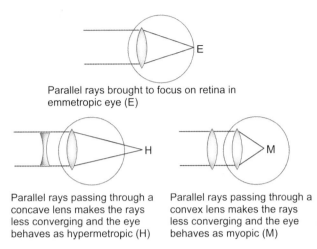

Parallel rays brought to focus on retina in emmetropic eye (E)

Parallel rays passing through a concave lens makes the rays less converging and the eye behaves as hypermetropic (H)

Parallel rays passing through a convex lens makes the rays less converging and the eye behaves as myopic (M)

Figure 8.28: Effect of concave and convex lenses on emmetropic eye

The dioptric value of an emmetropic eye is +60D that focuses (converging) parallel rays on the retina. If plus lenses are put in front of emmetropic eye, it starts converging more and the eye becomes relatively myopic. Similarly, if minus lenses are put in front of an emmetropic eye, the eye becomes relatively hypermetropic (Fig. 8.28).

Optics of Retinoscopy

1. Optics involved in any form of retinoscope (refer Fig. 8.23), i.e. mirror or self-illuminate are same.

2. In retinoscopy, an area of retina is illuminated by light from the retinoscope.

3. The illuminated area, which is otherwise not visible on oblique illumination acts as object for the retinoscope.

4. The light coming from this illuminated area that is commonly called retinal reflex/glow forms, an image at the far point of the eye under observation.

5. The far point may be:
   a. In front of the patient as in emmetropia or myopia.
   b. At an imaginary point behind the eye in hypermetropia.

6. The distance of far point from the eye indirectly gives the refractive status of the eye under observation.

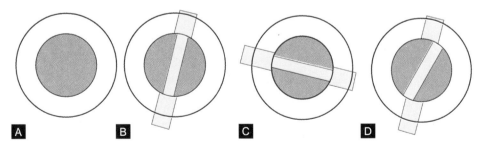

Figures 8.29A to D: Stage of illumination in mirror and streak retinoscope. **A.** Retinal glow in mirror retinoscope; **B, C and D.** Retinal glow in streak retinoscope; **B and C.** Spherical error—retinal glow aligned in all meridians; **D.** Retinal glow in astigmatism—retinal glow off the axis.

7. The light reflected in case of mirror retinoscope and spot retinoscope are circular and cover the whole of the pupil in spherical error and an oval spot is produced in high astigmatism.

8. In emmetropia, the whole of the pupillary area is illuminated by the retinal glow.

9. In streak retinoscope, the retinal glow is in the form of a streak that is called intercept. It occupies only a part of the pupil.

10. The steps of retinoscopy have three stages:
    a. Stage of illumination.
    b. Stage of reflex.
    c. Stage of projection.

Stage of illumination: It (Figs 8.29A to D) consists of understanding the movement of pupillary reflex in relation to movement of the mirror (Fig. 8.30):

1. MM1 is a plane mirror. L is the bulb used for retinoscopy. The image formed by mirror MM1 of L is L1. The distance LM = ML1.

2. Now, the mirror MM1 is tilted to the position M2M3. The image will move against, i.e. L1 will move to the opposite direction at L2. When L1 moves down, the illuminated spot moves up. If the plane mirror is substituted by a concave mirror, the movements are reversed.

Stage of reflex: This includes:

1. The illuminated area of the retina is taken as an object.

2. It is situated at the far point of the patient.

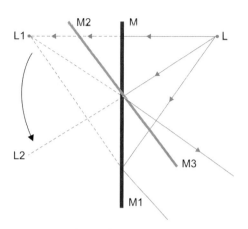

Figure 8.30: Relation between movement of the plane mirror and immediate source light (ISL); MM1 is the plane mirror; M2M3 is the moved plane mirror; L is the source of illumination; L1 is its image, which acts as immediate source of illumination, i.e. ISL; L2 is the moved image of L1 when the mirror is moved.

Stage of projection: The light reflected from the illuminated area of the fundus forms a reflex shadow in the pupillary area, which is projected in the eye of the observer. It becomes visible on aligning the eye of the observer in the path of the ray (Fig. 8.31).

Path of Rays During Retinoscopy

General principle of movement of glow:

1. If the far point is either behind the patient's or observer's eye, the glow will move with.

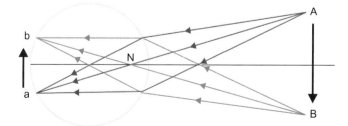

Figure 8.31: Relation between movements of illuminated spot on the retina with movement of ISL. A is the immediate source of light (ISL); a is the spot illuminated by A on the retina; B is the changed position of ISL below A. b is the changed position of a above a: The point a on the retina moves up (on the opposite direction), but in the same direction as the mirror and forms b on the retina.

2. If the far point is between the observer and the patient, the glow will move against.

The path of light rays differs in emmetropia and ametropia.

Path of light rays in emmetropia (Fig. 8.32): As follows:

1. The rays starting from the emmetropic eye are parallel.
2. They reach the observer's eye without deviation.
3. The illuminated spot seems to come from behind the patient's eye.
4. The rays coming from the patient's eye being parallel are focused without putting any lens in front of the eye.
5. The pupillary reflex moves with the movement of the plane mirror.
6. This movement with the mirror needs to be differentiated from hypermetropia.

Path of light rays in hypermetropia (Fig. 8.33): As follows:

1. The rays coming out of patient's eyes are diverging.
2. They appear to come from behind the eye of the patient.
3. The pupillary light reflex moves in the direction of the mirror (with the mirror).

4. Putting plus lenses in front of the patient's eye in increasing gradient will neutralize with the movement and a stage will come when the movement becomes against. This indicates point of neutralization.
5. This is the hypermetropic power of the patient's eye.

Path of light rays in myopia: The behavior of the light rays in myopia is little complicated as compared to emmetropia and hypermetropia. Different powers of myopia behave differently. On the basis of the power of the myopia, the path of the rays will take one of the following:

1. When myopia is less than 1D.
2. When myopia is 1D.
3. When myopia is more than 1D.

Path of rays when myopia is less than 1D (Fig. 8.34): As follows:

1. The rays emerging from the eye are convergent.
2. They meet at a place more than 1 m (working distance), but are intercepted by observer's eye before they meet.
3. The observer feels them to be coming from the observed eye, in the same manner as in emmetropia and hypermetropia. Hence, the pupillary reflex moves with

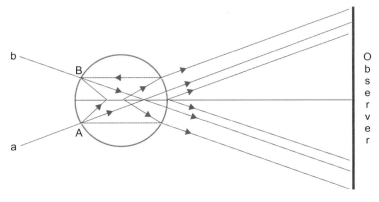

Figure 8.32: Path of light rays in emmetropic eye in relation to the observer. A and B are the two spots on the retina that seem to come from a and b, the far point of the observed eye. The rays emerging from the observed eye are parallel, which are intercepted by the observer in the path of parallel rays.

the movement of the mirror. So the reflex moves with the movement of the mirror, not only in emmetropia and hypermetropia but also in myopia less than 1D.

Path of rays when myopia is 1D (Fig. 8.35): As follows:

1. The rays emerging from the observed eye will no doubt be convergent.
2. Instead of meeting behind the observer's eye, they will meet on the pupillary plane of the observer.
3. The reflex will fill the whole of the pupillary area.
4. The light reflex will not move with the movement of the mirror.

Path of rays when myopia is more than 1D (Fig. 8.36): As follows:

1. In case of myopia more than 1D, the rays will also converge.
2. The rays will meet in front of the observer's eye at a distance less than 1 m.
3. The image formed is real.
4. It moves against the movement of the plane mirror.

The movement of the glow in relation to plane mirror in various errors of refraction is summarized in Figure 8.37.

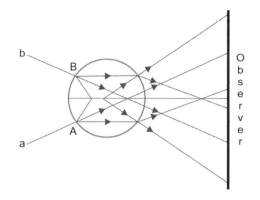

Figure 8.33: Path of light rays in hypermetropic eye in relation to the observer. A and B are two points on the retina that seem to come from a and b respectively, which are at the far point of the observed eye. The rays coming from the observed eye are divergent, which are intercepted by the observer.

If the reflex moves in the same direction as the plane mirror, the far point of the observed eye would either be behind the eye, in hypermetropia, behind the observer in emmetropia or myopia less than 1D. If the reflex moves against the eye, the eye is moderate to high myopia.

Movement in Concave Mirror

1. When concave mirror is used, the movement is reversed except in myopia of 1D where there is no movement with both plane or concave mirrors.

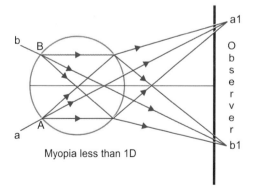

Figure 8.34: Path of light rays in myopic eye in relation to the observer

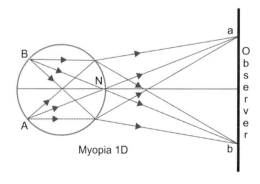

Figure 8.35: Path of light rays in myopic eye in relation to the observer

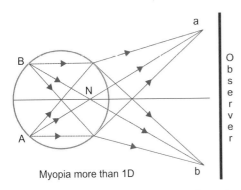

Myopia more than 1D

Figure 8.36: Path of light rays in myopic eye in relation to the observer

2. If the image moves with the movement of the concave mirror, it is myopia more than 1D. If the image moves against the movement of the concave mirror, it can be any of the following—emmetropia, myopia less than 1D or hypermetropia.

Concave mirror is far less commonly used than plane mirror in clinical practice.

It is used in case of high errors of refraction where the pupillary reflex is too dull to appreciate its movement.

Points to be Noted in Retinoscopy Glow

1. While using a retinoscope, right eye of the observer is used to refract the right eye of the patient and vice versa.
2. Size of the glow: Does it cover whole of the pupil?
   a. If it fills whole of the pupil, it denotes neutralized movement.
   b. It is large in lower degrees of refraction.
   c. It is small in high errors of refraction, both plus or minus.
3. Edge of the glow:
   a. Sharp in low errors of refraction.
   b. Blurred in high errors of refraction.

   c. Crescent in spherical refraction.
   d. Straight in astigmatic refraction.
4. Direction of movement of the glow in plane mirror:
   a. Moves with:
      i. Emmetropia.
      ii. Myopia less than 1D.
      iii. Hypermetropia.
   b. Moves against:
      i. Myopia more than 1D.
   c. No movement:
      i. Myopia 1D.
5. Brightness of glow:
   a. It is brightest in neutrality.
   b. It is bright in small errors.
   c. It is dull in high errors.
6. Speed of movement of glow:
   a. Fast in small errors.
   b. Slow in high errors.
7. Uniformity:
   a. Glow and its movement are uniform in all meridians in spherical error.
   b. Movement is different in different meridians in astigmatism.
8. Neutralization:
   a. All the meridians are neutralized by same power in spherical error.
   b. There is difference between power in two meridians in astigmatism.
   c. If there is difference in power in two meridians with same sign, the condition is compound astigmatism.
   d. The movements are in opposite direction in two meridians, the condition is mixed astigmatism.
   e. If there is power in only one meridian, the condition is simple astigmatism.

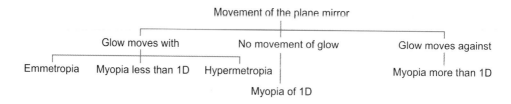

Figure 8.37: Movement of glow in relation to plane mirror in various errors of refraction

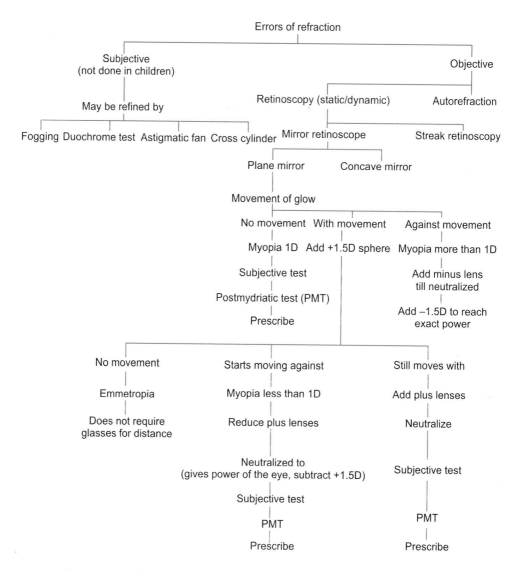

Figure 8.38: Subjective and objective methods of determining errors of refraction

How to Find the Type and Extent of Error of Refraction?

1. Retinoscopy can be done under cycloplegia static, without cycloplegia dynamic.
2. Commonly it is done at an arm's length, i.e. 2/3 of a meter.
3. More accurate is to do retinoscopy at 1 m.
4. Retinoscopy at a distance more than 1 m is more accurate, but creates difficulty in manipulation of lenses by the observer.

Subjective test may be done by putting lenses at random that gives better vision, fogging, duochrome test, astigmatic fan, cross cylinder (Fig. 8.38).

Dynamic Retinoscopy

Dynamic retinoscopy is an objective method to find out near point. This is done with normal pupil. The patient is asked to fix a distance object and plane mirror retinoscopy is done with reduced light. Then the patient fixes a near object and retinoscopy is repeated. The second part is difficult because the pupil instantly constricts when looking at near object. This is obviated by using weak drop of mydriatic without cycloplegia, i.e. phenylephrine 5%. The whole method is cumbersome, hence, is no more in clinical use.

Autorefraction

Autorefraction is electronic computerized device used in retinoscopy. All these instruments use infrared light to measure retinoscopic reflexes in multiple meridians and compute them to give the power in the principal meridian. The method can be applied with undilated pupil as well.

Concave Mirror

All the movements in concave mirror are opposite as compared to plane mirror.

Relation between retinoscopy finding and final power (Table 8.6):

1. The value of lens in myopic power prescribed to the patient will be more than retinoscopic power.
2. Value of lens in hypermetropic power prescribed to the patient will be less than retinoscopic power.

The PMT findings are not always same as retinoscopic findings under mydriasis.

Self-illuminated Retinoscopes (Refer Streak Retinoscope)

These instruments are miniature self-illuminated projectors. The average size of a self-illuminated retinoscope is generally the same as handheld direct ophthalmoscope. The instrument works either on dry battery cells or mains through a step down transformer, which is generally housed in the body of the instrument. The projected light can either be a streak or a spot. The streak is more favored than the spot because the streak can locate the meridian of the astigmatism. The streak is the image of the specially constructed bulb, which has a straight linear filament

Table 8.6: Relation between retinoscopic finding and final power of the glass

Sl No	Retinoscopic finding		Add	Power of the glass
1.	−2	−2	Add −1.5D sphere	−3.5D sphere
2.	+2	+2	Add −1.5D sphere	−3.5D sphere

that gives a streak when projected. The filament is stationary, but the convex lens above the bulb (refer Fig. 8.27) can be moved up and down to make the emerging rays parallel, converging or diverging. The beam is then reflected at right angles through a plane mirror imposed at an angle of 45° above the beam of light emanating from the bulb. The streak can be rotated by turning the sleeve of the instrument through 360° horizontally. Another sleeve can be moved up and down to project divergent parallel or convergent rays. This sliding sleeve contains planoconvex lens with convexity upwards. Thus, a single instrument can be used in place of two separate instruments, i.e. plane/concave as in mirror retinoscope. There is an aperture in the mirror to see the pupillary reflex. The streak is called intercept. It spans across the whole width of the cornea.

The instrument can be used with or without dilated pupil. While using the instrument in an undilated pupil, the brightness of the streak is lowered least a bright beam causes constriction of pupil, which may obscure the pupillary reflex. Better and more accurate results are obtained with dilated pupil. The added advantage of streak retinoscope is that it can be used both in ambulatory and non-ambulatory patients, infants and even in operation theater. It does not require an elaborate dark room or a separate immediate source of illumination (ISL).

Usually, while using the streak retinoscope, the patient sits upright at an arm's length from the examiner like in mirror retinoscope.

To use the streak retinoscope, the streak is first focused on the forehead of the patient and then the streak is lowered in the pupillary area. The lens in the vertically moving sleeve is adjusted to give a plane mirror effect. If there is no error of refraction, the whole of the pupillary area lights up with a uniform pink glow. Otherwise, a streak of reflex is seen in the pupil, depending upon the position of the axis of the streak. The streak can be horizontal or vertical. The streak over the iris is wider than the streak in the pupillary area. In case of spherical error, all the three parts of the streak, i.e. in the pupil, above and below the pupil are in the same line. An angulation between the two denotes astigmatism (refer Figs 8.29A to D).

It is common practice to use the vertical streak first and move it across the pupil in the same manner as with a mirror retinoscope. To note the movement of the retinoscope, i.e. with, against or no movement and then the streak is rotated by 90°. Spherical lenses are used to neutralize the movement. As the neutral point is reached, whole of the pupillary area starts glowing, instead of a linear glow. The two meridians are neutralized and the difference in power gives the power in astigmatism. The difference in power of two meridians is the power of the cylinder.

In case of regular astigmatism, traditionally the axis of the cylinder is determined first and the power later.

Steps of Streak Retinoscopy in Astigmatism

The steps in astigmatism (Fig. 8.39) consist of the following types.

Break Phenomenon

Break phenomenon is observed when the axis of the intercept and the reflex of the streak do not overlap. They are angulated to each other. To overcome this, the sleeve of the streak retinoscope is rotated to bring the two reflexes over each other. The points to be noted are:

1. Width of the pupillary reflex and the intercept: It is narrowest when the streak and the true axis are well aligned.

2. Brightness of the streak: The streak is brightest when aligned with the true axis.

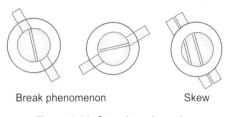

Break phenomenon   Skew

Figure 8.39: Steps in astigmatism

Skew

Skew is oblique motion of the streak in case of small cylindrical value. It is seen in presence of break phenomenon. The intercept and the pupillary reflex do not seem to move in the same direction. They are scissored. When the axis is properly aligned, the movements of the two reflexes are similar.

Straddling

Straddling is used to refine the cylindrical axis when the axis is off the correct position slightly. The retinoscope streak is turned by 45° off the axis both ways. If the axis is correct, the width of the reflex is same in both positions. In case of unequal width, the narrower side denotes the correct axis.

Correcting cylindrical power: Once the axis has been located correctly, the attention is shifted to correcting the power of the cylinder in a method similar to in mirror retinoscopy.

Subjective Method of Correcting Astigmatism

Subjective check of spherical correction is simple. It consists of adding or subtracting spherical lenses in front of the eye with diminished vision till best vision is achieved. In case of retinoscopy, this can be achieved by adding or subtracting plus or minus lenses to the retinoscopic finding after 24 hours.

Correcting astigmatism is more difficult than this, which requires patience and skill because it needs correction of power as well as axis in astigmatism. As a rule, axis correction gets priority over power correction.

Suspension of accommodation is essential to determine refractive state of an eye accurately barring myopia, aphakia and pseudophakia. Abolishing accommodation is more important in younger persons. The best way to eliminate accommodation is use of effective cycloplegia. Use of cycloplegia becomes less with advancing age and is almost not required after age of 40, when cycloplegia is replaced by use of plus lenses, which does not have disadvantages of cycloplegia. Putting plus lenses in front of any eye irrespective of error of refraction shifts the image forwards, i.e. in front of retina and a state of relative myopia is created producing a circle of blur on the retina. This phenomenon is utilized in simplest way of checking spherical and cylindrical power before and after retinoscopy. This procedure is called fogging.

This may be preceded by changing the axis by 5°–10° on each side of the axis present in the trial frame and the best axis is taken as most suitable.

Fogging

1. For spherical correction.
2. For astigmatic correction.

For spherical correction: As follows:

1. Note the vision for distance in the eye under observation occluding the other eye.
2. Put sufficient plus lenses to reduce the vision from 6/36 to 6/24. Add plus lenses over this and observe:
   a. If the vision improves, add plus lenses till best vision is reached.
   b. If vision decreases, add minus lenses till best vision is reached.
   An eye is not fogged when using a cross cylinder.

For correction of astigmatism: As follows:

1. Add plus lenses to bring the vision from 6/36 to 6/24. This will convert all hypermetropic astigmatism, may it be simple, compound or mixed to compound myopic astigmatism and enhance myopic astigmatism.

2. The patient is asked to look at astigmatic dial and asked to locate sharpest and darkest line. Suppose the axis 180° is sharpest and darkest, add minus cylinder in increasing strength with axis at 90° to the previous axis, i.e. 180° till all lines become sharp and dark.

3. This process neutralizes the astigmatism, but the spherical blur still persists.

4. Ask the patient to look at distant chart. Note the vision and reduce plus sphere or add minus sphere till best vision is acquired.

Rule of Thirty

Rule of thirty requires two astigmatic dials, one divided into segments of 30° and the other is divided in four equal segments (Fig. 8.40). The second dial is revolvable around the central point.

To use the dial, find out the darkest and sharpest line on the first dial. Add minus cylinders in increasing strength to the sharpest and darkest line at 90° to it, till all lines appear equal.

Now use the second rotatable dial, aligning the principle meridian. Note the axis, not in degrees, but as clock positions on the dial. Multiply the lower number in clock by 30. This will give the axis of minus cylinder.

For example, multiply 1 by 30 = 30°. Multiply 3 by 30, i.e. 3 × 30 = 90° and 6 by 30, i.e. 180°.

Landolt's Fan

Landolt's fan (Fig. 8.41) is a simple device that may be incorporated in distant vision chart or may be available separately. It is a black on white chart that is kept at 6 m from the patient like any distant vision chart. It comprises of a horizontal line from the middle of which lines of equal thickness and brightness radiate upwards in fashion of a fan. The lines are 10° apart. The line at 12 O'clock is 0° and the straight line below is 90° to it.

While using fan, the patient is asked to look at the fan with the eye under examination. If all the lines are equally bright and of same thickness, there is no astigmatism. Now, a plus sphere is put in front of the eye blurring all the lines. The blurring denotes absence of astigmatism. If some of the lines become bright, the patient has astigmatism in the axis, which will be at right angles to the bright line. For example, if the vertical line is brightest, the axis of the cylinder will be 180° and vice versa.

Maddox V

Maddox V (Fig. 8.42) is modification over Landolt's fan. This consists of two homocentrical circles with gap in between the two circles. The space between the two circles is divided into 360°.

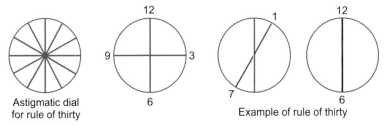

Astigmatic dial for rule of thirty   Example of rule of thirty

Figure 8.40: Illustrating rule of thirty

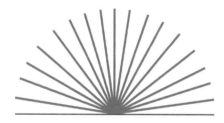

Figure 8.41: Landolt's astigmatic fan

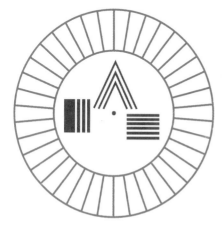

Figure 8.42: Astigmatic dial

Inside the circles are:

1. A V: The narrow end pointing out. This V can be rotated by 180°.

2. A block with horizontal lines at equal distance of equal thickness and equal brightness.

3. A similar block with vertical lines.

4. The blocks and the V can be rotated through 180°.

To find out the axis of the cylinder, the steps are as follows:

1. Best vision with spherical lens is noted.

2. A plus sphere is superimposed over the sphere already present.

3. The value of the superimposed sphere should be half the estimated power of the cylinder. For example, if the estimated power of the cylinder is 1, the power of the superimposed sphere will be 0.5D

sphere to convert the power into myopic astigmatism.

4. The patient is asked to point the most, brightest and sharp radiating line.

5. Draw the attention of the patient to the V.

6. Move the apex of the V (arrow) away from the clearest radiating line. This should blur the radiating line.

7. The apex of the V is rotated till both the limbs become equally bright.

8. The axis of the cylinder to be prescribed will be at right angles to it.

9. Shift the attention of the patient to the blocks and put minus cylinder at correct axis till lines in both the blocks become equally bright.

10. Now add +0.5D sphere in the trial frame. This should blur both the blocks.

Stenopaic Slit

Stenopaic slit (Figs 8.43A and B) is most inexpensive device to find out the axis of astigmatism. It is supplied with all trial sets. The slit should be longer than the interpalpebral aperture and 1.2 mm wide. The length is variable, but should not be less than the average diameter of cornea. The slit is cut in an opaque disk, which is mounted in a metal frame like any other lens in a trial frame. It is nothing, but a series of pinholes kept side by side. As the basic principle of the stenopaic slit is pinhole, it improves vision in ametropia as well, but is not used for that purpose. It is best used to find out the axis of astigmatism in irregular astigmatism.

To use the stenopaic slit, following steps are used:

1. Record distant vision in eye under examination.

2. Occlude the other eye.

3. Put the stenopaic slit in the trial frame and note if the vision improves.

4. If the vision does not improve, rotate the slit till the vision is improved.

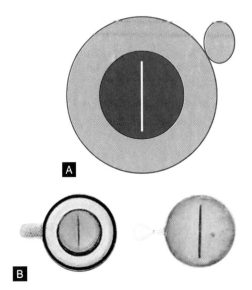

Figures 8.43A and B: Stenopaic slit. **A.** Schematic diagram of stenopaic slit; **B.** Photograph of stenopaic slits.

5. Add spherical lenses over the stenopaic slit till best vision is reached. This will give the power of the cylinder.
6. The axis of the cylinder will be at right angles to the long-axis of the stenopaic slit that gives best vision.

Pinhole (Refer Single Pinhole Test or Modified Scheiner's Test)

Pinhole improves vision in ametropia (refer Figs 8.3A and B). If vision improves by putting the pinhole over the final power of the lens, then it denotes that some ametropia is left, which needs to be corrected. For example, if the patient's vision does not improve beyond 6/18 with best correction, a pinhole should be put over the spherical lens in the trial frame. If vision improves with the pinhole, some ametropia is still left. Pinhole will not find out the axis of the cylinder. It may be used to find out presence of astigmatism.

Let us consider an eye with 6/36 vision that improves to 6/9 or 6/6 through a pinhole.

This denotes that the eye has only spherical error. If the vision with pinhole improves to 6/18 or 6/12 only, then astigmatism should be suspected provided there is no other lesion responsible for non-improvement of vision. Another finding worth noting is the value of the cylinder to give best vision is always more than spherical value to give same result. For example, an eye with 6/12 vision will be most probably corrected to 6/6 by 0.5–0.75 sphere, but an astigmatic eye will require 1.25–1.5 cylinder to reach the same level.

Jackson Cross Cylinder (Crossed Cylinders)

Jackson cross cylinder (Figs 8.44A and B) is a versatile, handy, cheap, optical device to find out the most suitable axis and power of astigmatism.

The device comprises of a sphere and a cylinder of opposite signs put together in a metal frame with a handle. The long-axis of the handle makes an angle of 45° to both the plus and minus cylinders. The value of the cylinder is twice the value of the sphere. It is available between ±0.1 and ±2.00. Commonest combination is a –0.25D sphere with +0.5D cylinder.

The equation (Fig. 8.45) explains the construction of a cross cylinder.

Generally, power and sign of the cylinders are etched on the lens. Some instruments have a white and a red dot painted on the lens. The white dot denotes plus power and red dot denotes minus power. In other words the cross cylinder consists of two planocylinders of same power, but opposite signs with their axes at right angle to each other.

The test is subjective hence depends on ability of the patient to discern between two positions and clarity. The test is performed with active accommodation. Like any other test for cylinder, correcting axis gets precedence over the power of the cylinder.

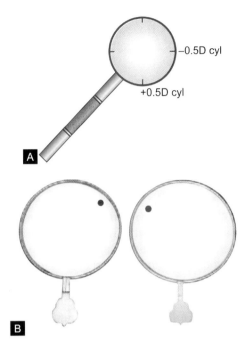

A

B

Figures 8.44A and B: Jackson cross cylinders. **A.** Schematic diagram of cross cylinder; **B.** Photograph of cross cylinder without usual handle with red and white marking.

Steps: The steps in use of Jackson cross cylinder are as follows:

1. Refract the eye by retinoscope.

2. Subtract usual plus sphere from retinoscopic reading depending upon distance at which retinoscopy was done and type of cycloplegic used.

3. Find out the value and axis of the cylinder.

4. Find out the improvement of vision as per retinoscopy.

5. If it is 6/6 or 6/5 there is no need to verify the power of the cylinder or axis of the cylinder.

6. If improvement is unsatisfactory, put a pinhole over the lens already present in the trial frame.

7. Improvement of vision by pinhole denotes that some ametropia is still left uncorrected and requires further adjustment, most probably by adding a cylindrical value.

8. Non-improvement of vision with pinhole over the glass means fault either in media or in fundus.

9. The cross cylinder is used generally during PMT.

To correct the axis of the cylinder: The steps are as follows:

1. A moderately strong cylinder, i.e. +0.5D or +1.00D is placed before the eye that already has sphere and cylinder as per retinoscopy.

2. Place the cross cylinder in such a way that each axis lies alternatively at 45° to each axis. For example, if the axis in the trial frame is 90°, the cross cylinder is placed in such a way that 1 axis is at 45° and the other at 135°.

3. The cross cylinder is flipped by 180°. This mutually changes each axis to the other, i.e. the axis 45° becomes 135° and vice versa.

4. If the patient tells that the vision is equally bad in either position, the axis of the cylinder in trial frame is correct.

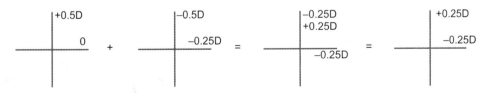

Figure 8.45: Equation for construction of a cross cylinder

5. If the vision is better in one of the two positions, the axis of the cylinder is not correct and the axis of the cylinder is moved toward the better axis.

6. When using a plus cylinder, the axis of the cylinder in a trial frame is moved toward the plus side of the cross cylinder.

7. In case of minus cylinder, the reverse is done.

To verify the power of the cylinder: The steps are as follows:

1. Lenses are put in the trial frame as per retinoscopy.

2. One of the axis of the cylinder of the cross cylinder is put over the lens in trial frame with the axis in the same direction as in the trial frame.

3. Then the direction of the axis in the cross cylinder is changed to make it perpendicular to the axis in trial frame.

4. One of the positions enhances the power of the sphere in cross cylinder and the other reduces the power by same number.

5. If the vision is unchanged in either position, the power of the cylinder is correct.

Duochrome Test (Bichrome Test)

Duochrome test (Fig. 8.46) is based on the principle of chromatic aberration of optical lenses. It has been discussed earlier that white light is composed of seven colors of different wavelengths with different refractive powers (VIBGYOR). Rays with less wavelength come to focus earlier than those with longer wavelength. The rays on the violet end bend more than the red end.

In the eyes the green rays are refracted more than the red. The green rays are focused in front of the retina, hence are more myopic. The red rays are focused behind the retina, hence are relatively hypermetropic. The yellow rays come to focus on the retina, hence is considered to be emmetropic. The distance between the focus of red and blue

is called chromatic interval. This may be as much as 1.25D. However, the difference is as less as 1/8th of a diopter; can be appreciated. In practice, this test is not done in vision less than 6/9.

The chromatic aberration is more marked in optical instruments like telescopes, microscopes, cameras than the eyes.

The ideal device to do duochrome test is cobalt blue filter that allows only red and blue rays to pass. But in practice, red and green colors are used.

The test is not symptomatic; it is diagnostic to find out the correct spherical power in the trial set. It is mainly done to avoid over correction of myopia. The other use of the test is to ensure that the eyes have been made emmetropic.

The appliance to perform duochrome test consists of a self-illuminated rectangular box. The upper half of the front panel is red and the lower green.

Snellen's letters of the size 6/12, 6/9 and 6/6 are written in black in descending order from left to right on each panel.

The examination does not require red-green glasses.

The test is not influenced by color vision and it does not detect color vision defect.

To perform the test: Consider the following:

1. The patient sits at usual distance of 6 m.

2. The procedure is explained to the patient. Children under 10 may not be able to comprehend the test.

3. One eye is tested at a time, the other eye is occluded.

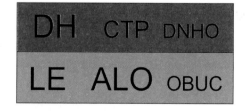

Figure 8.46: Panel of duochrome test

4. Lenses as per PMT are put in the trial frame.

5. The eye is slightly fogged.

6. The patient is asked to read letters on the duochrome panel.

7. If the lines, i.e. black on red and black on green are equally visible, a state of emmetropia has reached with the lenses and no change in the spherical value is required.

8. If the black on red is better visible, the eye is myopic and myopic power is increased to make both the lines equal.

9. If black on green is better, the eye is hypermetropic and more plus lenses are needed to be added.

This is analogous to traffic signal where green means go ahead, which means adding and red means stop or go back, which means subtracting.

In absence of duochrome panel, a friend panel can be used where red and green letters are written on black background.

Transposition of Spherocylinders

Transposition is defined as change of power from one type to another, but equivalent to original power. There are three types of transposition:

- Simple
- Toric
- Vertex.

Simple transposition: This is the commonest form of transposition used. It is more frequently used in presbyopic correction where plus spheres are added to minus cylinder or spherocylinder with different signs in two meridians. It consists of:

1. Change the sign of the sphere.
2. Change the sign of cylinder.
3. Change the axis of cylinder by 90°.

For example, to transpose the following prescription, i.e. +1.00D sphere with –2D 90°:

- Step 1: –1.00D sphere with –2.00D cylinder 90°
- Step 2: –1.00D sphere with +2.00D cylinder 90°
- Step 3: –1.00D sphere with +2.00D cylinder 180°.

Thus, +1.00D sphere/–2D cylinder 90° = –1.00D sphere/+2.00D cylinder 180°.

Toric transposition: This is required when the lenses have a back curve. The formula is noted in a fraction, where numerator is the sphere and the denominator is the base curve with cylinder. For example,

+1.00D sphere/–2D cylinder 90°

- Step 1: Do a simple transposition +1.00D sphere/–2.00D cylinder 90° = –1.00D sphere/+2.00D cylinder 180°
- Step 2: Algebraically subtract base curve of –6D from the sphere, i.e. –1.00D sphere – (–6D sphere) = +5D sphere
- Step 3: Add cylindrical power to the basecurve, i.e. +2D cylinder 180° + (–6.00D cylinder 180°) = –4D cylinder 180°
- Step 4: Change the axis of the cylinder from 180° to 90°.

Thus, the toric transposition will be +5.00D sphere/–6.00D cylinder 90° with –4D cylinder 180°.

Vertex transposition: This is required in thick and meniscus lenses. The steps are:

- Step 1: Simple transposition of the front surface
- Step 2: Calculate focal length in millimeters
- Step 3: Measure thickness
- Step 4: Divide thickness by refractive index
- Step 5: Find out focal length of front surface by adding steps 2 and 4
- Step 6: Find out the reciprocal of focal length of the front surface.

ACCOMMODATION AND CONVERGENCE IN RELATION TO REFRACTIVE STATUS OF THE EYE

Far Point

Far point has been discussed earlier. In emmetropic eye parallel rays are brought to focus on the retina without changing the refractive status of the eye. For all practical purposes, the rays are said to be parallel when they originate at infinity. In clinical practice, it is taken as 6 m or 20 ft. This point is called far point or punctum remotum and referred to as 'r' for calculation. The far point for an emmetropic eye is infinity in front of the eye; in myopic eye; it is a finite point in front of the eye. In case of hypermetropia, the far point is a hypothetical point situated behind the eye. This is also considered to be a point beyond infinity and taken as negative for calculation.

Depth of Focus

As the object moves nearer than far point, the rays do not remain parallel. They begin to diverge and are brought to focus behind the retina, but still clearly visible for a short range without the change in refractive power. This range is called depth of focus. The depth of focus is increased by constricting the pupil or placing a pinhole in front of the eye at anterior focal plane that is 17 mm from the cornea in front. A pinhole increases depth of focus far more than miosis, hence, used as a tool to differentiate between error of refraction and organic causes of diminished vision. This is true for both far and near vision. The depth of focus decreases with dilatation of pupil. The depth of focus also varies with distance of the object from the eye. More is the distance, better is the focus.

Near Point

A point very near to the eye at which the vision becomes blurred is the 'near point of the eye'. In other words, smallest distance at which small objects can be seen clearly is considered to be this point and called near point of vision or punctum proximum and is referred as 'p' for calculation. The near point for an emmetropic, non-presbyopic eye is 25–30 cm. This is the distance at which an adult under 40 years keeps the paper to read.

ACCOMMODATION

Accommodation is an inherent reflex that enables the eye to see the small objects clearly at near point of vision. It is under parasympathetic control that causes constriction of ciliary body, which in turn results in increase in curvature of the lens, thus increasing the converging power of the lens.

Constriction of the ciliary body → Increase in curvature of the lens → Increase in converging power of the lens.

Parallel rays are brought to focus on the retina to give a sharp and clear vision when accommodation is at rest (Fig. 8.47A).

In an eye without accommodation rays arising from near point P are brought to focus at P1 behind the retina (Fig. 8.47B). Unless this point falls on the retina, the near vision will remain poor.

There are some probabilities by which the point P1 can be placed on the retina. They are:

1. Elongating the eye so the retina reaches the point P1. This is not possible in normal eyes, but is possible in high myopia.
2. The corneal curvature is increased producing curvature myopia shifting the point anteriorly as in keratoconus.

None of the two are possible in normal eyes. It can be possible, either by increasing the index ametropia as happens in central nuclear sclerosis or by activating accommodation (Fig. 8.47C).

During accommodation, the increase in curvature of the lens is mostly in the anterior surface of the lens. This increases the total anteroposterior thickness of the lens, shallowing the anterior chamber minimally. The other two more marked changes brought about by accommodation are:

1. Miosis.
2. Convergence.

Miosis

During miosis, the pupil constricts; there is no direct relation between amount of miosis and accommodation. Miosis can be abolished by use of simple mydriatic retaining accommodation. Use of cycloplegic will abolish both miosis and accommodation.

Convergence

Convergence is a disjunctive movement of eyes where the two eyes move toward the nose. It can be voluntary or non-voluntary (reflex). Accommodation is associated with reflex convergence. When, a person fixes a distant object, the eyes are slightly divergent. To maintain parallelism, the eyes must converge slightly. This is physiological. This physiological state of convergence is known as tonic convergence. It is separate from more marked accommodative and fusional convergence. In such a case, accommodation and convergence are synergistic. Unlike accommodation, convergence does not change with age.

The convergence can be increased by orthoptics.

The accommodation cannot be increased and must be supplemented by plus sphere to increase it.

Convergence can be enhanced by suitable prism.

Convergence is measured in meter angles or prism diopters. The meter angle depends on the distance of the object from the eyes mostly and interpupillary distance slightly. Nearer the object, larger is the angle of convergence. To measure convergence, a small target is held in front of the eye and

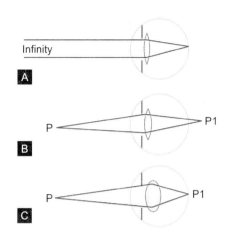

Figures 8.47A to C: Affect of accommodation on parallel rays. **A.** Parallel rays brought to focus on the retina when the accommodation is at rest; **B.** Diverging rays from near point P are brought to focus behind the eye at P1 when there is no accommodation; **C.** Diverging rays arising from near point P is brought to focus on P1 that is on the retina when the eye is accommodating.

the patient is asked to fix it. The target is gradually moved toward the nose and the patient is asked to maintain the fixation till the object becomes blurred due to diplopia.

The precise measurement is done by RAF gauge, Livingstone's gauge and Krimsky near point accommodation rule.

Royal Air Force Gauge

The Royal Air Force (RAF) gauge is a very handy, cheap instrument to measure subjective and objective amount of accommodation. This consists of a quadrangular bar 50 cm long on which distance in cm, accommodation in diopter and convergence in meter angle are etched. On one end is the handle and the other end is forked to rest under the nose. The handle points downward. Quadrangular bar is a small four-sided rectangular box, which can slide on the bar. The four sides of the box are used to measure near point, accommodation and convergence. To use the appliance, the forked end is put over the upper lip and the handle is away and downwards. The patient keeps both the eye open. The box is moved toward the eye till the smallest letter in near vision chart becomes blurred. The reading on the bar gives the reading distance and the others show amount of accommodation and convergence automatically and corresponding age (Fig. 8.48).

Livingstone's Gauge

The principle of Livingstone's gauge is similar to RAF gauge. The constructions of the two are similar except few alterations. Accommodation rule in black-painted metal comprises square section bar, moving cross target, swivelling occluder and V-shaped face rest.

Krimsky Near Point Accommodation Rule

The Krimsky near point accommodation rule consists of a plastic sheet that is wider at one end. The wider end is kept toward the eye. A near point target can be moved along the surface of the sheet. It has got two types of markings—the outer marking measures accommodation in diopters and corresponding age. The inner V-shaped scale is colored black. It measures the convergence near point centimeters.

The normal point of convergence is 8 cm like accommodation; convergence has two measurements, i.e. range of convergence and amplitude of convergence.

The range of convergence is defined as the distance between the far and near points of convergence and amplitude of convergence is the distance between maximum convergence and convergence at rest. The part of convergence between infinity and near point of convergence is called positive convergence and the part beyond infinity is called negative, which is in fact not convergence, but divergence.

The amplitude of convergence is measured in meter angles and prism diopters. The normal amplitude of convergence

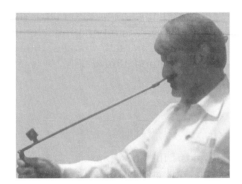

Figure 8.48: Patient using RAF gauge

is 10.5 meter angle. The convergence is measured by base-out prisms. The strongest converging prism that does not cause diplopia is the power of convergence (Table 8.7).

Table 8.7: Various parameters and their units of measurements

Parameters	Units
Far point	Meter/Centimeter
Near point	Centimeter
Range of accommodation	Meter
Amplitude of accommodation	Diopter
40 year and above	Centimeter
Range of convergence	Meter
Amplitude of convergence	Meter angle/Prism diopter
Physiological accommodation	Myodiopter
Physical accommodation	Diopter

Physiological and Physical Accommodation

Accommodation is the ability of the eye to bring the divergent rays arising from near point on the retina.

Accommodation has two components, physiological accommodation and physical accommodation.

Physiological accommodation represents the contraction of ciliary muscle, which initiates the second part, i.e. physical accommodation, which changes the refractive power of the eye. The physiological part of the accommodation is measured in myodiopters, while physical accommodation is measured in diopters that is arrived at, by dividing 100 by p.

Range of Accommodation

The distance between punctum proximum (p) and punctum remotum (r) is called range of accommodation (a) this makes, a = r – p.

The range of accommodation varies with age. The position of punctum remotum depends on static refraction in emmetropia and myopia, where it is in front of the eye and in hypermetropia, it is behind the eye. The punctum proximum changes with age and level of static refraction. The punctum proximum in a child is about 7 cm, at 30 years, it is reduced to 14 cm and at 40, it becomes 30 cm. The dynamic refraction in child with near point 7 cm is 100/7 = 14D.

Amplitude of Accommodation

The amplitude of accommodation is the difference between the refractive status of the eye with accommodation fully relaxed and refractive status with maximum accommodation. The refractive power of the eye when accommodated for r is designated as R and P denotes refractive status when eye is accommodated to p (the near point).

Amplitude of accommodation is difference between p and r and is measured in diopters.

The amplitude of accommodation varies with type of error of refraction.

Let us consider:

1. An emmetropic with punctum proximum (p) at 10 cm and punctum remotum (r) at ∞. The calculated amplitude will be:

$$a = p - r = 10 - \infty = \frac{100}{10} - \frac{1}{\infty} = 10 - 0 = 10D$$

2. A myope of –5D will have r at 20 cm and near point p at 10 cm. The amplitude of accommodation will be 10D – 5D = 5D.
3. A hypermetrope of +5D has its far point at a hypothetical point behind the eye and the sign for calculation for this point is taken as minus (–). Thus in case of hypermetropia of +5D the far point will be 20 cm behind the eye, which for calculation is taken as –20 cm. Thus, amplitude of accommodation will be:

$$\frac{100}{20} - (-\frac{100}{20}) = 5 - (-5) = 10D$$

The following table shows near point in various ages in different types of error of refraction (Table 8.8).

If we see the difference that takes place with age, we will find:

1. An emmetrope at 40 has only 3.5D of accommodation left in contrast to 7D at 30. His/her near point will be 33.3 cm against 25 cm at 30 years.

Table 8.8: Relation between type of error, age and near point of the eye

Type of error	Age	Near point
Emmetropic	20 year	20 cm
Myope –2D sphere	20 year	14.3 cm
Hypermetrope +2D sphere	20 year	33 cm

2. A hypermetrope of +2D at 40 years will be left with accommodation of 1.5D and his/her near point will recede to 75 cm.
3. A myope of –2D at 40 using 1D of accommodation will be able to see at 33 cm.

Relation of Accommodative Convergence to Accommodation

Accommodative convergence to accommodation (AC/A) is the amount of convergence measured in prism diopter (PD = Δ) that takes place for every diopter of accommodation D.

Accommodation in diopter is numerically equivalent to convergence in meter angles. An emmetrope fixing an object at 25 cm will be required to exert accommodation of 4D and convergence of 4 ma. A hypermetrope will require more accommodation and a myope require less. A hypermetrope uses accommodation in excess to convergence. A myope uses convergence in excess of accommodation. Accommodation in excess of convergence is called positive and less is called negative.

This relation between accommodative convergence and accommodation has important bearing in convergence and squint. It is influenced by type of error of refraction. In normal orthophoric persons, it is flexible and changes with type of error of refraction.

The normal AC/A is 3–5. Reduced amplitude of accommodation as met in presbyopia leads to an increase in AC/A ration. Binocular accommodation is more than uniocular accommodation. A person who cannot read small prints by one eye can read the same print at the same distance when both eyes are open. This additive effect on accommodation is due to stimulus derived from convergence. This is part of triad of miosis, accommodation and convergence. The complex is neural and called triad of synkinetic near reflex.

Near point of convergence (NPC) is the shortest distance required to see an object single.

Far point of convergence is not a real point. It is taken as relative.

Angle of convergence is the angle formed by two visual axes when a person fixes a near object and is measured in meter angles.

Meter Angles

When the two eyes fix an object at 1 m, the lines of sight meet each other in midway and form an acute angle. This is called meter angle. This is denoted as ma. The convergence exerted by each eye is inversely proportionate to the distance in meters. It would be 1 ma at 1 m, 1/2 ma at 2 m and 2 ma at 1/2 m (Fig. 8.49).

In emmetropes, each meter angle equals number of diopters of accommodation to see an object clearly. 1D of accommodation is associated with 1 ma of convergence for each eye.

Convergence in Prism Diopters/Meter Angle

Convergence needed for an eye to have single vision of an object at 1 m requires a prism of 1D and the convergence is taken as 1Δ convergence. It is not equal to 1 ma. 1 ma is equal to 3Δ convergence.

Near Correction

1. In normal eyes, parallel rays are brought to focus on the retina with fully relaxed accommodation (Fig. 8.50A).
2. The rays arising from near object are divergent and are brought to focus behind the retina when accommodation is at rest (Fig. 8.50B).
3. To bring the divergent rays to focus, the eyes accommodate as per distance of the object. The eyes need to accommodate more for an object nearer the eye (Fig. 8.50C).
4. Accommodation starts declining after 40 years, hence require supplementation in the form of plus lenses.

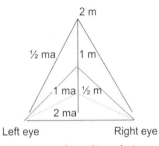

Figure 8.49: Meter angle and its relation to distance from the eye

5. These plus lenses are added to distant correction (Fig. 8.50D).

6. The lenses are added to distant correction. As emmetrope has no error of refraction, it requires no distant correction, it only needs near correction.

7. Other errors of refraction with diminished near vision require addition of plus lenses to distant correction.

8. Near correction depends on age of the patient, which is given in the Table 8.9.

   The figures are arbitrary and are variable as per occupation, error of refraction, ambient light at working place and overall well-being of the patient.

9. Besides age, the near correction depends on:

   a. Error of refraction—myopes require less addition than emmetropes and hypermetropes.

   b. Available accommodation.

   c. Near point of accommodation.

Available accommodation at various ages and corresponding near point of accommodation in an emmetropic eye are given in Table 8.10.

The loss of accommodation over years is gradual, but not uniform. The Table 8.11 shows loss of accommodation as per age.

Thus maximum loss of accommodation occurs between 40 and 50 years.

Table 8.9: Near correction as per age in emmetropic eye

Age (year)	Addition [diopter (D) sphere]
40	+1.00
45	+1.50
50	+2.00
55	+2 to +2.5
60	+2.75 to +3
More than 60	Near correction stabilizes and does not need more than +3D addition

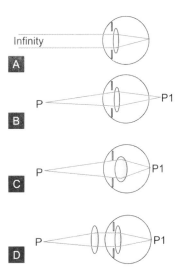

Figures 8.50A to D: Optics of near correction. **A.** Parallel rays brought to focus on the retina when the accommodation is at rest; **B.** Diverging rays from near point P are brought to focus behind the eye at P1 when there is no accommodation; **C.** Diverging rays arising from near point P is brought to focus on P1 that is on the retina when the eye is accommodating; **D.** Diverging rays arising from near point P is brought to focus on P1 that is on the retina by interposing a plus lens in front of the cornea at the anterior focal plane.

Table 8.10: Relation between available accommodation at various ages and corresponding near point of accommodation in emmetropic eye

Age (year)	Accommodation (diopter)	Near point (cm)
10	14.0	7
20	10.0	10
30	7.0	14
40	4.0	25
50	2.5	40
60	1.0	100

Table 8.11: Loss of accommodation as per age

Age (year)	Loss
8–40	1D
40–50	1.5D
50 upwards	2.5D

Measurement of Near Point of Accommodation

Measurement can be done roughly by asking the patient to read the finest line and observing the distance at which he/she can read the finest line on near vision chart (Figs 8.51 and 8.52).

Normal non-presbyopic patient can see the smallest print at about 30 cm. A presbyope keeps the chart at a distance more than this.

If a patient in pre-presbyopic age keeps the near chart at a distance shorter than 30 cm without distant correction, then he/she is definitely myope.

A pre-presbyope who keeps the near chart at a distance longer than 30 cm is most probably an uncorrected hypermetrope.

The more accurate method of determining near point of accommodation (NPA) is by an appliance called RAF gauge.

To measure near point of accommodation:

1. One eye is tested at a time and then with both eyes open. The patient should wear distant correction if needed.
2. The patient is given RAF gauge.
3. Patient holds the bar slightly inclined to the ground by the handle, puts the U-shaped prong over the nose.

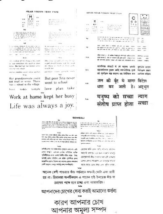

Figure 8.51: Various types of near vision charts for literates

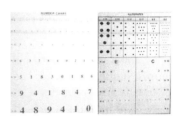

Figure 8.52: Various types of near vision charts for illiterates

4. The vision box is moved from periphery toward the eye.
5. The patient is asked to state when the letters become blurred. This is the endpoint.
6. The endpoint is read on the scale etched on the bar.
7. The amplitude of accommodation can also be read on the other surface.

Amplitude of accommodation at various ages is given in Table 8.12.

From the above chart, it is seen that amplitude of accommodation is high below 10 years and gradually decreases as age advances.

Table 8.12: Amplitude of accommodation at various ages

Age (year)	Amplitude of accommodation (diopters)
10	14
20	11
30	8
40	6
45	5.5
50	2.5
60	1.5

PRESBYOPIA

Presbyopia is neither a disease nor an error of refraction. It is a physiological condition and inevitable. Every person has to undergo this irrespective error of refraction after 40 years of age. It is equal among both the sexes. In presbyopia, the near point recedes beyond comfortable distance. It is almost equal in both eyes except in anisometropia, where it may differ in two eyes. The condition is progressive, but stabilizes in 2 decades from onset, i.e. in 6th decade, but lingers for rest of the life. The exact cause of condition is not known, but there is overwhelming evidence that it is brought about by hardening of the lens making the lens capsule less elastic. The hardening of the lens is due to chemical changes in the lens protein. The hardening of the lens makes the lens less malleable hence, less converging, i.e. power of the lens to accommodate becomes less. It has been discussed earlier that accommodation has two components, i.e. lenticular and ciliary. The under action of ciliary body in producing presbyopia is questionable.

It sets in early in some races. It is said to set in early in women and short-statured persons. Presbyopia sets in early in hypermetropia and undercorrected myopia. Due to reduced amplitude of accommodation, person working in dimly lit rooms develops symptoms early. Persons who have shorter working distance like goldsmiths, engravers, darners complain more and early difficulty in near vision. Illiterate, villagers who need not read or write never complain of presbyopia. The mechanism involved in onset of presbyopia is gradual decrease in amplitude of accommodation at 40. At 40, the amplitude of accommodation is reduced to 5D–6D from 10D at 14 years. The symptoms of presbyopia develop only when amount of accommodation required exceeds more than half of the total amplitude.

Symptoms of Presbyopia

Presbyopia is highly symptomatic. The symptom that makes the patient seek ophthalmic help is diminished near vision at about 40 years of age. This diminished near vision follows a set pattern.

First the patient finds it difficult to do near work in usual ambient light and moves toward a more lighted place. Patient learns to move the near work, i.e. book for example, away from the eye or moves the head backwards from stationary work like writing, drawing, etc. Then he/she comes to conclusion that his/her hands are too short to read fine prints.

A hypermetrope may complain of diminished near vision at pre-presbyopic age as he/she uses most of the accommodation for distant vision and is wrongly prescribed near correction, while all that is required to correct distant vision is by plus lenses. Similarly, astigmatism is relieved in pre-presbyopic age by only astigmatic correction. The loss of near vision is gradual, not painful and almost equal in both eyes. But the patient may develop asthenopia that leads to chronic conjunctivitis. Patient may develop exophoria or frank exotropia. Uniocular myope does not complain of diminished near vision as uses myopic eye for near vision and the other eye for distant vision. There are no signs of presbyopia except diminished near vision.

Management

There is no treatment, preventive or curative. All that is available is palliative and optical. The rationale behind management is to supplement amplitude of accommodation by plus glasses over distant correction. The steps in management of presbyopia consist of:

1. Record distant vision in both the eyes separately.
2. Correct any error of refraction, if present.
3. Find out near vision for both the eyes separately.
4. Find out amplitude of accommodation by RAF gauge/Livingstone's gauge.
5. Enquire about profession and usual distance of near work.
6. Ascertain age.

7. Exclude diabetes, chronic simple glaucoma can be treated.

8. Ideally it will be better to correct two eyes separately, but for all practical purposes, an average power is added to the distant correction when there is difference in near point between the two eyes.

9. There are many formulae for near correction based on age and distance of near work (Tables 8.13 and 8.14).

A patient may not be satisfied by the above formulae. The patient must be given most comfortable near vision with satisfactory range of near work. This happens only when one-third of amplitude of accommodation is left in reserve.

Example

A person's working distance is 25 cm; he/she requires 4D of accommodation.

At 45, near point has receded to 33 cm.

This gives an amplitude of accommodation of 3D.

As one third of accommodation is left in reserve, he/she is left with 2D of accommodation. Hence, he/she requires +2D as add, i.e. 4D – (+2D) = +2D.

He/she may be satisfied with +1D to +1.5D addition.

Table 8.13: Age wise addition of distant correction

Age (year)	Add (diopters)
40	+0.75D to +1.0D
45	+1.5D to +2.00D
50	+2D to +2.5D
55	+2.5D to +2.75D
60	+3.00D

Prescribing Near Correction in Presbyopia

Every emmetrope by the age of 40 finds it inconvenient to do near work at a distance he/she was accustomed to. This is more marked in dim light. He/she learns to keep the reading material away from the eye and prefers brighter light for reading small prints. This is corrected by adding plus lenses to distant correction.

Before embarking on prescribing near addition, following points should be noted:

1. Age: More is the age, larger is the addition.

2. Working distance: Those who have to keep the material of work at a distance less than 30 cm require more addition. Those persons whose working distance is between 30 cm and 1 m require less correction.

3. Commonly given addition as per age is given in Table 8.13.

4. Theoretically, the two eyes are to be tested separately and given different near addition if necessary. This is not always accepted by the patient. It is common practice to prescribe either a power in between the two eyes or lower power in both eyes.

Table 8.14: Distance wise addition over distant correction

Distance (cm)	Add (diopters)
25	+2.5D
33	+1.5D
40	+1.00D
50	+0.5D

Rule of thumb

Keep one-third to half amplitude of accommodation in reserve.

Comfort to patient gets priority over clarity.

Various Modes Available for Correction of Presbyopia

There is no medical treatment available for treatment of presbyopia. Those who claim that their near vision has improved without any treatment have in fact either developed central nuclear sclerosis that shifts the refraction of the eye toward minus power neutralizing the presbyopic addition or are uncontrolled diabetics.

The most practical satisfactory and comfortable treatment is optical method. The optical method consists of:

1. Spectacle correction.
2. Contact lens.
3. Surgical procedure.

Spectacle Correction

Single vision glasses for near work: The whole of the spectacle glass has uniform power that consists of total add. The patient has good near vision, but poor distant vision with glasses. The patient has to remove glasses for normal distance vision. This method is good for emmetropes who may slide the spectacle down the nose and see the distant object from upper part.

Bifocals: The spectacle has two types of power:

1. Large upper part for distant correction that may be plain in case of emmetrope or contain distant correction in case of ametropia.
2. A small lower segment that has add over distant correction, this is meant for near vision. The advantage of bifocals is that the person need not remove the glasses to see far (Fig. 8.53).

Trifocals: Some patients like tailors, carpenters, computer operators, librarians require different adds for intermediate distance. The intermediate correction is incorporated in between the far and near vision as a narrow strip. The intermediate add is generally half the near add (Fig. 8.54).

Progressive: The bifocals and trifocals have a visible line between the far and near correction, which is not cosmetically accepted by many. They require a glass that has advantage of vision at various distances without visible add. These glasses are called progressive glasses

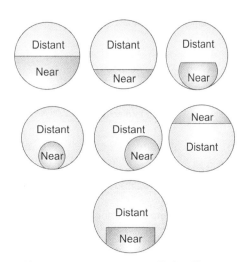

Figure 8.53: Various types of bifocal lenses

or varifocals where power gradually diminishes from bottom to top (Fig. 8.55). The disadvantage with these glasses is that they have greater peripheral distortion as the eye look down for near vision through a narrow channel. This also narrows the field of vision. The vision is distorted on horizontal movement. To avoid this distortion, the patient has to move the head, rather the eyes from side-to-side.

Monovision:

1. Unilateral myopes who can see near things without correction with myopic eyes and distance by ametropic eye is not prescribed with any glasses for near.
2. Using one eye for distance and the other eye is given near correction either in monocles or in spectacle correction.

Contact Lens for Presbyopia

Contact lens can be given as monovision where only one eye is corrected for near or in the form of bifocal contact lens. Refer Chapter on Contact Lens.

Surgical Treatment

Surgical treatment is good for monovision where one is corrected for near and the

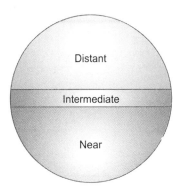

Figure 8.54: Trifocal lens

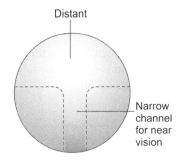

Figure 8.55: Diagrammatic representation of progressive lenses

other for distance. The surgical procedures (Fig. 8.56) are basically of three types:

1. Corneal procedures.
2. Lens related procedures.
3. Sclera surgery.

Note: Details of surgical procedures are beyond the scope of this book. They may be referred from books meant for refractive surgeries.

Practical Consideration in Prescribing Near Correction in an Emmetropic Presbyope

1. Let us consider a person of 50 years who has difficulty in reading newspaper in usual light.
2. The near distance is 25 cm.

3. The near point has receded to 33 cm.
4. Person can read the same letter by keeping at 40–45 cm away from the eyes, but not at 25 cm.
5. With 33 cm of near point, amplitude of accommodation is 3D.
6. By keeping one-third of amplitude in reserve, i.e. 1D, he/she has 2D of accommodation left for use.
7. For working distance of 25 cm, he/she requires 4D of accommodation.
8. Out of this 4D, he/she has 2D usable accommodation. Thus, the person needs 4D – 2D = 2D as near add.
9. Amplitude of accommodation in a person with –5D is 5D and for the same power that is +5D hypermetropia. This will be 15D.

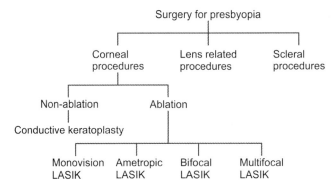

Figure 8.56: Various kinds of surgical treatment for presbyopia (LASIK, laser-assisted in situ keratomileusis)

10. Hence, near add will have to be adjusted according to error of refraction. Hypermetropes require more add than emmetrope and a myope may be comfortable will have less add.

Decentering for Near Vision

To maintain a single binocular vision when looking at a near point, the eyes converge. This convergence depends upon the distance between the near point and eye and type of error of refraction. Nearer is the object, more will be convergence. A myope converges more than emmetrope and hypermetrope. This convergence does not produce any prismatic effect in absence of lenses at the anterior focal plane. In presence of a lens for near, there will be prismatic effect when converging. To avoid this, near vision lenses need to be decentered. Otherwise, the patient will require prism; base out prism for myopia and base in prism for hypermetropia.

Decentering should be done during the manufacture of the lens and its fitting in frame in the spectacle frame. Decentering mostly depends on interpupillary distance and frame shape and dimensions.

The details of decentering are beyond the scope of this book. For details larger books on optometry may be consulted.

9 Contact Lenses

Contact lenses are optical devices (lens), which when put on cornea, improve the vision replacing the spectacle. History of contact lens is almost as old as spectacles. The credit of elucidating the basic principle of optics involved in contact lens is attributed to Leonardo da Vinci about 400 years ago. Vinci observed that while taking a dip in a pool of water, if one opens the eyes still submerged in water, the vision becomes foggy because the cornea-air interface is replaced by a huge water-cornea interface. Centuries after Vinci and enormous amount of research, it was realized that when cornea is immersed in water, 90% of power of cornea is reduced, i.e. from +43D to almost +4.3D, thus making an eye highly hypermetropic. There are two alternatives to make such an ametropic eye emmetropic:

1. Water in front of the cornea may be molded to change its vergence.
2. Trap the water within a transparent substance (medium) and the cornea, and give power to the substance.

The first is impossible, but the second alternative is feasible in the form of a small, transparent sheet on which the power can be grounded. This solid transparent device is the forerunner of present day contact lens.

People use contact lenses to see without being seen with glasses.

OPTICS OF CONTACT LENS

The purpose of both spectacle and contact lens are to bring rays arising from far point to focus on the retina to improve vision. However, the optics involved in each differs from the other. The spectacles do not change overall refractive status of the eye. They only change the vergence of the incidence rays, so as to make them behave as if they were parallel, i.e. originating from far point. In contrast to this, the contact lenses change the refractive power of the eye by removing cornea from the refractive media complex. The cornea is replaced by a new refractive complex comprising of air, contact lens and tear film. The refractive index of air is 1; contact lens is 1.496, tear is 1.338 and cornea is 1.376.

To make the contact lens optically effective, the power is grounded on the anterior surface of the contact lens. If a plain contact lens, i.e. without power is put on the cornea, it will also eliminate cornea from the refractive media complex. This will make the emmetropic eye hypermetropic because the cornea, which has a refractive power of +43D, is removed from the media complex and the eye is left with lens as a main refractive medium. It will make a hypermetropic eye more hypermetropic and a myopic eye less myopic.

The purpose of the tear film besides optical is to keep the lens in place, prevent the contact lens from falling out and glide smoothly over the cornea. All these functions are attributed to surface tension of the tear.

The contact lens is a saucer-shaped circular transparent, thin optical device, which when kept over the cornea, improves the vision. The concavity faces the cornea. The two surfaces of the contact lens have different radii of curvatures. The posterior curvature is almost same as that of anterior corneal surface. The anterior surface has a curvature less than corneal curvature.

A contact lens with anterior radius of curvature shorter than cornea increases the refractive power of the contact lens and curvature greater than cornea reduces the power.

The dioptric power of the cornea is inversely proportional to curvature of cornea.

The total power of the contact lens is achieved by the back curvature of the contact lens, base curve of the contact lens and actual power of the contact lens. The actual power of the contact lens is derived from the difference between the anterior and the posterior curvature. Only the second alternative is influenced by the refractive index of the contact lens material. The base curve is determined accurately by keratometry and roughly by trial lens. This is followed by calculation of front curvature by refraction over the trial lens or from patient's power in the spectacle giving due allowance to back vertex distance.

Back Vertex Distance

Back vertex distance is the distance between the back surface of the spectacle and the cornea. Thus, the back vertex distance in contact lens is zero. While in spectacle, it is between 14 mm and 16 mm. The power of the spectacle lens or contact lens can be changed by changing the back vertex distance. This effectively moves the focal length forward or backward. The calculation of the vertex distance is important to convert the spectacle power to the power of contact lens. The vertex correction is calculated by the following formula:

$$F_c = \frac{F}{1-xF}$$

where, F_c is the corrected lens power, F is the original lens power and x is the change in vertex distance in meters.

This is best explained with a thick plus lens.

Let consider a +13D at 11 mm (0.011 m) to be placed at 9 mm (0.009 m).

Here, F = +13D, x = 0.011–0.009 = 0.002 m,

$$F_c = \frac{13}{1-0.002 \times 13} = \frac{13}{1-0.026}$$
$$= \frac{13}{0.974} = \frac{13,000}{974} = 13.34$$

If the same lens, i.e. +13D is to be replaced by a contact lens where distance between lens and cornea is zero, the power will be 15.169D (Paul Riodan et al).

The power of plus contact lens is always more than spectacle power and power of the minus contact lens is less than the power of the lens in myopic spectacle. This is due to magnification caused by contact lens in comparison to spectacle lens.

Magnification in Contact Lens

Persons who are starting to use contact lenses or switching from spectacles to contact lens, find difficulty in distant adjustment, due to change in image size brought about by the change in the effective power of the contact lens, secondary to change in back vertex distance.

The spectacle lens causes magnification of 1.5%–2% per diopter. This is reduced to 0.5%– 0.8% in contact lens.

As the myopic contact lens is away from the far point, it reduces the overall power of the contact lens, as compared to spectacles. In hypermetropia, including aphakia, the contact lens is nearer the far point. Hence, has more power than plus lens in the spectacle. We have seen that magnification depends on the dioptric power and distance. Nearer the lens to the far point, greater is the magnification. A +13D lens in spectacle will require a contact lens of +15D to have same vision.

As discussed earlier:

1. Cornea has the maximum vergence.
2. A contact lens changes the vergence power of the anterior surface of the cornea by an optical complex, comprising of tear fluid and contact lens.
3. For this, the contact lens must have a posterior curvature similar to the anterior corneal curvature.

In initial days, contact lenses were developed more for cosmetic reason than for optical.

It was realized that good cosmetic results depend on good fitting and tolerance, which indirectly depend on its optical properties. It is no secret that in spite of four centuries of assiduous research, a perfect contact lens is far from reality. For this reason, the industry has an array of contact lenses, each with own merits and demerits.

Types of Contact Lenses

There is no single classification that fits to encompass all the available contact lenses. The contact lens can be classified variously based on:

1. Anatomical relation to the globe: Scleral and corneal.
2. Size: Small and large.

3. Shape: Focal and afocal.
4. Consistency: Hard, soft and semisoft.
5. Material used: Glass and plastic.
6. Water content: High and low.
7. Oxygen permeability/transmissibility: Good/Poor.
8. Wettability of contact lens.
9. Duration of wear.
10. Color.

Based on Anatomy and Size

The classification of contact lenses based on anatomy and size is shown in Figure 9.1.

Based on Variation in Shape

The lenses are mainly two types (Fig. 9.2):

- Focal
- Afocal.

Based on Consistency

According to consistency, contact lenses are classified into rigid, non-rigid and rigid gas permeable (Fig. 9.3).

Based on Material Used

1. Glass (no more in use).
2. PMMA: Polymethylmethacrylate (rigid).

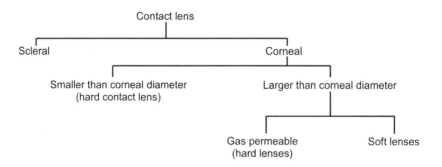

Figure 9.1: Classification according to anatomy and size of contact lenses

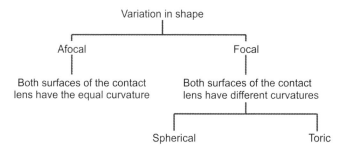

Figure 9.2: Classification of contact lenses as per shape

3. HEMA: Hydroxyethylmethacrylate (soft).
4. CAB: Cellulose acetate butyrate (rigid gas permeable).

Based on Water Content

Soft contact lenses have pores that imbibe water from the tear and increase water content. Water content of a contact lens denotes percentage of water in a contact lens. The functions of water (tear) in contact lens are:

1. Increase oxygen transmissibility—more the water content, more is the oxygen transmissibility.
2. Increase in water content multiplies oxygen permeability twice, i.e. 20% increase in water content increases oxygen permeability by 40%.
3. Increases the thickness of the lens.
4. Increases the physical strength of the lens, more the water content—more is the thickness and more is the physical strength.

Contact lenses with high water content are called hydrogel lenses or hydrophilic lenses. They may have:

1. Low water content (< 40%).
2. Intermediate water content (40%–55%).
3. High water content (> 55%).

Based on Oxygen Permeability/Transmissibility

Oxygen permeability/transmissibility is measurement of oxygen permeability in relation to thickness of lens that is influenced by water content. It is measured by a fraction DK/L where, D is the diffuse coefficient, K is the solubility coefficient and L is the thickness of the lens. Usually thickness of a –3D contact lens is taken as standard L. This is measured as 'DK' where, D represents coefficient of diffusion and K represents coefficient of solubility.

The unit of measurement of DK value is Fatt unit that is expressed as:

$$\frac{[cm^2\ mL\ (STP)\ O_2] \times 10^{-11}}{[sec\ mL\ mm\ Hg]}$$

where, STP is standard temperature and pressure.

Increase in temperature increases DK value. D and K are not related to passage of O_2 through lens material.

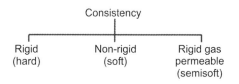

Figure 9.3: Classification according to consistency

Oxygen permeability is increased two folds, if water content is raised by 20%.

Based on Wettability of the Contact Lens

Wettability is adherence of tear to the surface of the contact lens. It represents the ability of the tear (fluid) to spread over the contact lens. Better the wettability better is the spread of fluid on the surface. It is measured in wetting angle. Wetting angle is the angle formed by the solid surface and tangent to the fluid that ranges between 0° and 150°. Better the wetting, less is the wetting angle. Thus, a complete wet surface has a wetting angle of 0°, while non-wetting surface has wetting angle of 150°. HEMA, which is hydrophilic, is more wettable than PMMA, which is hydrophobic.

As Per Duration of Wear

• Daily wear
• Extended wear
• Disposable.

Based on Color

• Transparent
• Transparent with various colors
• Opaque.

Desirable Properties of Contact Lens Material

The comparison between some of the salient features of hard, rigid gas permeable and soft contact lenses is shown in Table 9.1:

1. Transparency: This is most important optical property of the contact lens. The lens can be opaque or colored—for cosmetic purpose only.
2. Refractive index: Same as tear film.
3. Tolerance: Tolerance depends on:
   a. Biocompatibility: Free of toxins and allergic substances.

   b. Gas permeability.
   c. Wettability.
4. Ease of sterilization and disinfection.
5. Mechanical stability: Curvature, size and thickness should remain stable.

Specific Types of Contact Lenses

There are two types of contact lenses:
• Scleral
• Corneal.

Scleral Contact Lenses (Haptic)

Originally, almost all contact lenses were sclera supported and may be considered to be forerunner of present day haptic lenses. The haptic lenses are large contact lenses, which have a scleral part that can either be transparent or colored and a corneal part, which again can be transparent or colored, to hide disfigurement of the cornea.

In the past, scleral contact lenses were made of transparent glasses, which were non-permeable to oxygen, hence not very well-tolerated, making them obsolete. The corneal part does not directly rest on the cornea like other lenses. There is a clear gap between the posterior surface of the contact lens and the cornea. This space is so large that it cannot be filled with usual tear produced by the eye and require artificial tear to fill the gap. The present day scleral contact lenses are made of PMMA; some gas permeable lenses with high DK are also available. Latter are more difficult to manufacture.

The scleral lenses, due to their shape and size, bulge forward. To increase the oxygen supply to the cornea, the lenses are fenestrated or channeled on the periphery. The fenestrations are made on the temporal side in the interpalpebral aperture. The distance between the limbus and lateral edge of a scleral lens is more, than on the nasal side. The lens is so constructed that it does not press over the limbus. They are being used more frequently now even to improve vision, where standard corneal contact lenses are not tolerated. The other indications are to reduce pain and photophobia, microphthalmos, severe keratitis, corneal ectasia, Stevens-Johnson syndrome, aniridia, chemical injuries, lid deformity, post-LASIK problem and ptosis crutches.

Corneal Contact Lenses

According to size of the corneal contact lenses, they are divided into two types:

1. Smaller than the cornea.
2. Larger than cornea, but smaller than sclera.

The lenses smaller than cornea are called hard contact lenses due to their hard consistency. The contact lenses larger than the cornea are called soft contact lenses and rigid gas permeable lenses.

Hard contact lenses

Hard contact lenses are the first generation of the contact lenses that replaced the glass contact lenses and are made up of plastic polymer called Perspex, the chemical name of which is PMMA. The hard contact lenses are also called acrylic lenses. The lenses rest on the cornea, hence are known as corneal lenses also. They have diameter less than average corneal diameter of 11 mm. They are available

Table 9.1: Comparison between some of the salient feature of hard, rigid gas permeable and soft contact lenses

Sl No	Features	Hard contact lens	Rigid gas permeable lens	Soft lens
1.	Size	Smaller than cornea (7.5–9.5 mm)	Larger than cornea (9.00–10.00 mm)	Very large (13.5–16.50 mm)
2.	Consistency	Hard	Semisoft	Soft
3.	Commonest material used	PMMA	CAB	HEMA
4	Oxygen permeability	Nil	Moderate	High
5.	DK	0	10–100	Up to 140
6.	Optical properties	Very good	Good	Moderate
7.	Neutralizing astigmatism	Better	Best	Poor
8.	Duration of wear	Daily (8 hour)	Daily (24 hour or more)	Many days
9.	Comfort	Least	Better	Best
10.	Adaptation period	Longest	Intermediate	Very short
11.	Overwear syndrome	+++	+	Nil
12.	Corneal edema	++	+	Nil
13.	Chances of infection	Least	±	++
14.	Maintenance	Easy	Fairly easy	Difficult
15.	Expected duration of use	8–10 year	1–2 year	Not more than 1 year

in diameters of 7–10.5 mm. They are hard in consistency; hence do not change their shape, which happens in soft contact lenses. They can be molded and fenestrated. The average life span of a hard contact lens is longer than soft and semisoft lenses. It may be as long as 8–12 years. However, it is advised to change them every 4–5 years. The hard contact lenses do not absorb water. They are called focons, i.e. their water content is poor. They have zero DK. One of the advantages of hard contact lenses is that they correct corneal astigmatism to some extent, but not exceeding 2D cylinder. For higher degree of astigmatism, rigid toric lenses are recommended as they are not oxygen permeable, hence prone to cause hypoxia of corneal epithelium. Due to poor oxygenation, they cause more spectacle blur, forming Sattler's veil. The hard lenses cause glare, photophobia and flare.

Common complications in hard contact lenses

Spectacle blur

Normal tear film without contact lenses contains sufficient oxygen for proper metabolism of corneal epithelium. This is hampered by hard contact lens that forms a barrier between the atmospheric oxygen and cornea. The hard contact lens is impervious to oxygen. In this changed situation, the cornea depends solely on the oxygen present in the tear trapped between the hard lens and the corneal epithelium that is not sufficient enough to maintain corneal metabolism. This creates a state of hypoxia. This hypoxia in turn depletes the glycogen present in the corneal epithelium, leading to edema of the epithelium and stroma resulting in swelling of anterior stroma, shifting the refractive index towards myopia. Surprisingly that becomes more evident after the contact lens is removed. This is the cause of spectacle blur. The symptoms of epithelial hypoxia and edema are blurred vision, pain of short duration after removal of lens. The symptoms become evident few minutes to few hours after the

removal of the lens, especially when one changes from contact lens to spectacles. This happens almost in all contact lenses.

Sattler's veil (Fick's phenomenon)

The corneal edema caused by hypoxia secondary to hard contact lens, results in colored halos around the light. This is called Fick's phenomenon and the effect is called Sattler's veil. The loss of vision in Sattler's veil is not very high.

Flare (Ghost image)

This is not to be confused with flare in AC.

Flare refers to poor vision round the objects at night due to two small central zones. This happens when the size of the pupil is larger than the optical zone in twilight, when light enters the pupil from the peripheral zone.

Creeping myopia

It is presumed that children using soft contact lens have a tendency towards increase in myopic power. This gets eliminated by discontinuing the lens. This is an overwear syndrome of hard contact lens, but may be seen in extended wear contact lenses also due to microedema in the epithelium. It may be as high as 1.00D–1.5D. Reversibility depends on early diagnosis.

Soft contact lenses

Soft contact lenses are made up of substances called hydrogels. The commonly used hydrogel is HEMA. The soft contact lenses are flexible enough to take up the corneal curvature, making them unsuitable to correct corneal astigmatism are larger than corneal diameter. Their diameter ranges between 13 and 14.5 mm, spreading over the limbus. They have DK ranging between 10 and 40. The water content ranges between 30% and 80%. The daily wear soft contact lenses have about 30% of water contents that rises to 80% in extended wear. The increased water content enhances the thickness of the lens. The greatest advantage is that oxygen permeability is very good in soft contact lenses. Increased oxygen permeability increases with water content. The soft contact lenses are easy to fit and comfortable to wear. One of the drawbacks with the soft contact lenses is that they give less sharp vision as compared to rigid lens. Some of the advantages of soft contact lenses include short adaptation time, absence of spectacle blur and flare that is too common with hard lenses, because the edge of the lens never crosses the pupillary margin. The soft lenses neither pop out of the eye nor vault over the cornea. Thus, they have least chances of being lost. The greatest disadvantages of the soft lenses are their short lifespan. They are difficult to clean and store with high incidence of microbial contamination. Immune reaction and deposits on the back surface of the lens are more frequent in soft lenses, so is giant papillary conjunctivitis. They are prone to develop chemical reaction to preservatives. Corneal edema and corneal neovascularization is also possible.

Rigid gas permeable contact lenses

Their position among the contact lenses is between the rigid and soft lenses. They share the advantage and disadvantages of both. They are basically hard lenses with good oxygen permeability with DK value of 15–100. They are made up of CAB, silicone acrylate, silicone styrene, but the commonest substance being CAB. The surfaces of the lens are water wettable like soft lenses. They are suitable for daily wear. They are more comfortable to use. The adaptation time is shorter than the rigid lenses and correct astigmatism better, hence are contact lenses of choice for keratoconus and irregular corneal astigmatism.

Other types

Toric contact lenses

These lenses are either modified hard contact lenses or modified semisoft lenses with all their properties and shortcomings. They are meant to correct astigmatism well. To correct astigmatism, they have to be stable on the cornea and not move during blink. Toric contact lenses are difficult to fit. All patients do not tolerate them. These patients prefer spherical ametropia to be corrected by contact lenses, and use spectacles to correct astigmatism and presbyopia when present. Nowadays, soft toric lenses are also available.

Bifocal contact lenses

Correcting presbyopia in persons using contact lenses is difficult. There are two alternatives. The first step is correcting near vision by spectacle over contact lenses and second is to correct presbyopia by contact lens only. This too has two alternatives, the first is monovision and the second is bifocal contact lenses. In monovision, one of the eyes is corrected for distant and the other for near, both by contact lenses. The bifocal contact lenses can either have power for distance in the centers and near on the periphery or have distant power on the periphery and near power in the center. Both the types have some inherent flaws. Both of them rotate with each blink and are difficult to fit (Fig. 9.4).

Disposable lenses

Disposable lenses are soft lenses. They are meant to be discarded before problem arises. They may be disposed every week or every fortnight. They are ideally disinfected by hydrogen peroxide. They have few advantages over non-disposable lenses.

The advantages of disposable contact lenses are reduced chances of preservative related toxicity, keratitis, less chances of lens deposit and less incidence of giant papillary conjunctivitis. Chances of deposit are almost zero; they are most suitable for children.

Therapeutic contact lenses

These are in fact soft contact lenses that have no optical properties. They can be left in the eye for 7–10 days. Drugs permeate through them. The extended wear lenses are soft or

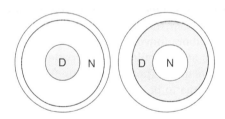

Figure 9.4: Bifocal contact lens

ultrasoft and ultrathin with 80% water content, very good oxygen permeability. They can be worn during sleep. They need not be removed as long as 24 hours. The extended wear lenses are good for aphakic eyes; however, not all eyes are suited for extended wear lenses. This makes patients selection a prerequisite. They act as splints to the cornea and form a barrier between the lid and the cornea. They are not meant to improve vision, but to give comfort.

According to water content, bandage contact lenses are divided into three types, i.e. high, intermediate and low water content. The high water content lenses are thickest and low water content lenses are thinnest. Thin lenses are called ultrathin or membrane lenses. The functions of the therapeutic contact lenses are:

1. To act as a barrier between tarsal conjunctiva/lid margin and cornea.
2. They prevent the lashes to rub against the cornea in trichiasis and entropion.
3. They encourage wound healing in corneal ulcer, threatening to perforate, leaking wound, bullous keratitis and recurrent erosion.
4. They keep the corneal surface wet by trapping tear between the lens and the corneal epithelium.
5. They also act as reservoir of drugs.

Bandage contact lenses

They are soft contact lenses. They are large with high water content. They do not have optical properties. They may be useful as extended wear lenses. Common conditions where bandage lenses are used are ocular pemphigus, Stevens-Johnson syndrome, keratitis sicca, bullous keratopathy, neurotrophic keratitis, sterile indolent ulcers, alkali burn and deformity of the lid.

The common indications for bandage lenses are:

1. Bullous keratitis of all types, i.e. phakic, aphakic, pseudophakic and idiopathic.
2. Corneal perforation not healing with usual treatment prior to penetrating keratoplasty.
3. Postkeratoplasty status.
4. Descemetocele.
5. Leaking corneal wound.
6. Recurrent corneal erosion.
7. Filamentary keratitis.
8. Trophic ulcer.
9. Alkali burn.
10. Keratoconus (piggyback contact lens).

Piggyback lenses

Piggyback lenses were developed in late 60s of last century. They are a combination of soft lens and a rigid gas permeable lens. They are commonly used when rigid gas permeable lenses are not tolerated. The piggyback lenses are used commonly in keratoconus, pellucid corneal degeneration, irregular astigmatism due to scarred cornea and astigmatism requiring high cylinders. They are difficult to fit and costly.

Specific Physical Properties in Relation to Contact Lens

Specific physical properties in relation to contact lenses are:

- Water content
- Wettability
- Oxygen transmissibility
- Oxygen permeability.

They are all interlinked and depend on each other to some extent.

Water Content

Soft contact lenses have pores that imbibe water from the tear and increase water retention in the lens. The functions include increased oxygen transmissibility and permeability, increase in thickness and physical strength of the lens.

Wettability

Wettability, (as discussed earlier in this chapter) denotes ability of the fluid to spread over the contact lens and is measured in wetting angle. HEMA, which is hydrophilic, is more wettable than PMMA, which is hydrophobic. The wetting angle is more than 90° in hydrophobic lenses and less, i.e. acute angle (less than 90°) in hydrophilic lenses.

Oxygen Transmissibility

Oxygen transmissibility is the measurement of oxygen transmissibility in relation to thickness of the lens that is influenced by water content. It is measured in a fraction DK/L where D is the diffused coefficient, K is the solubility coefficient and L is the thickness of the lens.

Materials Used in Manufacture of Various Types of Contact Lenses

Originally, contact lenses were made up of glass. They were very rigid, very difficult to fit and uncomfortable. With discovery of synthetic plastics, use of glass was abandoned and interest shifted to plastic polymers, which were found to be superior to glass as contact lens materials. Over the years, many polymers have been developed to manufacture perfect contact lens.

The polymers used can be classified into two groups:

1. Those used in hard contact lenses.
2. Those used in soft contact lenses.

The first group comprises of PMMA and the second comprises of HEMA alone or in combination with others.

The materials used can be broadly divided into two groups:

1. Focon (hydrophobic): Used for rigid lenses and some gas permeable rigid lenses.
2. Filcons (hydrophilic): They are used in soft hydrogen lenses.

Properties of Ideal Contact Lens Material

1. Refractive index of the contact lens should be nearer the refractive index of the cornea.
2. The contact lens should remain transparent.
3. They should be physically, chemically and biologically competent.
4. They should be hard enough to remain in shape and soft enough, not to hurt the cornea.
5. They should possess the property to get hydrated when worn.
6. They should be wettable.
7. They should be oxygen permeable.
8. They should be safe to wear.
9. They should be resistant to chemicals in storing and clinical fluids.
10. They should be microbial resistant.
11. They should be moderately priced.

Materials Used in Manufacture of Hard Contact Lenses

The materials are basically plastic, commonest used material is PMMA. Its optical qualities are very good. It rarely causes allergic reaction. The lenses are smaller than any other contact lenses. Usual size varies between 8.5 and 10 mm. They last longer. They give fairly good vision.

The disadvantages are:

1. It being hard is capable of hurting the cornea, while inserting and removing.
2. DK value is zero: It means that the lenses do not allow oxygen to permeate.
3. Absence of wetting, however, tear film formed over the lens is fairly stable, neutralizing the absence of wetting to some extent.

Materials Used in Manufacture of Rigid Gas Permeable Contact Lenses

The rigid gas permeable lenses have rigidity of PMMA lenses, but are gas permeable, hence are also wrongly termed as semisoft lenses.

The commonly used materials are:

1. Cellulose acetate butyrate (CAB).
2. Silicone acrylate.
3. Silicone and PMMA.
4. Silicone.
5. Fluoropolymers.
6. Tertiary butylstyrene (T-butylstyrene).

Materials Used for Manufacture of Soft Contact Lenses

They are made from substances called hydrogels that have a hydroxyl group in them. They are cross-linked polymers. They are made of HEMA. They are the most commonly used contact lenses. They are 1–2 mm larger than the cornea.

Optical Purposes of Contact Lens

The most important use of a contact lens is its optical property that make the parallel rays come to focus on the photosensitive layer of the eye. This can also be achieved by a spectacle. Correction of ametropia requires placing of spectacle lens or contact lens at such a place in front of the eye that makes the parallel rays to coincide with the far point of the eye under consideration.

Parameters Required for Contact Lens Fitting

- Refraction of the eye
- Corneal curvature
- Diameter of the contact lens.

Refraction of the eye

Refraction of the eye should be determined in minus cylinder and corrected to make allowance for spectacle vertex distance to vertex distance of contact lens, which is obviously zero.

For example, let the power of the lens in spectacle be –8.25D with +0.5D at 90°. This, when converted to minus cylinder form, becomes –7.5D with –0.5D at 180°. The vertex distance of spectacle is 15 mm. The vertex distance of the contact lens is zero. Thus, correcting for vertex distance to zero, the power will come to –6.75D with –0.50D at 180°. This requires modification according to vertex distance.

Diameter of the contact lens

Diameter of all contact lenses are not the same. It is maximum in soft contact lens, i.e. 13–15 mm. The diameter is shortest in hard contact lens (PMMA) where it ranges between 7.5 and 8.8 mm. The diameter of rigid gas permeable lenses lies in between the two, i.e. 9.00–9.8 mm. The diameter of the contact lens is not twice the radius of curvature. It is the distance across the lens at the middle of the lens. The diameter is taken in millimeters (mm); the diameter is equal in all meridians, irrespective of the type of the lens, i.e. hard/soft/semisoft.

Corneal curvature

Examination of curvature of the corneal surface

Dimensions of the corneal curvature are most important measurements for perfect fitting of contact lenses. There are many ways of measuring the corneal curvature. Some of them are very crude and lost clinical significance in present day setting; others are very sophisticated. The appliances can be divided into two groups:

- Keratoscopes
- Keratometers.

The optics involved with both is the fact that the cornea acts as a convex mirror. The image formed by it is erect, virtual, small and 4 mm behind the cornea. In fact, the image formed is nothing, but the first Purkinje image. The image is distorted, if the anterior surface of the cornea is irregular or oblong. The size depends on the curvature of the cornea. More is the curvature, smaller is the image.

The keratoscopes have limited role in contact lens practice except photokeratoscopes. The non-photokeratoscopes are being discussed here for academic interest only.

Window reflex

This is the simplest example of image formed by the anterior surface of the cornea without any role in contact lens practice. To elicit the reflex, the patient stands in front of grill of a window. The observer places himself/herself between the patient and the window and observes the image of the grill on the cornea without any torch or loop. A true replica of the window means regular (normal) corneal surface. Wavy or irregular image means irregular surface, absence of image denotes total corneal opacity (Figs 9.5A to C).

Placido's disk

This is an ancient appliance that is very handy, cheap and easy to use. The instrument is more useful than window reflex, but far less accurate than keratometer. The instrument consists of a hard circular disk, about 10 inches wide with a central peephole that has a +2D lens incorporated in it, the purpose of which is to relax the accommodation of the observer. The peephole is encircled by circles of black and white, 8–10 in number at equidistant from each other. The circles are of equal

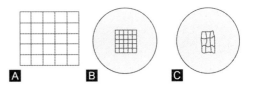

Figures 9.5A to C: Window reflex on cornea. **A.** Image of window; **B.** Normal corneal surface; **C.** Irregular corneal surface.

width. To use this, the patient faces the disk, the back towards a source of light in such a way that the disk is well illuminated. The disk is held about 10 inches from the patient and the observer looks at the image of the circles on the cornea through the peephole (Figs 9.6A to D):

1. If the cornea is bright without any irregularity, the circles are not distorted, look sharp and bright (refer Fig. 9.6B).
2. Both the eyes are examined for comparison.
3. Distortion of the circles means irregular surface (refer Fig. 9.6C). The causes of distorted circles are pterygium, limbal growth, irregular opacities, tight sutures, iris prolapse, keratoconus.
4. Oblong images mean high astigmatism (refer Fig. 9.6D). They will be horizontally oval in case of astigmatism with the rule and vertically oval, in case of astigmatism against the rule.
5. An unusually small image means more curved cornea and large image in flat corneas.
6. Deficiency in circles denotes corneal opacity.

Better than usual placido's disk are similar circles incorporated in the head of the direct ophthalmoscope where the circles are internally illuminated. The instruments are used like standard direct ophthalmoscope and a +40D can be put in the peephole for magnification.

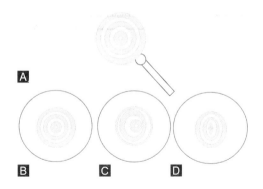

Figures 9.6A to D: Placido's disk and its images on the cornea. **A.** Placido's disk; **B.** Image of placido's disk on normal cornea; **C.** Image of placido's disk on irregular cornea; **D.** Image of placido's disk in high astigmatism.

Keratometers (ophthalmometers)
and keratometry

On a cursory examination or even with a slit lamp, the cornea seems to be equally curved all over. This assumption is not compatible with keratometric examination (Fig. 9.7).

The cornea is asymmetrically aspheric. The central 3–4 mm is almost spherical. 90% of refractive power of the anterior surface is located in this area, which is called optical zone.

The rest of the cornea all around gradually flattens.

The keratometer is a device that measures the corneal curvature. Keratometry is the process of measuring the corneal curvature. The principal of keratometer is based on the fact that the anterior surface of the cornea acts as a convex mirror and the images of the objects (target-mires) kept at any distance in front of the cornea forms an image 4 mm behind the cornea. The image is virtual, erect and small (Fig. 9.8).

The size of the image depends on curvature of the anterior surface of the cornea. More curved corneas give smaller images than flatter corneas.

The cornea looks circular from front, in fact it is not so. Neither the diameters nor the curvatures are same in all meridians. It is wider horizontally.

Average measurements of the normal cornea are:

1. Average measurement is horizontally 12 mm and vertically 11 mm.
2. Anterior surface is less curved than the posterior surface. They are 7.8 mm and 7.00 mm respectively.
3. This makes the center of the cornea thinnest.
4. This thinning is not involved in contact lens fitting, but has a bearing in refractive surgeries on the cornea.
5. Difference in vertical and horizontal diameters is due to changed curvature in the two meridians.
6. The vertical meridian is more curved than the horizontal meridian.
7. This increases vertical curvature, makes it more myopic than horizontal.
8. This induces a small amount of astigmatism that is called physiological astigmatism or astigmatism with the rule.
9. Though the posterior surface is more curved, for all practical purposes of contact lens fitting, it is taken as parallel

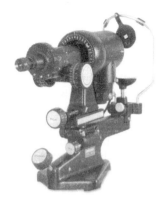

Figure 9.7: A keratometer

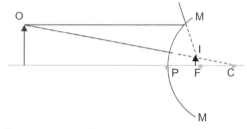

Figure 9.8: Image formation in the anterior surface of the cornea. O is the object. MM represents the anterior surface of the cornea, which acts as a convex mirror. P is the pole, F is the focus and C is the center of curvature. I is erect, virtual and minified image of O.

to the anterior surface. In contact lens practice, refraction at the posterior surface is not taken into consideration. The refractive index of the cornea, which accounts for three-fourth power of the eye, is 1.376 and causes +43D refraction.

10. The rest of the power, i.e. +17D is attributed to lenses, aqueous and vitreous, which are not taken into account in contact lens fitting.

11. The greater refractive power of the cornea is due to large difference between the refraction of cornea, (1.376) and air (1.00).

12. Earlier, we have seen that deviation of rays when passing from rarer to denser medium depends on the difference between refractive indices. Greater is the difference, more is the deviation, thus cornea is more converging than lens, aqueous and vitreous put together.

13. The radius of corneal curvature can be determined by the following formula:

$$r = 2d \frac{I}{O}$$

where,

r is the radius of curvature.

d is the distance of the object (mire).

I is the size of the image formed on the cornea.

O is the size of the object.

14. Determination of dioptric power of the cornea.

The dioptric power of the cornea can be calculated by the formula, i.e.

$$d = \frac{n-1}{r}$$

where,

d is the refractive power measured in diopters.

n is refractive index of cornea, which is 1.3375.

r is the radius of curvature measured in millimeter.

Measurement of the corneal curvature: The most accurate measurement of corneal curvatures obtained by keratometers that use the principle of first Purkinje image.

$$d = \frac{n-1}{r} = \frac{1.3375-1}{r}$$

$$= \frac{0.337.5}{r\,(m)} = \frac{337.5}{r\,(mm)}$$

All the measurements are taken in the central optical zone of 3 mm.

The mires are separated by a distance of 1.25 mm.

KERATOMETERS

The keratometer essentially consists of:

1. Body of the instrument.

2. Mires.

3. A low power telescope.

4. Doubling device.

5. A rotating device for alignment of the axis.

6. The distance between the cornea and mire is 75 mm.

7. This is considered to be very large in terms of keratometry.

8. The size of the image is 3 mm. This is magnified six times by the telescope. This magnification is in no way related to corneal curvature.

Uses

1. Determine the curvature of the cornea.
2. Calculation of intraocular lens (IOL) power.
3. Management of intraoperative astigmatism.

Most of the keratometers measure the corneal curvature between 6.5 mm and 9.38 mm, which correspond to 52D and 36D refractive power, which are good enough for most of the contact lens fittings. Difficulty arises when the cornea is too curved or too flat. In such cases, a planoconvex lens of 1.25D is fitted over the aperture of the keratometer with its convex surface facing the cornea. This extends the range to 61D, i.e. 5.53 mm. In case of flat cornea, fixing a planoconcave lens of –1D can change this to 30D or 11.25 mm. In case of very irregular astigmatism, a soft contact lens of known power is placed over the cornea and readings are taken. The power of the soft contact lens is subtracted later. The power of the contact lens differs from the power of the lens in spectacles.

Types

There are two types of keratometers:

• Manual
• Automatic.

The manual keratometer can be either one point keratometer or two point keratometer. The basis of both is the same. They use the principle of image doubling to avoid problem of eye movement. The doubling is done by prism incorporated in the instrument. Both types use moving mires and use telescope to magnify the cornea image.

The mires in the automated keratometers are digitalized and use infrared rays that are bounced from the cornea and measure the corneal curvature at different points. They are generally handheld and compact instruments.

One Point Keratometers

In this instrument, the size of the object does not change, but the size of the image changes. The corneal image starts acting as objects for telescope. The mires are in front of the objective and form an erect, small image. The mire is a circular disk with a central aperture with plus and minus signs on it. The instrument can be divided into two parts:

• Mechanical
• Optical.

Mechanical part consists of a sturdy base on which the optical part rests. The components of the mechanical parts are:

1. Height adjustment.
2. Chin rest.
3. Forehead rest.
4. An ocular.
5. A locking device.

Optical part consists of the following:

1. Image enhancing device: A low focus, low-powered telescope that can be moved along its long axis; this is the focusing device the telescope enlarges the image of the target six times. The corneal image formed by the mires acts as the object for the telescope.
2. Mire forming device: This portion is placed in front of eyepiece of the telescope and has following parts:
   a. Mires: They are printed on a circular disk on the periphery, with a central circular aperture for light to pass and a circular circle in between. The mires are marked as + and – signs at right angles to them. The mires are illuminated by an illuminating

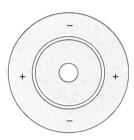

Figure 9.9: Diagram of mire forming device in one point keratometer

device consisting of a mirror and a bulb (Fig. 9.9).

b. The aperture diaphragm: There are four circular apertures in a disk. The apertures are arranged in diamond pattern to vertical meridian and are placed at right angles to each (Figs 9.10A to G).

c. The doubling prisms: The doubling prisms are two in number; one is placed with base-up and the other base-out. The prism with base-out shifts the image horizontally, while the prism with base-up shifts the image vertically. The prisms divide the light passing only through the horizontal hole. Light passing only through the upper and lower quadrants do not pass through any of the prisms. They form an image. The plus signs are superimposed to measure horizontal curvature and minus signs are used to measure vertical curvature.

Method of using one point keratometer is as follows:

1. Adjust the focus of the instrument on a flat white paper, with a black line drawn on it.

2. Calibrate the keratometer on the steel ball of known curvature, supplied with the instrument.

3. Adjust the height of the instrument, as per patient's requirement.

4. The patient is made to sit in front of the instrument, with chin on the chin rest and forehead against the head bar.

5. Only one eye is examined at a time. The other eye is occluded by an occluder fitted in the instrument.

6. Now, adjust the height of the instrument to the level of pupil.

7. The patient is asked to look into the instrument.

8. The observer views the mires as shown in Figures 9.11A to E.

9. To measure the horizontal curvature, the adjacent plus sign of the central and left mires are superimposed.

10. To measure the vertical curvature, the adjacent minus mire of the vertical and the central mire are superimposed.

11. If the two plus signs are not aligned, the cornea has oblique astigmatism.

12. The instrument is rotated to align the plus mires.

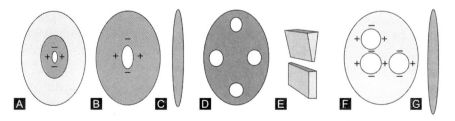

Figures 9.10A to G: Line diagram showing optics involved in one point keratometer. **A.** Mires on cornea; **B.** Mires in keratometer; **C.** Objective; **D.** Apertures; **E.** Doubling prisms; **F.** Doubled mires seen by observer; **G.** Observer.

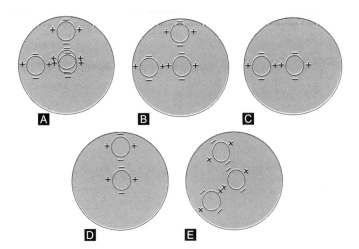

Figures 9.11A to E: Mires in the cornea as seen by the observer. **A.** Mires not focused properly; **B.** Mires focused properly; **C.** Measurement of the horizontal curvature; **D.** Measurement of the vertical curvature; **E.** Example of oblique astigmatism.

13. In spherical cornea, all the mires are perfect circles.
14. In case of astigmatism with the rule, the mires are horizontally oval.
15. In case of astigmatism against the rule, the mires are vertically oval.

Characteristics of finding in one point keratometer are as follows:

1. Normal stigmatic cornea:
   a. The mires are circular.
   b. The principle meridians have same power.
2. Astigmatic cornea:
   a. The mires are oval instead of circular.
   b. In astigmatism with the rule, the mires are horizontally oval.
   c. In astigmatism against the rule, the mires are vertically oval.

Two Point Keratometer

Two point keratometer is based on the principle of variable object size and constant image size using Woolston of visible doubling by principal prism.

Like one point keratometer, the instrument too has a sturdy base on which the optical system is mounted. The instrument differs from one point keratometer, due to the fact that the mires in two point keratometer are not built in the optical system and can be moved synchronously. The mires are mounted on an arc that can be rotated round the long axis of the optical system. The arc itself is calibrated in millimeters and diopters (Fig. 9.12). The mires are housed in two internally illuminated boxes. One mire is colored red and the other green.

The optical system consists of a low power telescope to enlarge the mires formed on the anterior surface of the cornea. As far as keratometry is concerned, image formed only within optical zone are taken into account.

The shape of the mires in different models is different with common purpose.

The most commonly used two point keratometer is Javal-Schiotz keratometer that has one mire in vertical rectangle and the other is a stepped triangle (Fig. 9.13A).

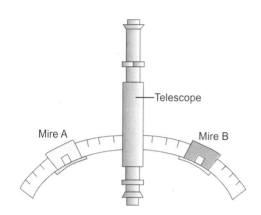

Figure 9.12: Line diagram of two point keratometers

The mires are adjusted to give a composite picture touching each other. The arc is rotated by 90° and a similar reading is taken. In spherical cornea, the mires will have appearance as in first position and the size of the mires will remain unchanged (Fig. 9.13B).

In astigmatic cornea, the mires look smaller due to increased curvature and will overlap as the mire A is stepped; each step represents 1D. The amount of astigmatism can be read off by counting the steps overlapped. The principle remaining the same in other models, the mires are of different shapes.

One mire is stepped with base against each other, but separated by a straight gap. The other mire is a pair of squares separated by a gap. The two squares and the gap give the mires a shape of a rectangle. The height and width of both the mires are same. The stepped mire is green and the rectangular mire has a red filter.

To find out keratometric measurement, the radius of curvature in one meridian is noted first. Then the arc is rotated through 90°, to note the curvature in new meridian.

In non-astigmatic cornea, the size of the mires in the two meridians will be same without overlap. In case of astigmatism, more curved meridian will have smaller mires and there will be overlap of the mires. The area of

overlap has a mixture of red and green color and almost looks gray. Each overlap step represents 1D of astigmatism.

TOPOGRAPHY OF CONTACT LENS

Contact lens is a concave saucer-shaped transparent device, which is placed on the cornea with convex surface away from the cornea. It has a diameter, surfaces, various curvatures, thickness, edge and power.

Diameter

Diameter does not affect the dioptric power of the lens, but influences the depth of the lens. Wider the diameter, greater will be the sagittal depth. Larger diameters have flatter curved surface. The diameter of the contact lens is proportionate to corneal curvature. Less curved corneas will require larger diameter.

Surfaces

Contact lens has two surfaces. The anterior surface is convex and the posterior surface is concave. A very thin layer of tear covers the anterior surface. The layer of tear between the contact lens and the cornea, when large in volume, abolishes the corneal irregularity and neutralizes mild-to-moderate astigmatism. It reduces the irregularity of the cornea in irregular corneal astigmatism. The posterior surface of contact lens should confirm with the anterior surface of the cornea.

Curvature

Curvature of the contact lens is divided into two parts—the anterior curve and the posterior curve (Fig. 9.14):

1. The anterior curve has two parts, the central curve and the peripheral curve. The central curve represents the anterior curvature of the optical zone. The power of the contact lens depends on the anterior central curve. Peripheral anterior curve is

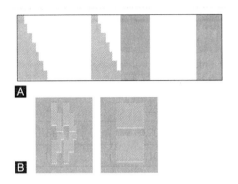

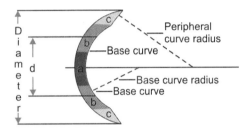

Figures 9.13A and B: Different types of mires in two point keratometer

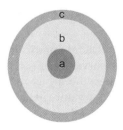

Figure 9.14: Curvatures of a contact lens. **a.** Optical zone; **b.** Intermediate zone; **c.** Peripheral zone; **d.** Back curve zone.

gradual, flattening of the curvature from the anterior central curve to the edge of the lens. In high-powered lenses of both signs, an intermediate curve may be needed (Fig. 9.15).

2. The posterior curve is also referred to as base curve. It also has two variations:
   a. Central posterior curve: This fits on the central optical zone of the cornea. It varies between 7.0 and 8.5 mm.
   b. Peripheral curve: This is divided into an intermediate posterior curve and peripheral posterior curve.

Thickness

This represents the difference between the anterior and the posterior curves. Measurement in the central zone is only relevant. The thickness increases with enhanced water content.

Edge

Edge of the lens is the polished, gradually merging of peripheral posterior curve and peripheral anterior curve of the lens.

Power

Power is measured in diopter, representing the posterior vertex power.

CONTACT LENS FITTING

Comfort of wearing an optical device, greatly depends on the contact lens fitting.

Parameters

The parameters required for fitting the contact lenses are:

- Power
- Base curve
- Diameter.

Power

The power is determined following retinoscopy. The patient's astigmatism should be determined in minus cylinder, thus a power –8D sphere with +0.5D cylinder of 90° should be taken as –7.5D sphere with –0.5D cylinder at 180° and corrected as per vertex distance (Figs 9.16A and B).

Figure 9.15: Various parts of anterior curve. **a.** Central optical zone; **b.** Intermediate zone; **c.** Peripheral zone.

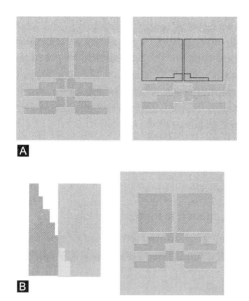

Figures 9.16A and B: Mires in uncorrected and corrected astigmatism

Base Curve

The corneal curvature is found out by keratometer. The anterior curvature of the normal cornea is not equal in horizontal and vertical meridian. The vertical curvature is more curved (steeper) than horizontal curve Hence, this makes the vertical curvature more myopic than the horizontal. This is known as physiological astigmatism or astigmatism with the rule.

The keratometer readings give curvature in millimeters and its corresponding value in diopters. The flattest curvature is called K. Thus, a keratometer reading of 44.25D/46.5D at axis 90° will mean 44.25 at 180° and 46.5D at 90°. In this case, 46.5 will be called K.

The central posterior curve (CPC or base curve) is the curvature on the posterior surface of the contact lens that conforms with the front surface of the cornea. A contact lens with CPC more than 44.25 will be called steeper than K and lens would be called flatter.

Remember: Dioptric power of the cornea is inversely proportional to curvature of cornea.

The following informations are required for fitting of contact lens:

- Retinoscopy
- Keratometry
- Determining central posterior curvature (CPC).

The diameter of the trial contact lens is given in a table, accompanying the trial contact lens set.

For K reading 43.00/44.50, the starting lens diameter will be 8.8 mm, CPC would be 43.50D and a lens with above information will be ordered. Less cumbersome method is fitting by trial, from a contact lens trial set, with standard peripheral and intermediate curves.

Astigmatism is the difference between the keratometry readings in the two meridians.

To fit a contact lens in astigmatic cornea, the guidelines to be followed are given in Table 9.2.

Table 9.2: Guidelines for fitting contact lenses in astigmatism

Astigmatism	Power	
Less than 0.05D	On K	
0.05D–1.00D	Add 0.25D to K	
More than 2D	Half of the difference added to K	

Curvature	Difference	Add
45.00/45.5	0.5	Nil (on K), i.e. 45.0
45.0/46	1	Add 0.25 to K, i.e. 45.25D
45/48	3	Add half of difference, i.e. 3/2 = 1.5 = 46.5

Summary

- On the basis of keratometry
- On the basis of trial contact lenses
- Combination.

Qualities of a Good Contact Lens Fitting

1. Physically accepted:
   a. No discomfort.
   b. No toxic reaction.
   c. No allergic reaction.
   d. No watering.
   e. Lens should move without being felt.
   f. There should be no excess blinking.
2. Optical:
   a. The vision should be either better or at least equal to spectacle vision.
   b. There should be no distortion of vision.
   c. There should be no creeping myopia.
   d. No spectacle blur.
   e. No flare.

Some of the Difficulties Met with Contact Lens (Refer Complications in Hard Contact Lenses)

- Spectacle blur
- Flare (ghost image)
- Creeping myopia.

Checking Contact Lens Fitting

After first fitting of contact lens, 15–20 minutes are allowed to pass to overcome initial reflex watering. This is almost universal. A drop of 1% fluorescein is put in the conjunctival sac (not on the contact lens). Two minutes later, the cornea is examined either on a slit lamp under cobalt blue light or handheld ultraviolet light. Following points are noted:

- Position
- Movement
- Fluorescein pattern.

Position

The lens should be centered in the optical axis of the eye. The lens should be positioned slightly up with sufficient visible cornea in the remaining part. A large or too steep lens will ride low. A small or flat lens will ride up. Other causes of low rides are:

1. Faulty intermediate or peripheral curve.
2. Plus lenses ride low.
3. Astigmatism against the rule, the lenses shift in the horizontal plane. The causes of high ride are:
   a. High minus lenses.
   b. Astigmatism with the rule.

Movement

The lens should move effortlessly with each blink and movement of the eye. A lens with good fitting moves downward, when the lid comes down and moves up as the lids move up and then settles in the original central position.

Fluorescein Pattern

Corneal touch stands out as dark spot. Loose areas show pooling of fluorescein. Normal fluorescein pattern shows pooling under the center. A narrow strip represents intermediate curve and a widening shows peripheral curve (Figs 9.17A to C and 9.18A to D).

Causes of acquired poor vision following good fitting and satisfactory vision may be as simple as interchanged lenses, i.e. right lens is put on the left cornea and vice versa. This can be eliminated, if the manufacturer puts different marks indicating right and left. The marks can be put in the marked storing boxes. The causes may be as complicated as excessive watering, poor wettability, corneal edema and damage to the lens edge or substance, flare, spectacle blur.

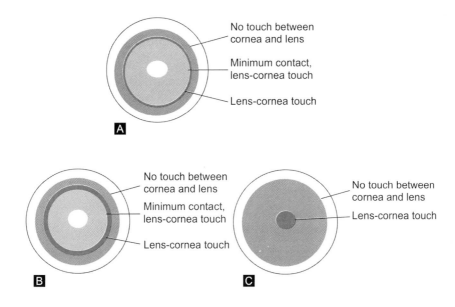

Figures 9.17A to C: Fluorescein pattern in contact lens fitting. **A.** Perfect fluorescein pattern in spherical cornea; **B.** Steep fit; **C.** Imperfect fluorescein pattern in spherical cornea (flat fit).

Indications for Contact Lens

As has been pointed out earlier, the contact lenses were originally developed to see without being seen with them. This remains the main desire till today, but while listing indications, it is better to give optical indications over cosmetic reasons. Thus indications of contact lens prescription are:

- Optical
- Therapeutic
- Cosmetic
- Occupational.

Optical

Contact lens can be logically prescribed in any error of refraction from very small to high ametropia. In clinical practice, they are prescribed above refraction of 2D of either sign because patient with less than 2D power have sufficient vision to move about and carry on usual day-to-day work with or without usual spectacles. The optical indications are as follows.

Errors of refraction

1. Isometric: Moderate to high errors of refraction with a difference less than 1D.

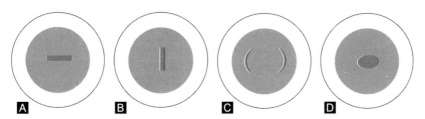

Figures 9.18A to D: Fluorescein pattern in astigmatic cornea. **A** and **B.** Perfect fit; **C** and **D.** Imperfect fit.

2. Anisometropia:
   a. Uniocular errors: High errors of re-
      fraction without error of refraction in
      the other eye. The commonest exam-
      ple is uniocular aphakia.
   b. Binocular errors: Difference is more
      than 2D–3D between the two eyes,
      but of the same sign.
   c. Two eyes have different signs. One is
      myopic and other is hypermetropic.
3. Astigmatism: Irregular astigmatism.
4. Keratoconus.

Therapeutic

1. Corneal disorders:
   a. Bullous keratitis.
   b. Filamentary keratitis.
   c. Recurrent corneal erosion.
   d. Non-healing corneal ulcer.
   e. Postkeratoplasty and post-LASIK
      complications.
2. Lid deformity:
   a. Recurrent trichiasis and entropion.
   b. Moderate coloboma of the upper lid
      over the cornea.
   c. Moderate exposure keratitis.
3. Some conjunctival conditions. To prevent symblepharon.
4. Drug delivery: Constant delivery of drugs
   especially in glaucoma.

Cosmetic

- Ugly corneal scar (painted contact lenses)
- Small eyes (phthisis and microphthalmos)
- Others:
  - Aniridia
  - Large coloboma of iris
  - Albinism.

Occupational

- Public speaker
- Actors
- Sportsman.

Contraindications for Contact Lens

Lack of Motivation

1. Low errors of refraction.
2. Simple presbyopia in absence of other errors (they require special lenses).
3. Large angle squint (will not improve vision).
4. Addition of prism more than three in
   spectacle.

Ocular

- Dry eye
- Poor blinking
- Allergy to:
  - Contact lens material
  - Contact lens solution
- Chronic conjunctivitis:
  - Allergy
  - Infective
- Recurrent stye, chalazia and blepharitis
- Limbal growth
- Progressive pterygium
- Corneal anesthesia.

Systemic Causes

- Uncontrolled diabetes
- Thyrotoxicosis
- Tremors
- Rheumatoid arthritis
- Mental instability.

Advantages and Disadvantages

Advantages of Contact Lenses Over Spectacle

1. Cosmetic.
2. Ocular:
   a. High errors of refraction require thick
      glasses, giving a non-acceptable ap-
      pearance, which is eliminated by
      contact lens.
   b. Large field: The lens moves with the
      gaze.

c. Almost no prismatic aberration.

d. No spherical aberration.

e. No chromatic aberration.

f. No fogging due to sudden change in temperature.

Disadvantages of Contact Lens Over Spectacle

1. Cost.

2. Long adaptation period.

3. Intolerance:

    a. Hard lenses are less tolerated, but of correct astigmatism and lasts longer.

    b. Soft lenses are better tolerated, but have poor visual correction, especially moderate to high astigmatism and have short lifespan.

4. Maintenance and upkeep: The contact lenses require regular cleaning, disinfection and storage.

5. Accommodation:

    a. Myopic correction requires more accommodation.

    b. A pre-presbyope has to keep book away to read clearly with contact lens correction.

6. Bilateral aphakes may not be able to insert and remove contact lenses without help.

7. There is always a chance of infective keratitis with contact lens.

Advantages of Soft Contact Lenses

1. Better adaptation.

2. More comfortable.

3. Long period of wearing time.

4. Almost no risk of extrusion.

5. Less corneal edema.

6. Good for sportsman.

Disadvantages of Soft Lenses

1. Costly.

2. Short lifespan.

3. Difficult to maintain.

4. Meticulous disinfection required.

5. Chances of deposits are more over long periods.

6. Relatively poor visual outcome.

7. Astigmatism not well corrected.

8. Corrects spherical part only.

9. Possibility of peripheral corneal vascularization.

10. More papillary hypertrophy.

Advantages of Disposable Lenses

1. Easy to fit.

2. Good for children.

3. Complications due to long wear time are less.

4. No deposits.

5. No infection.

6. No allergy.

7. Less chances of papillary hypertrophy.

8. Easy to get spare lenses.

Complications of Contact Lenses in General

Complications can arise due to many factors, which are listed below:

1. Due to ill-fitting:

    a. Non-improvement of vision.

    b. Intractable watering.

    c. Vascularization of peripheral cornea.

    d. Injury to cornea.

    e. Vaulting.

    f. Decentering.

    g. Discoloration.

    h. Extrusion.

    i. Foreign body trapped under the lens.

2. Errors of power calculation:

    a. Overcorrection.

    b. Undercorrection.

    c. Spectacle blur.

    d. Creeping myopia.

3. Non correction of astigmatism.
4. Changes related to accommodation.
5. Corneal changes:
    a. Corneal hypoxia.
    b. Corneal vascularization.
    c. Recurrent erosion.
    d. Superficial punctuate keratitis.
    e. Reduced corneal sensation.
    f. Microcystic epitheliopathy.
6. Allergic reaction:
    a. Giant papillary hypertrophy of conjunctiva.
    b. Superior limbic keratopathy.
    c. Keratoconjunctivitis.
7. Toxic reaction to contact lens solution.
8. Immobile lens syndrome.
9. Keratitis: Less frequent, but most severe of all complications. They can be microbial or still less commonly sterile. The two organisms that are dreaded most are *Pseudomonas* and *Acanthamoeba*. Both keratitis due to any of them is of ophthalmic emergency.

First thing to do on mere suspicion of infection should be to remove the lens and start instillating 'preservative-free broad-spectrum antibiotic' on hourly basis and consult ophthalmologist as soon as possible.

10

Low Vision Aids

The problem of low vision is a public health concern that puts a great strain on national exchequer. It is an important cause of loss of man-days, especially when it is present in children and people in their prime. Besides economic aspect, low vision is a major cause of personal inconvenience and social embarrassment.

Low vision is found world over in all races, in both sexes, spread over all age groups. In underdeveloped countries, it goes mostly unattended. Its incidence is showing an upward swing due to increase in population, increased unpreventable prevalence of congenital anomalies in children. More children with gross congenital anomalies of the eyes are living longer to face the difficulties. Overall increased longevity has compounded the problem many folds in old age. The causes of low vision in old age are mostly untreatable ocular and central nervous system (CNS) pathologies.

CLASSIFICATION OF LOW VISION

Like definition of blindness, which used to differ from country-to-country before, World Health Organization (WHO) gave a comprehensive definition for blindness, which consists of:

1. Total absence of light.
2. Visual acuity not exceeding 6/60 in better eye with best correcting glasses.
3. Limitation of field of vision, subtending an angle of less than 20°.

The classification for visual impairment, as per International Classification of Diseases by WHO, 1977 is given in Table 10.1.

The low vision too has been defined variously in different countries.

The latest classification of visual impairment is shown in Figure 10.1. It has separated low vision from blindness. The two require different strategies to manage. The flowchart shows that low vision has been divided into two broad categories of moderate and severe loss, which again require different strategies to manage.

Management of low vision has not received the status in management that has

Table 10.1: Classification of low vision as per WHO, 1977

Type of impairment	Category of visual impairment	Visual acuity (best corrected)
Low vision	1	6/18 to 6/60
Low vision	2	Less than 6/60 to 3/60
Blindness	3	Less than 3/60 to 1/60 or count fingers (CF 3 m–CF 1 m) or Field of vision between 5° and 10°
Blindness	4	Less than CF 1 m to light perception or Field of vision less than 5°
Blindness	5	No light perception

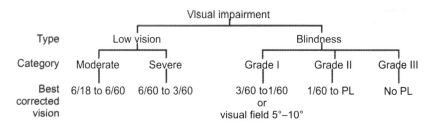

Figure 10.1: Classification of visual impairment (PL, perception of light)

been given to blindness. The funds allotted to treatable blindness far exceeds than allotted to low vision.

For all practical purposes, low vision is that residual vision, which persists to prevent a person to carry out routine work in his/her usual place of work, i.e. house or travel unaided.

According to, Government of India, Persons with Disabilities Act 1995, 'person with low vision' means a person with impairment of visual function, even after treatment or standard refractive correction, but is potentially capable of using vision for the planning and execution of a task with appropriate assistive device.

The other terms used in visual impairment are:

1. Totally blind: Individuals with no light perception are legally and functionally blind.
2. Functionally blind: Individuals with light perception, but no useful vision even with vision enhancement techniques are legally blind.
3. Partially sighted: Low vision.

Persons with best corrected visual acuity, less than 6/18, but better than 6/60 or a field restricted to 20° all around is not considered to be legally blind.

Characteristics

Low vision is:

a. Not blindness.
b. It has some salvageable vision.

c. Salvaged vision does not exceed 6/18 in better eye.
d. It is a bilateral condition.
e. It can only be central loss of vision, i.e. macular lesion.
f. It can be peripheral loss of vision, i.e. peripheral retinal lesions.
g. Peripheral loss can be:
   i. All around as in retinitis pigmentosa (RP), advanced glaucoma.
   ii. Partial:
      • Bitemporal hemianopia
      • Binasal hemianopia
      • Bilateral altitudinal field loss.
h. It may start in childhood and continue in adulthood, may be stationary or progressive.
i. The causes can be in the eyes or CNS, or both.
j. All persons with low vision will not benefit with low vision aids.
k. Vision may improve with low vision aids, but the patient may not accept the low vision aid due to:
   i. Lack of motivation.
   ii. Long adaptation time.
   iii. Cumbersome posture to use the low vision aid.
   iv. The person is sufficiently accustomed to his/her immediate surroundings without low vision aids.
   v. Good family support.
   vi. High cost.

CAUSES OF LOW VISION

Causes of low vision vary in different age groups. It may start in childhood and remain stationary or spread over adulthood and old age. Some low visions are exclusively seen in the elderly; the most important out of them is age-related macular degeneration.

Broadly, the causes of low vision have been divided into three age groups:

1. Below 15 years.
2. Between 15 and 50 years.
3. Beyond 50 years.

Causes in Children

1. Congenital anomalies in the eye.
2. Retinopathy of prematurity.
3. Albinism.
4. Nystagmus.
5. Heredo-familial optic neuropathy.
6. Optic atrophy of childhood.
7. Buphthalmos.
8. Bilateral toxoplasmosis.
9. Unattented bilateral dense cataract.
10. Untreated or partially treated trauma.
11. Bilateral extensive keratomalacia.

Causes in Adolescence and Presenile Persons

All the causes in children will spread to this group also. To this, are added:

1. Retinitis pigmentosa.
2. Sympathetic ophthalmia.
3. Macular dystrophies.
4. Unattended bilateral retinal detachment.

In old age, the most important cause is age-related macular degeneration; the others are diabetic retinopathy and advanced glaucoma (that has remained either untreated or partially treated or repeated surgeries have failed) bilateral central vein thrombosis, bilateral anterior ischemic optic neuropathy, primary and secondary optic atrophy, and choroidal dystrophies.

MANAGEMENT OF PATIENTS WITH LOW VISION

1. Management of patients with low vision is a complex procedure that requires patience and perseverance on the part of patient, patient's family members and optometrists.
2. Low vision aids should only be prescribed when all therapeutic, surgical and optical methods have failed.
3. Management requires proper selection of patients and proper selection of low vision aids, which in turn needs proper understanding of the optics of low vision aids, their mechanism of work, method of handling and utility to particular person.
4. The prescription of low vision aid is a very personalized matter.
5. All patients with low vision will not improve with low vision aids as expected.
6. Patients who benefit most with low vision aids are pathological myopia, aphakia, primary optic atrophy, chorioretinal degenerations and age-related macular degenerations.
7. Patients who benefit less are: diabetic retinopathy, hypertensive retinopathy, retinal detachment, retinitis pigmentosa and glaucoma.
8. Persons who have low vision for a long time do not respond, so well as compared to low vision of short duration.
9. Children do not accept low vision aids, so well as compared to adults.
10. Absence of immediate visual gain is a hurdle in acceptance of low vision aids. A single low vision aid will not be useful in improving central and peripheral loss of vision at the same time.

11. An aid that improves central vision, both for distance and near will not be of much help in improving peripheral vision.

12. Loss of central vision improves better by low vision aids than peripheral vision.

13. History plays an important role in selection and anticipating possible acceptance by the patient.

HISTORY TAKING IN LOW VISION

As the existence of low vision is of gradual onset and of long duration, the person may not be very precise with the history.

The history should consist of:

1. The age by which the patient became aware of his/her low vision.

2. Does have any knowledge of the pathology that is responsible of low vision and the investigations done to clinch the diagnosis?

3. Is condition stable or still deteriorating?

4. Has he/she used any optical or non-optical device for low vision in the past or is using any at present?

5. Is he/she satisfied with the device? If not, What is the explanation for poor satisfaction?

6. Level of his/her literacy.

7. Does he/she require better distant or near vision or both?

8. Is vision better in bright light or dim light?

9. Higher illumination is needed for central fundus lesions.

10. Elders require twice as much of illumination as person half his/her age. A person of 60 years will require illumination that is twice the illumination required by a person of 30 years for similar lesion under same condition.

11. Does he/she require higher magnification than the present one he/she is using?

12. Lower magnification suffices in opacities of media.

13. Can he/she move about with ease in known surroundings?

14. Is he/she required to travel alone?

15. Medical history.

CLASSIFICATION OF LOW VISION AIDS

The broad classification of low vision aids is shown in Figure 10.2.

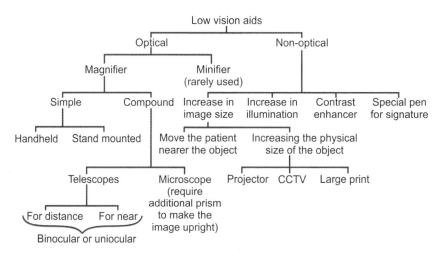

Figure 10.2: Classification of low vision aids

PRINCIPLE/OPTICS

Principle Involved in Functioning of Optical Low Vision Aids

1. The central retina (macula) has best resolving power.
2. In low vision, the resolving power in the macular area is reduced.
3. The paramacular area has relatively low resolving power.
4. The low resolving power of the paramacular area is sufficient to salvage and enhance paracentral vision.
5. The purpose of low vision aids is to utilize paramacular region.
6. This is brought about by giving a magnified image that will not only cover the non-seeing macula, but spill over paramacular area, enhancing vision sufficiently. The patient will be able to do his/her daily routine unaided, will be able to read large prints and watch TV.
7. The reading ability can be enhanced by increasing the illumination on the reading material. This is more effective in elderly persons, who even with normal eye require more illumination for reading than persons half their age.
8. The distant vision can be enhanced by moving nearer the object (TV). This is called approach magnification. A reduction in distance from 3 to 1 m enhances the size by 3 times.
9. The disadvantage of the low vision aids that enlarge the central image are:
   a. They have short working distance.
   b. Reduced peripheral vision.
   c. The above two when put together, reduce peripheral field. Thus, magnifiers have no role in constricted field.
10. Minifiers like reverse Galilean telescopes theoretically increase peripheral field, but minify central image, hence they have very limited use in low vision.

Optics of Low Vision Aids

The aim of prescribing low vision aids lies in the ability of the low vision aid to explore the residual vision and convert it into best advantage position of subjective improvement.

This can be achieved by:

1. Relative distant magnification.
2. Angular (apparent magnification).

The principles involved in enlarging the image are:

1. By moving the image nearer.
2. By moving the person nearer the object.
3. Enlarging the image.

The mechanism involved in moving it nearer the patient is explained by the following example.

An object, 2 cm high, kept at 50 cm from the eye will produce a retinal image of 0.06 cm. Now the same object is moved to a distance that is only 5 cm from the eye. This forms an image of 0.6 cm high that is 10 times larger than the image when the object was at 50 cm. This works well only in persons who have good amplitude of accommodation. This is angular magnification. Here, image formed by the object when shifted nearer the eye is larger than it was when situated at a distance. Angular magnification is the principle involved in all optical low vision aids (Fig. 10.3).

$$\text{Angular magnification (M)} = \alpha'/\alpha$$

where,

α = angle ANB

α' = angle CND

M is directly proportional to vergence from 5 to 50 cm, i.e. 1st and 2nd positions in relation to the eye. This is inversely proportionate to distance 5–50 cm. But, this is not possible always and the second difficulty that arises is that, the object cannot be kept so near the eye for a long time. It is assumed that an object at arbitrary distance of 25 cm is the most comfortable distance of seeing a magnified image.

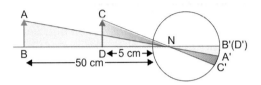

Figure 10.3: Angular magnification. Here, the image formed by the shifted object at 5 cm (CD), forms a retinal image (C'D'), which is larger than the retinal image (A'B') formed by AB, which is 50 cm from the eye; $\angle$ A'NB' = $\angle$ ANB = α; $\angle$ C'NB' = $\angle$ CND = α'.

It is also presumed that any object kept at this distance subtends a unit of magnification. This presumption is used in calculation of magnifications in optical magnifiers.

To overcome this difficulty of approach magnification, i.e. moving the object nearer the eye, magnifiers are introduced between the eye and the object to get the same effect of angular magnification. Let's consider that a convex lens of power L is kept at a distance of D from the eye, the magnification will be M that is equal to $1 + D/L$.

Now let us consider a simple form of magnification, which is produced by a single convex lens that may be a handheld magnifier or its table model (Fig. 10.4).

Let us consider an object AB that needs to be magnified is kept in front of the eye and subtends an angle α on the retina. To obtain magnification, a strong convex lens is introduced between the object AB and the eye (E). If the power of the convex lens is +10D, its focal length will be 10 cm. The +10D lens is kept in such a position that object AB falls within the focal length of the lens. From the previous Chapters we know that an object kept within the focus of the convex lens forms an erect, virtual and magnified image A'B' on the side of the object, but away from the lens.

The +10D lens itself is kept at O, at 15 cm away and in front of E. Thus, the anterior focal point of the lens (L) automatically becomes $15 + 10 = 25$ cm = 250 mm.

Magnification (M) = $1 + (15/10) = 1 + 1.5$ = 2.5 or α'/α.

Factor 1 in the above equation is arbitrary for distance 25 cm that results 1 unit of magnification.

Now let us consider another situation where the object is moved nearer the eye. The object at closer distance will increase the angular size of the image.

The object was at 25 cm in the first instance that was subtending an angle α on the retina. Now the object is moved nearer, i.e. at 10 cm. Now the object subtends an angle α'. Tangent α'/tangent α will be 25/10. So, M becomes 25/10, i.e. 2.5X.

In the third situation, an additional convex lens with magnification M' is introduced. The total magnification (m) will be M × M'. We have seen that M = 25/10 and M' is $1 + 15/10$. This makes m = 2.5 (1 + 1.5) = 2.5 × 2.5 = 6.25.

Some Terms Used in Optical Magnification

1. Relative distance magnification: This is magnification by a microscope.

2. Angular magnification: Produced by telescopes.

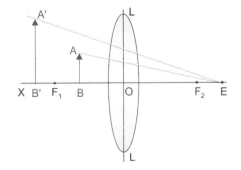

Figure 10.4: Angular magnification. LL is a +10D sphere, XE is its optical axis, O is the optical center, F_1 and F_2 are the focal points and $OF_1 = OF_2$ are the focal lengths, which are 10 cm. AB is the object and A'B' is the magnified, virtual and erect image of AB. OE is 15 cm and EF_1 is 25 cm.

3. Relative size magnification: This is obtained by enlarging the size of the object, i.e. large prints, distant vision charts projected on wall, large fonts in computers.
4. Transverse magnification: This is real image magnification required for very high level magnification without distortion, which is not possible by lens, which is available only electronically like CCTV.

MAGNIFIERS

Simple magnifiers are cheap, portable, easy to handle and maintain. However, sometimes a person may require more magnification than produced by a simple magnifier, which is provided by a compound magnifier like a telescope or a microscope. The telescope, as a low vision aid should be handy and light, that can be effective at various working distances with a comfortable field of vision. All requirements cannot be made available in a single magnifier. Higher magnification is handicapped with short working distances and reduced field. The telescopes used as low vision aids can be handheld—uniocular or binocular or spectacle mounted working distance. The short working distance may require additional illumination that can be inbuilt or supplied from side. The commonest type of telescope is a Galilean type of telescope that gives a magnified erect image in contrast to astronomical telescope that gives a magnified, but inverted image unless a prism has been added to make the image upright. This process of making the image upright by the prism is utilized in operating microscope and is not suitable as low vision aids.

The operating loupes are better alternatives that can act either as simple magnifier mounted in a headband or spectacle. The commonest example is a binomag that acts suitable for lower degree of low vision. The binomag gives a magnification of 1.5X. As they are binocular, they have stereopsis and larger field. Base in prisms can be incorporated in them to assist convergence.

Galilean Telescope

The low-powered Galilean telescopes mounted on a spectacle gives better magnification without astigmatic distortion and a flat-field. For near vision, additional plus lenses are incorporated in the frame.

The basic construction of Galilean telescope consists of (Fig. 10.5):

1. A minus eye piece (oculus).
2. A plus (objective).
3. They are centered on a common optical axis.
4. The power of the convex objective is the half the power of the concave oculus.
5. The focal length of the eye piece is shorter than the objective.
6. They are separated by the algebraic sum of their focal lengths.
7. The image formed is virtual, erect and magnified.
8. Magnification (M) = Diopter of the objective/diopter of the oculus.
9. The magnification offered by spectacle-mounted telescopes may be as low as 1.5X to as high as 6X.
10. By inserting plus addition for near work, the magnification is enhanced by the product of the magnification of the

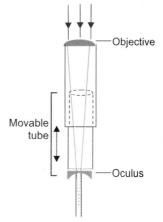

Figure 10.5: Outline of construction of Galilean telescope

reading power and magnification of the telescope.

11. The telescopes can be mounted either on upper part or center of the spectacle (Fig. 10.6), the angulation between the two telescopes can be changed, so can the interpupillary distance.

12. The magnification is inversely proportionate to working distance.

Various types of magnifiers used in low vision aids are shown in Figures 10.7 and 10.8.

NON-OPTICAL LOW VISION AIDS

Non-optical low vision aids are different for near and distant vision.

Non-optical Low Vision Aids for Near Vision

1. Enhancing illumination.
2. Focusing light on reading material.
3. Use large prints.
4. Correcting contrast (Fig. 10.9).

Non-optical Low Vision Aids for Distance Vision

1. Moving the person nearer the object.
2. Moving the object nearer the person.
3. Enlarging the letters, figures and pictures (refer Fig. 10.9).

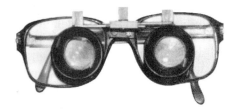

Figure 10.6: A typical spectacle-mounted Galilean telescope

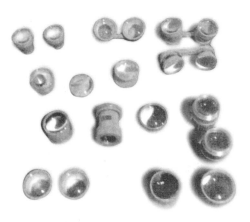

Figure 10.7: Binocular and uniocular magnifiers available in low vision trial set

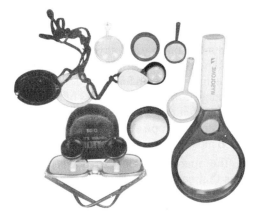

Figure 10.8: Various types of magnifiers used by patients as low vision aids

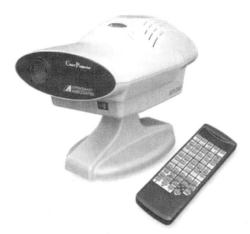

Figure 10.9: Auto chart projector with contrast sensitivity. The letters can be enlarged as per requirement [*Courtesy:* Appasamy Associates (with permission)].

RECORDING OF VISUAL ACUITY IN LOW VISION

Knowledge of vision in a person with low vision is of utmost importance in prescription of low vision aids. Both distant and near vision must be recorded separately in two eyes and both eyes together. This should be followed by recording of vision with best correction.

Examination of visual acuity in low vision differs from examination of usual vision. Not only this method differs but also the vision charts used in low vision are entirely different from usual Snellen's chart. A person with low vision may not be able to give clue regarding his/her visual status on ordinary Snellen's or its equivalent chart.

The usual protocol of recording visual acuity in low vision is:

1. Test distant vision on usual Snellen's chart.
2. Most of the persons with low vision may not be able to read the top letter except those who have peripheral vision.
3. A person may have some island of vision, which he/she tries to use by moving the head.
4. Move the patient towards the chart and note the vision.
5. Put a pinhole in the trial frame and note, if there is any improvement in the vision.
6. If the vision improves, it means that the patient may improve with optical devices.
7. Record best corrected vision and note down the power of the glasses.
8. Put the best correcting glass in the trial frame and put a single pinhole over the distant correction. Any improvement means that there is some residual vision that can be salvaged.
9. Sometimes multiple pinholes give better result than single pinhole (Fig. 10.10).
10. Sometimes, a patient may just have hand movement in straight gaze, but may be able to count fingers eccentrically.
11. Examine vision with special low vision charts.

The advantages of these special low vision charts are that they directly give:

1. Percentage of loss of vision.
2. Directly correlate loss of vision to extent of magnification that will benefit the person most.
3. The specially built charts are used at 1–3 m distance in a well-illuminated room.
4. The optical principle involved in construction of optotypes is the same as in standard Snellen's chart.

Commonly used Charts for Distance

1. Bailey-Lovie logMAR (Fig. 10.11).
2. Modified early treatment diabetic retinopathy study (ETDRS).
3. Bausch and Lomb.
4. Sloan.
5. Keeler (Fig. 10.12).
6. Staub.

Like all optotypes, distant and near features have difference in size. The commonly used charts for near (Fig. 10.13) are:

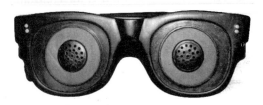

Figure 10.10: Multiple pinholes

1. Modified ETDRS charts.
2. Sloan's chart.
3. Keeler's modified charts.

Sloan's Chart

Sloan's chart is read at 40 cm. Like usual near vision chart, the patient is asked to identify the line with smallest letter. The usual Jaegers near chart do not have continuous story. The Sloan's chart has continuous matter in them.

Keeler's Chart

The Keeler's charts are marked A1–A20 to be read at 20 cm. It also gives magnification required for comfortable reading. There is a definite ratio between the optotypes. As the number increases, the percentage declines. For example, A2 = 80% of A1, A3 is 64% of A1 and A20 is only 1.4% of A1.

The charts are marked M1–M20. M1 is usual news print. It directly gives magnification, required to read. M10 means that the patient requires 10X more magnification than required to read M1.

Points to be Remembered in Prescribing Near Vision Aids

1. A well-motivated patient is the best patient.
2. A well-motivated patient tolerates a low vision aid better.
3. Low vision aids are very personalized.
4. A particular aid that is well accepted by a particular person may be rejected by the next.
5. Low vision aids should give best vision without hampering mobility of the patient.
6. Increased magnification has following disadvantages:

60 m/200 ft	F N P R Z	1.0
48 m/160 ft	E Z H P V	0.9
36 m/125 ft	D P N F R	0.8
30 m/100 ft	R D F U V	0.7
24 m/80 ft	U R Z V H	0.6
18 m/65 ft	H N D R U	0.5
15 m/50 ft	Z V U D N	0.4
12 m/40 ft	V P H D E	0.3
9 m/30 ft	P V E R H	0.2
6 m/20 ft	N U Z F E	0.0

Figure 10.11: Bailey-Lovie logMAR distant vision chart

a. Decreases working distance.

b. Reduces peripheral field.

c. Causes more optical distortion.

d. Requires more illumination.

7. The aid selected should be easy to use, simple in structure, easy to repair, easy to replace and light in weight.

8. The low vision aids, especially the telescopes are costly than ordinary spectacles, hence may not be suitable to persons with low economic status.

9. The best baseline is to give trial to spectacle mounted simple magnifier for both near and distance.

10. If the patient accepts such a simple device than only one should switch over to more sophisticated models.

11. Both eyes should be tested separately, not only for distance and near but also for magnification required separately by each eye. If the difference is small, both eyes are corrected with two separate magnifications.

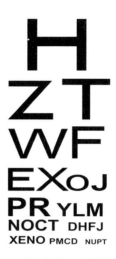

Figure 10.12: Keeler's modified chart for distance vision

12. If the difference is more, the magnification in the better eye is given to both the eyes.

13. Older patients, due to stiff body, cannot keep the reading material at close quarter for long duration. They are better given non-optical magnifiers.

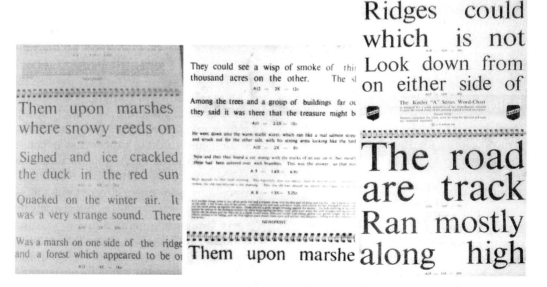

Figure 10.13: Various types of vision charts used in recording low vision

11 Refractive Surgeries

Refractive surgeries include a group of procedures that may be surgical or laser assisted, on cornea or lens. The refractive procedures do away with the need of spectacle and contact lenses. The surgeries on cornea are done far more frequently than on the lens. The principle involved in corneal refractive surgeries is to mold the corneal curvature to change its refractive power in contrast to contact lens, which eliminates cornea from the refractive media. Removal of lens reduces the converging power of the refractive media. It has been discussed earlier that cornea is the most important refractive surface and medium that imparts maximum refractive power to the eye. The maximum refractivity takes place at the air-cornea interface. The power of the cornea also depends on the curvature of the cornea. Increased curvature makes the eye more myopic and decreased curvature makes the eye more hypermetropic. Irregular curvature causes astigmatism.

PRINCIPLE

The principle involved in refractive surgeries of myopia is to make the central cornea flatter and periphery steeper. In hypermetropia, the reverse is the rule. While in astigmatism, flattening the more curved surface is the aim.

The refractive surgeries are elective surgeries; hence, the decision to undergo the surgery on the part of the patient and to do the procedure on the part of the surgeon should not be rushed through. Counseling of the patient regarding pros and cons of the surgery should be the first prerequisite. It should be emphasized that the procedure is almost permanent and the eye cannot be brought back to pre-procedural state, though some modifications are possible. It should also be emphasized that the patient may require some additional optical correction by way of spectacle or contact lens in spite of a successful surgery. Generally, presbyopia is not tackled by these procedures that correct refractive errors only. Hence, the patient in presbyopic age requires presbyopic addition, unless a specialized surgery for presbyopia too has been undertaken (refer refractive surgeries for presbyopia).

The surgery is done on anatomically and physiologically normal cornea. They only help to get rid of spectacle and contact lenses. The procedures are effective only on refractive medium (cornea and lens) without having any effect on already existing changes or that are likely to develop in future on the posterior segment. The surgeries do not modulate accommodation.

All eyes with error of refraction will not need refractive surgeries. Very high errors of refraction and low errors of refraction are not subjected to these procedures because very high errors of refraction do not benefit by the procedures and low errors can be corrected by safer spectacle or contact lens. Some of the eyes that may benefit visually by surgery cannot be operated due to existing contraindications. Even eyes, that require surgeries without contraindications may not benefit from procedures due to presence of changes in posterior segment. They will also not improve in case of amblyopia. In some cases, reoperation may be required to correct overcorrection or undercorrection.

CLASSIFICATION OF REFRACTIVE SURGERIES

Procedures to Correct Errors of Refraction

The procedures done to correct errors of refraction can be (Fig. 11.1):

1. Non-laser procedures (surgical):
    a. On cornea.
    b. On the lens.
2. Laser procedures.

Non-laser Procedures

Non-laser procedures available are:

1. Radial keratotomy for myopia.
2. Hexagonal keratotomy for hypermetropia.
3. Transverse/Arcuate keratotomy for astigmatism.

4. Intracorneal ring.
5. Keratomileuses.
6. Anterior ciliary sclerotomy for presbyopia.
7. Clear lens extraction.
8. Clear lens extraction:
    a. With intraocular lens (IOL).
    b. Without IOL.

Laser Procedures

Laser procedures available are:

1. Photorefractive keratotomy.
2. Laser-assisted in situ keratomileusis (LASIK).
3. Laser-assisted subepithelial keratectomy (LASEK).
4. Epipolis laser in situ keratomileusis (epi-LASIK).
5. Laser thermal keratoplasty.
6. Other newer methods:
    a. Femtosecond laser.
    b. Customized ablation.

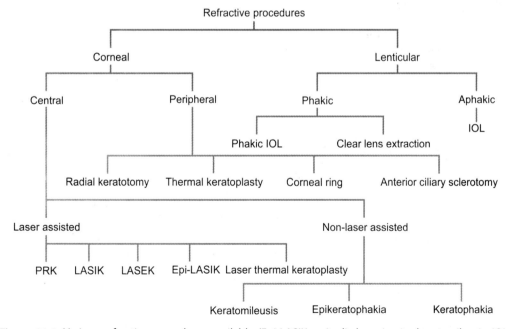

Figure 11.1: Various refractive procedures available (Epi-LASIK, epipolis laser in situ keratomileusis; IOL, intraocular lens; LASEK, laser-assisted subepithelial keratectomy; LASIK, laser-assisted in situ keratomileusis; PRK, photorefractive keratotomy).

Procedures Based on Errors of Refraction

Refractive procedures can also be grouped as per errors of refraction (Table 11.1).

SELECTION OF CASES FOR REFRACTIVE PROCEDURES

Unlike emergency procedures where there is limited scope to select cases, refractive surgeries being elective in nature have ample scope to select cases to give best result with utmost patient satisfaction. While selecting eyes for refractive procedure, the following points should be kept in mind.

Counseling

Many of the patients presume that refractive procedures are the last word in restoring vision in all subnormal visual statuses. Some persons with small errors of refraction may demand surgery without knowing the pros and cons of the procedure. Yet, a group of patient may not be able to differentiate between laser procedures on posterior segment, done mostly for vascular retinopathies and laser procedures done on the anterior segment for the errors of refraction. The best way to overcome such misconception is to counsel the patients and their guardians.

Motivation

A well-motivated patient is more satisfied patient. His/Her expectations are not in excess. The better motivated patients are stage and cine artists, and public speakers who want to improve their appearance and have contact lens intolerance.

Age of the Patient

The age of the patient is most important factor. It ranges between 20 and 45 years. The errors of refraction under 20 years have higher chances of being unstable and persons over 45 years have following drawbacks:

1. They are more likely to be overcorrected.
2. This is the age where presbyopia sets in that may be enhanced by refractive procedures. It should be explained to the patient that the procedure is being done to overcome errors of refraction, i.e. myopia, hypermetropia and astigmatism. Presbyopia requires another set of procedures or near correction by spectacle.
3. By 45 years, many of the patients will develop lenticular changes that will again unstabilize the power and the patient may blame the refractive procedure.

Table 11.1: Refractive procedures grouped according to errors of refraction

Error of refraction	Refractive procedures
Myopia	Radial keratotomy, photorefractive keratotomy (PRK), laser in situ keratomileusis (LASIK), laser subepithelialkeratomileusis (LASEK), custom laser in situ keratomileusis (CLASIK), clear lens extraction, phakic intraocular lens (IOL), clear lens extraction followed by IOL
Hypermetropia	Hexagonal keratotomy, laser thermal keratoplasty, hypermetropic PRK, hypermetropic LASIK, LASEK, epi-LASIK, conductive keratoplasty, wavefront guided LASIK, phakic intraocular lens, clear lens extraction with IOL
Astigmatism	Astigmatic keratotomy, limbal relaxation incision, PRK, LASIK
Presbyopia	Anterior ciliary sclerotomy, laser thermal keratoplasty, corneal inlay

Stabilization of Refraction

The procedures should be done only on eyes that have unchanged errors of refraction, at least 1 year prior to surgery. The causes of unstable refraction are:

1. Patients under 20 years.
2. Onset of keratoconus.
3. Untreated diabetes.

Contact Lens Users

It is recommended that the patient using contact lenses for error of refraction discards contact lenses prior to surgery. In case of soft corneal contact lens, the period should be 3 weeks and for rigid gas permeable lenses, 7 weeks. The disposable contact lenses are not used for 1 week prior to surgery.

Range of Error of Refraction

Moderate errors of refraction give better results with minimal complications. The range of errors of refraction that benefit from refractive procedures ranges between +6D sphere (Dsp) and −12Dsp. There are different procedures for different range of errors of refraction. Photo refractive keratotomy is suitable between +3Dsp and −6Dsp, while laser gives good results in a larger range of +4Dsp and −12Dsp.

Informed Consent

The informed consent is taken after proper and detailed counseling of the patient and his/her attendants/guardians. This minimizes the risk of unnecessary litigation later.

Indications

There are no absolute indications, but there are plenty of absolute and relative contraindications for refractive procedures.

Contraindications

Absolute Contraindications

Absolute contraindications are:

1. Uninformed patient.
2. Unwilling patient.
3. Infectious conditions of the eye and adnexa that are contraindicated for any intraocular surgery.
4. Keratoconus.
5. Keratectasia.
6. Systemic and local immune suppression: Prolonged use of steroids and immunosuppressive drugs.
7. Glaucoma.
8. Posterior segment anomalies that are bound to give poor visual result.
9. Amblyopia.
10. Amblyopic patient may be operated for cosmetic reasons and not for visual improvement.
11. Contact lens warpage.
12. Untreated corneal dystrophies.

Relative Contraindications

Relative contraindications are:

1. Dry eyes.
2. Allergic keratoconjunctivitis.
3. Diabetes mellitus.
4. Pregnancy.

SELECTION OF EYES FOR REFRACTIVE PROCEDURES

Selection of eyes is common for all types of refractive procedures, may be surgical or laser:

1. Vision:
   a. Without glasses.
   b. With pinhole.
   c. Best corrected.

All the visions are noted for distance and near in each eye, and recorded separately.

2. Cycloplegic refraction:
   a. This helps to avoid over- or under-correction, especially in younger children with active accommodation.
   b. Autorefractometry readings are not reliable.
3. Slit lamp examination:
   a. To find out subtle signs of present or past inflammation.
   b. Faint corneal opacity in the optical zone.
   c. Imperceptible deep vascularization.
4. Corneal sensation.
5. Schirmer's test.
6. Keratometry for:
   a. Subtle keratoconus.
   b. Degree of astigmatism and axis of astigmatism.
7. Videokeratography.
8. Ultrasonic pachymetry: The thin corneas are at more risk of perforation.
9. Pupillary size in bright and dim light with patient fixing a distant object, because mesopic pupil has to be smaller than optical zone.

INSTRUMENTS REQUIRED FOR REFRACTIVE PROCEDURES

1. Operating microscope: Coaxial with zoom. All procedures are done under operating microscope.
2. Instruments: The instruments are divided into two groups:
   a. For incisional procedure.
   b. For laser procedure.

Instruments for Incisional Procedure

Instruments used for incisional procedure are as follows:

1. Knife:
   a. Blade: Diamond, sapphire, ruby and high grade stainless steel. There are various types of cutting edges of the knife, i.e. oblique, vertical and mixed.
   b. Foot plate: Straight and angled.
   c. Handle.
   d. Micrometer.
2. Markers (Fig. 11.2).
3. Fixation forceps.

Instruments for Laser Procedures

The two important instrument in laser procedure are:

1. An excimer laser (for construction and optics of laser).
2. A microkeratome.

An excimer laser uses a combination of inert gases and a reactive gas under special condition of stimulation by electricity to create a dimer. The dimer exists in energized state giving rise to laser in ultraviolet range. The inert gases react with halogens—chlorine and fluorine.

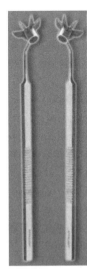

Figure 11.2: Corneal markers for radial keratotomy [*Courtesy:* Appasamy Associates (with permission)]

Various types of excimers and their respective wavelengths are depicted in the Table 11.2.

Table 11.2: Various types of excimers with their wavelengths

Excimer molecule	Chemical composition	Wavelength
ArF	Argon fluoride	193 nm
KrF	Krypton fluoride	248 nm
XeCl	Xenon chloride	305 nm
XeF	Xenon fluoride	351 nm

To summarize what has been discussed earlier, the laser is acronym for light amplification by stimulated emission of radiation. There are various types of lasers, i.e. solid, fluid and gas. The laser pulses may be delivered as short pulses or continuous pulse. The lasers have various uses from industry to medicine. Use of a particular laser in a selected condition depends from its wavelength and capabilities to produce power.

Commonly used materials in laser of medical use are argon, xenon, krypton, carbon dioxide, copper vapor, helium and neodymium-doped yttrium aluminum garnet (Nd:YAG).

Commonly used lasers in ophthalmology are excimer, argon, Nd:YAG and CO_2. The laser emits intense heat and power at a short distance. The laser instrument converts different frequencies of light in unified coherent collimated monochromatic beam. The commonly used laser in refractive procedure is excimer or exciplex (Fig. 11.3). The former is short version of excited dimer and the latter is short form of excited complex.

Dimer: A dimer is a molecule or molecular complex, which is a combination of two identical molecules that form a simple compound in the form of pseudo molecule.

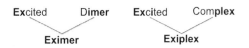

Figure 11.3: Commonly used laser in refractive procedure

The noble gases used in excimer laser are inert and do not form chemical compounds naturally, but when excited electrically or by high energy electron beam form a short lived compounds with halogens, i.e. fluorine and chlorine and form a new molecule. The molecule has two ground states, i.e. a bound (associated) and repulsive (disassociated). The excited compound undergoes stimulated emission giving a strong repulsive state, which in picoseconds disassociates into two unbound atoms releasing ultraviolet lights in wavelengths of 193 nm lasting for 10–15 nanoseconds with frequency between 10 and 50 Hz and energy up to 450 mJ.

The light from excimer laser is absorbed by organic matter. Excimer laser does neither burn nor cut the tissue. It only breaks the molecular bonds of the superficial tissue ablating the tissue in a very thin layer without involving the surrounding tissues. Lasers with longer wavelengths than 193 nm damage deeper tissues like Descemet's membrane and endothelium. In ophthalmology, the shorter wavelength of excimer laser, i.e. 193 nm is used for photorefractive keratotomy, LASIK and LASEK.

REFRACTIVE PROCEDURES FOR MYOPIA

Myopic eyes are the most frequently subjected eyes to refractive procedures that started more than a century ago when peripheral cornea was cauterized with heat. The procedure never became popular and passed into oblivion. This happened due to ever increasing popularity of contact lenses, which involved non-invasive protocol. It was in 4th decade of last century that interest was regenerated in the form of keratotomy by Sato (1940). In the present-day surgical procedures, only the anterior corneal surface is involved with incision not more than 16 in number. Sato's procedure required 80 incisions, equally divided in both the surfaces. Damage to endothelium in this process led to frequent development of corneal decompensation. This led to giving up the procedure. The next wave of procedures was developed between 1970 and 1980 in the form of anterior radial keratotomy. They remained popular till laser procedures pushed them to the backseat.

LASER PROCEDURES

Presently, the laser procedures are the most practiced method to deal with not only myopia but also other errors of refraction. The two commonly used procedures for myopia are:

1. Photorefractive keratotomy (PRK).
2. Laser in situ keratomileusis (LASIK).

The other less frequently used laser procedures are LASEK, epi-LASIK, femtosecond laser and customized ablation.

Photorefractive Keratotomy

Photorefractive keratotomy one of the earliest laser-assisted refractive surgeries. It has superseded radial keratotomy (RK) which was in vogue before laser became available for ophthalmic use. The PRK itself has since then been virtually replaced by LASIK. The procedure can be used in all errors of refraction, but best results are obtained in moderate myopia between –2D and –6D. In the process, the tissue is not cut, incised or burnt; it is only ablated. The ablation is limited to the superficial layer of the stroma. It requires de-epithalization of cornea. Following de-epithalization, the laser is set at 50 microns. The whole of the cornea is not ablated. Only a central zone of 6 mm in myopia is ablated. The ablated zone is always kept 0.5–1 mm shorter than de-epithalized

area. The surgery is done under topical anesthesia with microscope and excimer laser (Figs 11.4A and B).

Steps

The steps of procedure are:

1. De-epithalization.
2. Centration of ablation zone.
3. Ablation proper.
4. Immediate postlaser management.
5. Late laser management.

De-epithalization

De-epithalization can be achieved by any of the following, i.e. mechanical, chemical or laser.

Mechanical de-epithalization is achieved by scrapping the epithelium by a blunt spatula or back of a cataract knife. This leaves the surface irregular. The same result is also achieved by using a specially designed automated nylon brush.

Chemical de-epithalization is achieved by 20% isopropyl alcohol left over the epithelium for 30 seconds and washed with balance salt solution quickly.

Laser de-epithalization is achieved as follows:

1. The excimer laser is targeted up to 40 microns and activated. The remaining epithelium is scrapped mechanically.
2. Here, excimer is set at definite depth and activated till the end of autofluorescence.

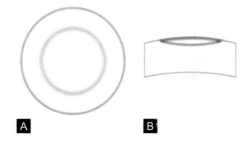

Figures 11.4A and B: Diagrammatic representation for photorefractive keratotomy for myopia. **A.** Front view; **B.** Lateral view.

Centration of ablation zone

While centering the ablation zone, the other eye is patched. The aim is to bring the fixation light in the microscope, surgeons and patient's line of vision in the same line. This is achieved by self-fixation and eye tracking device.

Ablation proper

1. The stromal ablation is done by excimer laser.
2. The excimer is programmed to ablate.
3. The ablation depends on:
   a. Type of error of refraction.
   b. Extent of error of refraction.
4. While doing ablation, the stroma is kept at normal hydrated state.
5. The time lapse between de-epithalization and ablation should be short.

Immediate postlaser management

1. The eye is patched after instilling broad-spectrum antibiotic, cycloplegic and non-steroidal anti-inflammatory drops.
2. The patch is replaced by a soft contact lens next day, which is used for 4–5 days.
3. Some surgeons start using soft contact lenses immediately after ablation.
4. The patient is advised to use a broad-spectrum antibiotic, a non-steroidal anti-inflammatory drop and lubricant 5–6 times a day for next few weeks.
5. If required, weak steroids like fluorometholone are added to the above.
6. No anesthetic drugs are recommended to combat pain.
7. In case of high error of refraction, mitomycin C 0.02% is applied for 90 seconds just after ablation.
8. Mitomycin has been used to minimize haze, but this has not received wide acceptance. It takes a few weeks to clean the postablation haze.
9. Pain is very common after ablation. For this, systemic analgesics may be required.

Late laser management

As it takes few weeks for the haze to clear, steroids, NSAID are used in weak solutions. The patient is examined every week. It takes few weeks for the vision to be stabilized. This makes the patient apprehensive. Reassurance and preoperative counseling minimizes apprehensions.

Complications

The surgery is safe and almost devoid of complications. Yet some complications do creep up. They may be intraoperative or postoperative.

The commonest complication during the procedure is decentering of ablation area that may lead to poor vision, diplopia, glare, halos and astigmatism. Other complications that become obvious are corneal haze, glare at night, halos, keratoconjunctivitissicca, epithelial erosion and diminished corneal sensation. Corneal haze is almost universal and more in high myopia. The other contributing factors are missed ocular surface disorder, pre-existing corneal opacity and presence of autoimmune disease. Corneal haze is maximum between 1 and 3 months, and disappears completely after that. Glares and halos are more common in ablation zone. This makes night driving uncomfortable. The complications that reduce postoperative best corrective vision are:

1. Regression.
2. Undercorrection.
3. Overcorrection.
4. Astigmatism.
5. Refractive instability.
6. Decentration of ablation zone.

The first four may require optical correction either by spectacle or contact lens, or may be required to be reoperated. Reopera-tion is advocated in marked undercorrection, but not before 6 weeks and steroids have been tapered off at least 3 months prior.

Laser In Situ Keratomileusis

At present, LASIK is most popular refractive procedure, which has left RK and PRK far back. This is more efficient than the above two. It uses high energy ultraviolet (193 nm) laser. The procedure is a form of subepithe-lial stromal ablation. It uses a highly sophisti-cated auto mated micro keratome to remove partial thickness epithelium of uniform thick-ness (180 microns) to create a circular flap that remains hinged to the parent cornea. The flap is deposited back after the stromal bed has been ablated. The flap does not need suturing. The healing is quick without much discomfort. The postprocedure recovery of vision is fast. The procedure does not leave corneal haze that is common in PRK. LASIK can be used as primary procedure in all errors of refraction and in presbyopia. With proper modifications it gives best result in moderate myopia though it has been used in very high myopia with fairly good result.

Patient Selection

Criteria for selection of eyes for LASIK is similar to any of the refractive procedures with special emphasis to:

1. Interpalpebral apertures (IPAs): Too small or too wide IPAs create problem for suction ring and functioning of mi-crokeratotome. The IPA should be within normal expected range.
2. Globe: The globe should neither be deep set nor very prominent.
3. Corneal thickness: It should be mea-sured by ultrasonic pachymeter. The cen-tral corneal thickness should be at least 450 microns. There should be no ectasia. The corneal thickness should be uniform within normal range.

4. Pupil: Eyes with large pupil require larger optical zone. Larger pupils result in glare and halos in the postoperative than small pupil. The pupil is constricted by pilo-carpine before starting the procedure. A constricted pupil helps in better center-ing of the optical zone.
5. Intraocular pressure (IOP): Patient with glaucoma are not suitable for LASIK, so are the cases with IOP less than 15 mm Hg. The IOP is required to be raised up to 65 mm Hg artificially by suction ring. The sudden rise causes transient blurring or absence of vision. As the procedure is done under local anesthesia, the patient becomes aware of sudden diminished vision and may panic unless he/she has been counseled well before the surgery about this unpleasant phenomenon dur-ing surgery. The vision returns to normal as soon as the suction ring is deactivated.
6. Contact lens: It should be discarded be-fore the surgery. The protocol followed is the soft lenses are required to be removed 2 weeks before and rigid lenses, 3 weeks.
7. Ocular disorders that are not suitable for LASIK are:
   a. Anterior segment pathologies:
      i. Thin cornea.
      ii. Active corneal ulcer.
      iii. Ocular surface disorder.
      iv. Corneal vascularization.
      v. Hypoesthesia cornea.
      vi. Limbal bleb.
      vii. Uncontrolled glaucoma.
      viii. Hypotony.
      ix. Proptosis.
      x. Blepharophimosis.
   b. Posterior segment pathologies:
      i. Proliferative diabetic retinopathy.
      ii. Retinal vascular disease.
      iii. Systemic vascular disease.
      iv. Widespread autoimmune disease.

Investigations

Essential investigations required prior to LASIK include:

1. Vision:
   - Distant:
     - Uncorrected
     - Corrected.
   - Near:
     - Uncorrected
     - Corrected.
2. Refraction under cycloplegia:
   - Spherical—specially in low myopes
   - Cylindrical:
     - Cylindrical refraction is converted in minus
     - Exact axis of cylinder.
3. Slit lamp examination for:
   - Lenticular opacities
   - Thickness of cornea
   - Corneal dystrophies and degenerations
   - Subtle deep vascularization.
4. Ultrasonic pachymetry.
5. Ophthalmoscopy: Direct/Indirect.
6. Keratometry:
   - Optical keratometry
   - Video keratography.
7. Intraocular pressure by applanation tonometer.

Instrument Required for LASIK

1. The procedure is done under topical anesthesia with operating microscope in absolutely aseptic conditions.
2. Micokeratomes: There are various types of microkeratomes available for the purpose. The microtome is powered by electricity. The activation of the microtome is controlled by a foot switch. The mechanical parts of the microtome are detailed in Table 11.3.

Table 11.3: Microkeratome—parts and its function

Parts	Functions
Head	Holds blade, blade holder and thickness plate
Handle	Contains micrometer
Console	Houses power regulator
Foot plate	Controls power that stabilizes the eye and pressurize the eye

The overall purpose of the microkeratome is to make an homogeneous corneal flap that should have uniform thickness all through to be cut in a predetermined dimension.

3. The suction ring: This operates on a suction pump. The purpose of the suction ring is to raise the IOP to 65 mm Hg, while making the flap. It fixes and stabilizes the globe and helps the microkeratome to move in a desired track. Other instruments used are shown in Figures 11.5A to F.

Preparation of Operation Theater for Laser Operation

1. The operation theater (OT) should be absolutely sterile and the surgery should be done under utmost aseptic and antiseptic methods.
2. The filters in air supply should be applied at least 2–3 hours before the commencement of the procedure.
3. The ambient air in the OT should be devoid of suspended particle.
4. The OT temperature should be between 15° and 20°.
5. Humidity should be less than 50%.
6. There should be standby power supply that takes over automatically in case of power failure.
7. All the equipments to be used in the procedure should be checked well in advance.

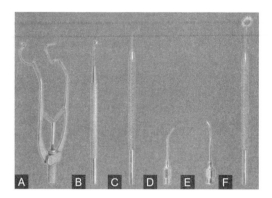

Figures 11.5A to F: Instruments required for LASIK. A. Lid Speculum; B. LASIK depressor; C. LASIK spatula; D. LASIK flap irrigator; E. LASIK irrigating canula; F. LASIK marker [*Courtesy:* Appasamy Associates (with permission)].

Preparation of Patient for Laser Operation

1. The surgery is daytime surgery and the patient is permitted to go 1 hour after the procedure.
2. The surgery is done under local anesthesia.
3. Apprehensive patients may require mild sedation.
4. Before the patient comes to the OT, he/she is given a complete face wash; the head is covered by a disposable cap.
5. Broad-spectrum antibiotic drops are instilled every 5 minutes for 4 times.
6. The lids are cleaned with 5% povidone solution.
7. Pupil is constricted by pilocarpine.
8. Usual surgical drapes are used.
9. The other eye is occluded.
10. The IPA is widened by wire speculum.
11. The patient is so positioned on the table that the laser beam is perpendicular to the cornea.

Laser Procedure

Creating corneal flap

1. The procedure starts after the patient has been draped and positioned under microscope.
2. The corneal periphery is marked by specially designed corneal marker with gentian violet or methylene blue. The corneal marker has one outer ring with diameter of 10.5 mm and an inner central ring of 3 mm diameter. From the inner ring, extend two parallel radial markers tangentially to join the outer circle (Fig. 11.6). The inner circle is placed concentric with the pupil as shown below. The outer circle makes the suction ring concentric with the pupil. The radial lines help to mark astigmatism, if the flap becomes free.
3. Fixing of suction ring: The pneumatic suction ring is fixed to the sclera and the suction is activated. The patient is warned about the blurring of vision that will take place as the intraocular tension rises to 65 mm Hg and assured that vision will return to normal once the procedure is over.

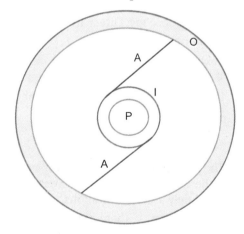

Figure 11.6: Typical corneal marker for laser. O is the outer ring, P is the pupil, I is the inner ring and A is the axis marker.

4. The IOP is measured by specially designed applanation tonometer following activation of suction.

5. The raised intraocular tension by suction ring facilitates fashioning of corneal flap that is optimal in respect of thickness, smoothness of surface and diameter.

6. Preparing corneal flap (Figs 11.7A to D):

   a. Moisten the cornea with balanced salt solution (BSS) and keep moistened for smooth passage of microkeratome.

   b. Insert the head of the microkeratome in the track of suction ring at the lower pole.

   c. Depress the forward foot plate of the microkeratome to make the microkeratome move across the cornea from one end to the other.

   d. Leave a part of the corneal flap attached to the cornea. This will act as a hinge on which the flap will be everted during laser application.

   e. Care should be taken not to cut the hinge. Once the microkeratome has traversed the desired distance, press the reverse foot plate. This makes the keratome to traverse back to original position.

   f. Most of the surgeons prefer to have a flap thickness of 180 microns with diameter of 8.5 mm.

   g. In case of high myopia and central corneal thickness, less than 530 microns thinner flaps are made. It may be as thin as 130 microns.

   h. Keep the cornea wet all through cutting of the flap. At the same time, excess of fluid from the stromal bed is sponged out to make it as dry out as possible to facilitate application of laser.

   i. Release the suction immediately. The eye should be exposed to high tension only for minimum time required to cut the flap.

7. Ablation is done by excimer laser.

8. Ablation should be done within 30 seconds of the preparations of the flap.

9. To ablate, lift the flap by special spatula.

10. Always keep the stromal bed absolutely dry.

11. The cornea should be moist, while raising the flap and the stroma should be dry, while ablating.

12. The actual ablation is done with predetermined correction of excimer.

13. Before starting ablation, check the centration of the eye by asking the patient to look at the fixation light.

14. All precautions are taken not to damage the hinge mechanically or by laser.

15. While ablating, the aim should be to leave 250 microns undisturbed.

Note: Remember the mnemonic "Cut wet ablate dry" for laser procedure.

Replacement of flap

Replacement of flap is as important as creating a flap. After ablation:

1. A drop of distilled water is put on the ablated area.

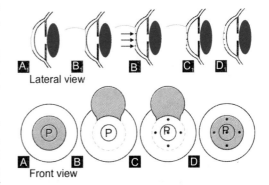

Figures 11.7A to D: Diagrammatic representation of LASIK. **A/A₁.** Outline of the flap; **B/B₁.** Everted flap; **B'.** Application of LASER; **C/C₁.** Post LASER flap still everted; **D/D₁.** Reposition of flap after LASER.

2. The flap is generally replaced back over the stroma.

3. The stroma is irrigated under the flap to remove postexcimer debris.

4. Excess of fluid is soaked by moistened sponge. The flap is allowed to dry for 2–3 minutes. The speculum is removed without touching the cornea.

5. The drapes are removed. The patient is asked to close the lids lightly and open gently.

6. A drop of clear solution of broad-spectrum antibiotics is instilled in the lower fornix.

7. The eye is covered by a plastic shield.

8. The patient is asked to stay in the hospital for an hour or so after which the placement of the flap is checked on the slit lamp.

9. The patient is asked to go home after 2 hours either with a patch or dark glasses and instructed:

   a. Not to rub the eye.

   b. Instill antibiotic drops six times a day along with NSAID.

   c. Use lubricant drop six times a day.

   d. Patient can resume usual routine activities from 2 days afterwards but not to go swimming.

   e. Avoid driving and prolong visual activity like reading or watching TV.

Complications of LASIK

LASIK is a safe procedure, yet complications are met with. The complications can be:

1. Intraoperative.
2. Immediate postoperative.
3. Delayed postoperative.

Preoperative complication

There may be preoperated problems such as:

1. Narrow IPA and deep set eyes. This requires modified suction ring.

2. Wide IPA with bulging globe. This results in suction loss.

3. Pinguecula or small pterygium causes suction loss.

4. Steep cornea causes button hole in a flap.

5. Flat cornea results in small thin flap.

Intraoperative complications

Intraoperative complications are mostly caused due to malfunctioning of suction ring, microkeratome or excimer machines in various combinations and less extent to wire speculum drape, hydration or dehydration. Thus, the complications can be suction ring related, flap related and laser related.

Suction-related complications: These are explained below:

1. Improper application of suction ring.

2. Failure to create high IOP.

3. Hypotonic due to suction-related ciliary shutdown.

4. Clogging of suction holes.

Flap-related complications: These are listed as follows:

1. Incomplete flap due to malfunctioning of microkeratome.

2. Irregular thickness of the flap.

3. The flap can be too thick or too thin.

4. Damage to flap may result in hole in the flap.

5. Free flap.

6. Damage to the hinge.

7. Dislocation of the flap.

8. Loss of flap.

9. Uneven stromal bed.

10. Hydration of stroma.

11. Dehydration of stroma.

12. Faulty reposition of flap.

13. Perforation of the cornea.

14. Wrinkling of the flap.

Most unwanted intraoperative complication is introduction of infection during any stage.

Laser-related complications: These are given below:

1. Problem with laser machine.
2. Laser damage to the flap.
3. Damage to the hinge.
4. Decentration of the ablation.
5. Unequal ablation.
6. Poor ablation.
7. Accidental intrastromal ablation.

Postoperative complications

Immediate complications: As follows:

1. Epithelial trauma.
2. Faulty adhesion.
3. Lost flap.

Late complications: These are given below:

1. Unwanted astigmatism: May be regular or irregular.
2. Undesirable correction:
   a. Undercorrection.
   b. Overcorrection.
   c. Regression.
3. Corneal ectasia.

LASEK

LASEK is acronym of laser-assisted subepithelial keratectomy. It is also known as laser epithelial keratomileusis. Excimer is used to ablate the subepithelial tissue after the basement membrane has been removed from the Bowman's membrane, leaving the stroma undisturbed. Unlike LASIK where a microkeratome is used to raise an uniformly thick flap, no microkeratome is required in LASEK. The corneal epithelial is peeled off the Bowman's membrane with the help of 18%–20% alcohol. A specially constructed trephine is used to make a circular ring in the superficial epithelium and the epithelium is soaked with alcohol for 20 seconds. Then the alcohol is washed off. The alcohol loses the epithelium as a sheet. This thin membrane is pushed toward the periphery and the bed thus prepared is ablated by excimer as per requirement.

The epithelium is nudged back. No sutures are required. Growing epithelium from the periphery replaces the loosened epithelium; a bandage contact lens is put for next 2–3 days. This helps the epithelium to go back. The limbal stem cells are liable to be damaged, if exposed for long. The patient is prescribed lubricants 4 times a day for 2 months along with a steroid in tapering dose. Some surgeons prefer to use mitomycin, 0.02% for 30 seconds. The procedure where mitomycin is used is called MLASEK.

Epi-LASIK

Epi-LASIK is a laser-assisted ablation procedure of central cornea that can be placed between LASIK and LASEK. Unlike LASEK, it does not require alcohol to de-epithalize. A specially designed plastic spatula used to fashion the epithelium sheet of 45–60 microns. The spatula is called epithelial separator. The subepithelial bed is ablated by excimer after which the epithelium is stroked back and the eye is irrigated with chilled BSS. The cornea is covered by a high DK contact lens and the patient is put on tapering protocol of local steroid, NSAID. Lubricants are added to the above drugs.

NON-LASER PROCEDURES FOR MYOPIA

Intercorneal Ring

Of all the refractive surgeries, this is the only reversible procedure. It is a non-laser procedure where an ultrathin polymethyl methacrylate (PMMA) ring is implanted at two-third stromal depth. The ring does not encircle the whole of the periphery. It is divided into two segments of 150° each. The thickness varies between 0.25 and 0.45 mm. The flattening of the cornea is mostly dependent upon the thickness of the ring. The procedure does not require any long learning curve. It has the least chances of perforation. Central cornea is left untouched where LASIK can be done in future, if need arises. The visual improvement is very fast, the cost is very low, the surgery is done under local anesthesia. In this process, two intrastromal channels are made inside the limbus, concentric with the limbus, on each side of midline. The two ends of the channel are made by radial cuts. A special stromal separator is introduced at one end and gently pushed through the two third of stromal depth till the spatula emerges on the other end. Once the tunnel has been made, the segment of the ring is inserted in the channel. The procedure is suitable for low myopia, between −1D and −5D. The procedure does not interfere with aspherocity.

Radial Keratotomy

Radial keratotomy (RK) is one of the first refractive surgeries in the fourth decade of the last century and was only available refractive surgery before the advent of laser. It is a non-laser-assisted incisional procedure done under local anesthesia with specially made knives. The knives can be diamond, sapphire and ruby. Even high quality stainless steel is used. This procedure gives good results in myopia between −1D and −6D (Figs 11.8 and 11.9).

Principle

The principle involved in the procedure to make the central cornea, i.e. the optical zone flatter in relation to the periphery that bulges following radial incision. The numbers of radial cuts vary between 4 and 16 on the epithelial surface; the incision involves 90% of the corneal thickness. Its peripheral end begin 1mm inside the limbus and the central end reaches the periphery of the optical zone that is situated in front of the pupil, concentric with the center of the pupil. The diameter of the optical zone varies between 3 and 6 mm depending upon the extent of myopia. The correction depends on number, length and depth of the radial incisions and diameter of

the optical zone. The number of incisions and diameter of the optical zone are determined on the basis of various nomograms available. An example of a commonly available nomogram is shown in Table 11.4.

Thus, from Table 11.4, it is obvious that correction of myopia depends upon number of incisions and size of the optical zone. Higher power requires more incision and smaller optical zone.

The first four incisions impart maximum reduction, the next four will reduce only half

Table 11.4: Nomogram for radial keratotomy in myopia

Myopia	Number of incisions (refer Fig. 11.8)	Size of optical zone
−1D to −1.5D	4	4.5 mm
−1.5D to −2.5D	4	4 mm
−2.5D to −3.5D	4	3.5 mm
−3.5D to −4.5D	4	3.5 mm
−4.5D to −5.5D	8	3 mm
−5.5D to −6.5D	8	3 mm
−6.5D to −7.5D	8	3 mm

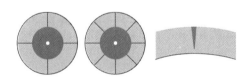

Figure 11.8: Optical zone, number of radial incisions and depth of radial incisions. The dot indicates center of the pupil, dark blue circle denotes the optical zone and deep blue lines indicates radial incisions.

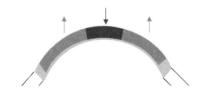

Figure 11.9: Mechanism of radial keratotomy

the amount of reduction achieved by four incisions and the remaining incisions will reduce one third of the power reduced by eight incisions.

Thus, to correct myopia of 5D, the first four incisions will correct –3D leaving –2D, which has to be corrected by further incisions. The next four incisions will reduce half the initial reduction, i.e. 3/2 = 1.5, remaining 0.5 will require eight additional incisions.

Regarding direction of incisions, there exists two diagonally opposite practices; one is called uphill and the other, downhill. The former is also known as centripetal and the latter, centrifugal.

Indications

There is no absolute indication because the surgery is done on normal cornea and the surgery is a cold surgery.

Contraindications

Absolute: There are many absolute contraindications. Some of them are:

1. Unwilling patient.
2. Ill-informed patient.
3. Non-counseled patient and relatives.
4. Thin cornea with irregular thickness as in keratoconus or subtle corneal ectasia.
5. Corneal vascularization.
6. Hypoesthetic cornea.
7. Contact lens warpage.
8. Local or systemic immunosuppression due to prolonged use of steroids and/or antimetabolites.
9. Connective tissue disorders.
10. Deep amblyopia.

Relative: List of relative contraindications is:

1. Ocular surface disorder.
2. Chronic blepharitis.
3. Allergic keratoconjunctivitis.
4. Diabetes.
5. Uncontrolled glaucoma.

Investigations

Essential ocular investigations required for RK are explained below.

Pachymetry: Ultrasonic pachymetry is perhaps the most important investigation required to rule out very thin corneas and corneas with irregular thickness, which are likely to perforate.

Keratometry and computerized video keratometry: In earlier days, lot of importance was given to optical keratometry. Now, its role has been questioned. Best results are between readings of 42D and 46D. Results are poor in corneas flatter than 41D. The computerized video keratometry is excellent method to detect early keratoconus, which may otherwise be missed and get operated with a battery of complications that may follow.

Cycloplegic refraction: It is helpful in avoiding overcorrection, especially in younger patients who still have some accommodation in excess.

Intraocular pressure: It is recorded by applanation tonometer.

Slit lamp biomicroscopy: It is done to exclude anterior segment disorders that may interfere with ultimate visual result.

Indirect ophthalmoscopy: RK for myopia is done in eyes that may have peripheral myopic degeneration, which may result in retinal detachment. It is better to give prophylactic treatment to the lesions that are prone to develop retinal detachment afterwards, prior the RK is done. Retinal surgeries in eyes that have undergone RK pose more problems than eyes without RK.

Outcome

The eyes undergoing RK have chances of good results in 80%–85%.

Factors influencing outcome

The outcome depends on many factors. The factors can broadly be divided into two groups:

1. Those that are influenced by surgical procedures.
2. Those that are influenced by factors in the patient.

Surgical factors

The surgical factors that influence the outcome are explained below.

Diameter of the optical zone: The diameter of the optical zone in RK for myopia varies between 3 and 4.5 mm. A change in diameter by 0.5 mm results in change of 1.0D of refraction.

Number of incisions: In earlier days, the number of incisions given were as many as 80. This made the cornea more pliable than required and chances of corneal decompensation were enormous. The number of incisions is reduced with better outcome; 4–8 incisions are supposed to be quite sufficient.

Depth of incisions: Deeper incisions reduce the power greater than shallower incisions. The exact relation of depth of incision to correct error of refraction has eluded mathematical calculations.

Intraoperative complications: The eyes with intraoperative complications have poorer vision and may require additional surgery.

Patient-related factors

The factors in patient that influence the outcome are detailed as follows.

Age: Younger patients have relatively poor correction than older people for the same amount of error of refraction.

Sex: Younger females have poorer correction for the same power done in the corresponding age group of males. This difference passes off and correction in both sex become equal with increased age.

Ocular factors: There are various ocular factors that influence the outcome of RK.

Corneal thickness: There is no relation between thickness of cornea and outcome. However, thin corneas are more prone to perforation, making preoperative pachymetry mandatory in RK.

Corneal curvature: In the past, it was supposed that steeper corneas have better reduction than flatter cornea for same degree of error of refraction. Presently, this belief has been questioned.

Corneal diameter: Larger corneas give better reduction. This too has not been substantiated.

Ocular rigidity: Eyes with higher ocular rigidity have better outcome.

Intraocular pressure: Eyes with glaucoma are not operated, but a mild rise of ocular pressure in the postoperative weeks are said to give better reduction. Preoperative IOP less than 10 mm Hg have poor reduction as compared to 20 mm Hg.

Instruments Required for RK

The instrument required for RK are shown in Figures 11.10A to K:

1. Operating microscope.
2. Keratometry knife.
3. Optical centering device.
4. Central zone marker.
5. Incision marker.
6. Fixation forceps.
7. Wound openers.

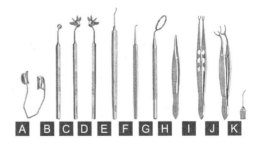

Figures 11.10A to K: Various instruments required for RK. **A.** Wire speculum; **B.** Zone marker; **C and D.** Radial marker; **E.** Visual axis marker; **F.** Incision depth gauge; **G.** Fixation ring; **H.** Corneal fixation forceps; **I.** Incision spreading forceps; **J.** Corneal fication forceps; **K.** Air ejecting cannula [*Courtesy:* Appasamy Associates (with permission)].

Surgical Procedure

The procedure is done under topical anesthesia. No attempt should be made to perform the procedure without a good microscope. The operation theater must be absolutely sterile; the surgery should be done under utmost antiseptic and aseptic methods as required for any intraocular surgery.

The patient lies on the table and is asked to fix straight ahead to mark the center of the optical zone. The center of the optical zone more or less corresponds to the center of the normal pupil. The center of the optical zone is better marked by a centering device. The other methods to mark the center include operating microscope and direct ophthalmoscope beam. The next step is to mark the clear central zone that will remain untouched during the process. This is done by a circular ring of variable size. From the periphery, radiate spikes that mark the position of the future incision. The eye is fixed with a special two pronged fixation forceps.

The actual incisions are given thereafter, preferably by a diamond knife, wither from the periphery to the center or from center to the periphery. The incision should be placed equidistant, have uniform depth and straight with sharp edges. They should stop 1 mm shorter of the limbus and reach just the periphery of the optical zone. The first four incisions are 90° apart and the next are in between, i.e. at 45°. The depth of the incision is 90% of thickness of cornea. Once desired incisions have been made, the cornea is gently washed with balanced salt solution to remove the debris from the incision. A drop of clear solution of broad spectrum is instilled and the eye patched lightly for 4–6 hours.

Complications of Radial Keratotomy

Surprisingly, complications are infrequent. Unfortunately, the complications when occur are magnified disproportionately by the patient because the surgery is done on an eye without redness or pain. The complications can be listed into four groups.

Intraoperative complications

1. Eccentric central zone.
2. Incision:
   - Too long:
     - Encroaching into clear central zone
     - Reaching the limbus.
   - Not perpendicular to the central zone
   - Unequal depth
   - Microperforation
   - Gross perforation
   - Loss of anterior chamber (AC)
   - Soft eye
   - Epithelial defect.

Immediate postoperative complications

1. Pain, lacrimation, photophobia.
2. Glare.
3. Ghost image.
4. Unstable vision.

Late postoperative complications

They are mostly refractive in nature:

1. Overcorrection.
2. Undercorrection.
3. Astigmatism.

Delayed complications

1. Difficulty in contact lens fitting.
2. Difficulty in cataract surgery.
3. Difficulty in calculating IOL power.
4. Possible complications during retinal detachment surgery.

Advantages of Radial Keratotomy

The greatest advantage of RK is its low cost as compared to laser procedures. To this may be added shorter recovery period and absence of haze because the procedure involves corneal periphery leaving a clear central optical zone.

Disadvantages of Radial Keratotomy

The disadvantages include corneal weakness, especially when too many incisions have been given. This enhances the possibility of corneal rupture following moderate blunt injury and during encircling surgery for retinal detachment in future. Presence of radial opacities may interfere with IOL power calculation. There is too much of scarring during healing. Irregular astigmatism is more common. Glare during driving is a frequent annoyance.

REFRACTIVE SURGERIES FOR HYPERMETROPIA

The results of refractive surgeries in hypermetropia are not as encouraging as in myopia. In myopia, the results of refractive surgeries are predictably accurate and give far more satisfactory visual improvement.

Like myopia, the refractive surgeries in hypermetropia can be incisional or laser assisted. The principle involved in both the methods is to cause the central cornea change its curvature, i.e. in myopia flatter and hypermetropia steeper. The incision method is a keratotomy. The procedure is identical to that used in myopia with a difference that the incisions are tangential to optical zone, rather radial as in myopia. The optical zone in hypermetropic keratotomy is larger than in myopia. In myopia, the optical zone varies between 3.00 and 4.5 mm, while in hypermetropia, it varies between 5.0 and 6.0 mm. Lower the hypermetropic power, larger is the optical zone. Thus, +1.00D sphere will require an optical zone of 6.0 mm and +3D will require a zone of 5.00 mm. The number of incisions is six, giving a configuration of hexagon; hence the procedure is also called hexagonal keratotomy (Fig. 11.11).

LASER-ASSISTED PROCEDURES

Laser-assisted refractive procedures include:
1. Laser thermal keratoplasty.
2. Conductive keratoplasty.

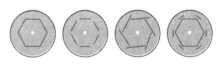

Figure 11.11: Showing various kinds of incisions in hexagonal keratotomy

3. Hypermetropic PRK.
4. Hypermetropic LASIK.

Laser Thermal Keratoplasty

Laser thermal keratoplasty (LTK) is suitable for low hypermetropia in persons between 40 and 50 years, presbyopia and astigmatism. It is a collagen shrinkage surgery. It takes very little time to perform and is claimed to have fast recovery. The infrared laser is directed by a contact fiber optics handpiece or non-contact slit lamp delivery. The wavelength of the laser is midinfrared at 2.06 micrometers with a pulse duration of 300 microseconds, repetition rate of 15 Hz and power 19 mJ. The laser used is holmium: YAG laser. The function of the laser procedure is to produce mild charring of midstroma, resulting in formation of a constricting band all round, forcing the central cornea to be steeped. As in other refracting procedures for hypermetropia, the optical zone is large, i.e. 6.00 mm. The laser beams are applied in two rows; one at 6.00 mm and the subsequent at 7.00 mm. Each ring of burns is generally eight in number. The complications are regression and introduction of astigmatism.

Hypermetropic PRK

Hypermetropic PRK, an ablation procedure using excimer laser, done on eyes with hypermetropia up to 4D. As in all hypermetropic procedures, the laser ablation is done beyond a large optical zone of 6 mm, which is surrounded by a transition zone of 9 mm. The number of laser spots is three times more than required for myopia of same order. The procedure produces a large doughnut-shaped ring of ablation all around with a large epithelial defect that requires longer healing time. Regression is common.

Hypermetropic LASIK

Hypermetropic LASIK, an ablation procedure, done under the corneal flap, similar to done in myopia. The process is used for moderate hypermetropia.

Principle

The principle involved is to create a central steeping by peripheral circular ablation. It requires larger flap than myopia. The diameter of the flap is 9.0–10.0 mm. The flap is mostly created by microkeratome. A better alternative is a femtosecond laser.

Advantages

Hypermetropic LASIK has some advantages over hypermetropic PRK. The advantages are:

1. There is fast visual gain.
2. Less regression.

3. Quick epithelial healing with minimal haze.
4. It can be performed with thinner cornea as compared to myopia.

Disadavantages

The disadvantages include:

1. Introduction of astigmatism.
2. Over- and under-correction.
3. Inter, face scarring.
4. Hypermetropic LASEK or epi-LASIK are also claimed to be viable alternative in hypermetropia.

Conductive Keratoplasty for Hypermetropia

Conductive keratoplasty is collagen shrinkage procedure. In this procedure, 350 kHz of radiofrequency is used. The energy is delivered to the stroma at multiple spots in a circular fashion. The energy is delivered through a contact delivery system comprising of a stainless steel probe. The energy, on reaching the stroma, causes a shrinkage of the collagen. The shrinkage results in steeping of central

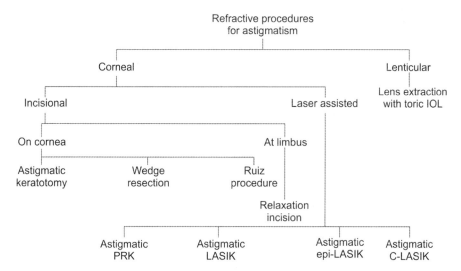

Figure 11.12: Refractive procedures for astigmatism

cornea. This procedure can also be used to correct presbyopia and keratoplasty-induced astigmatism. The common shortcomings of the procedure are initial overcorrection, regression and iatrogenic astigmatism.

REFRACTIVE PROCEDURES FOR ASTIGMATISM

The refractive procedures done in case of astigmatism are illustrated in Figure 11.12.

There are two sets of keratotomy:

1. For steep meridian:
   a. Ruiz procedure.
   b. Flag incision.
   c. Circumferential relaxing incision (Figs 11.13A to D).
2. For flat meridian:
   a. Wedge resection.
   b. Troutman sutures.

NON-LASER-ASSISTED PROCEDURES USED IN ASTIGMATISM

Astigmatic Keratotomy

In astigmatism, one meridian is either steeper or flatter than the normal. Flattening the steeper meridian makes this meridian less converging and the axis at 90° more convergent. In myopia, the steeper axis is flattened and in hypermetropia, the flatter axis needs

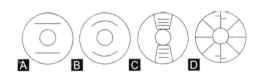

Figures 11.13A to D: Various types of incisions used to correct steeper meridian in astigmatism. **A.** A paired transverse incision; **B.** Paired curved incision; **C.** Ruiz procedure; **D.** Flag incision.

to be steepened. Radial incisions flatten the cornea and the transverse incisions steepen the cornea. Flattening of steep axes is accompanied by steepening of the flatter axes. This is called coupling effect. In coupling effect, the cylindrical value is changed without interfering the spherical value. Longer the incision, lower is the coupling effect. Deeper the incision, better is the correction (Figs 11.14A to D).

Better results are achieved when spherical equivalent is closer to zero and in regular astigmatism. Best results are seen in simple astigmatism ranging between 1D cylinder (Dcyl) and 6Dcyl. It is also good in regular astigmatism. The patients tolerate with the rule astigmatism, so many surgeons prefer to leave some astigmatism with the rule. The axis of the astigmatism should be marked with patient sitting erect on a slit lamp because reclining changes the axis of the astigmatism. Besides axis of astigmatism, the points 12 O'clock, 3 O'clock, 6 O'clock and 9 O'clock should also be marked.

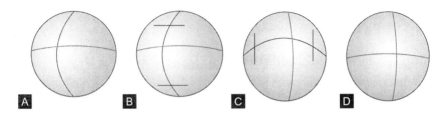

Figures 11.14A to D: Effect of transverse astigmatic keratotomy on cornea. **A.** Cornea with different curvature. Black line shows steeper meridian, cyan line shows normal meridian. **B and C.** Transverse keratotomy done on steeper meridian; **D.** Curvature of the steeper meridian reduced to normal curvature.

Selection of Cases

1. Primary corneal astigmatism.
2. Stable refraction.
3. Uniform thickness of cornea.
4. Regular astigmatism.

Instruments

1. The instruments required are almost same as in RK. It is better if the operating microscope has a built-in keratoscope.
2. The surgery is done under local anesthesia.

Types of Incisions

There are two types of incisions:

1. Transverse.
2. Arcuate.

Steps of Procedure

1. Axis of astigmatism and meridians at 12, 3, 6 and 9 are marked under local anesthesia on slit lamp with gentian violet.
2. Patient is placed on the table and draped in usual method.
3. A wire speculum is applied.
4. The patient is asked to fix the fixation mark in the microscope.
5. Optical center is marked.
6. Axis of astigmatism and optical zone are determined.
7. Any of the standard nomogram is consulted, determining the length of incision.
8. The incisions are best placed between 5 and 7 mm from the center of the pupil.
9. The incisions transverse or arcuate are given in pair. In high cylindrical error, an additional pair may be required. Before starting the incision, the globe is stabilized with special fixation forceps.

Postoperative Management

The eye is patched for a day with broad-spectrum antibiotic drops and steroid drops. Patients may require mild oral analgesics. After the eye is open, the patient is instructed to use broad-spectrum antibiotic drops for next 10 days. Initially steroids are instilled along with broad-spectrum antibiotics 6–8 times a day and gradually tapered.

Complications

Intraoperative complications: These are same as in RK, but less frequent. This happens because less numbers of incisions are used in astigmatic keratotomy than in spherical error.

Postoperative complications: These are listed below:

1. Undercorrection.
2. Overcorrection.
3. Regression.
4. Irregular astigmatism.
5. Change in axis from original.

Limbal Relaxation Sutures

Limbal relaxation sutures is simpler version of astigmatic keratotomy. It is not performed on cornea, but at the limbus; hence all the postoperative complications such as glare and smudged vision are absent. The only drawback with this procedure is that it is effective in low cylindrical error between 1D cylinder and 2D cylinder.

LASER-ASSISTED PROCEDURES USED IN ASTIGMATISM

The two commonly used laser procedures are:

1. Photorefractive keratotomy.
2. Astigmatic LASIK.

Astigmatic PRK

Astigmatic PRK is based on the same principle as that of spherical correction. The area ablated in astigmatic PRK is cylindrical rather than spherical as used in spherical correction. The axis of cylinder is marked as in spherical error, i.e. the patient is seated on a slit lamp. Rest of the steps are same as in spherical PRK. In case of compound myopic astigmatism, an elliptical ablation corrects both spherical and cylindrical errors. Cylindrical correction up to 4D gives satisfactory results in myopia. Hypermetropic astigmatism does not give as good result as in myopia.

Astigmatic LASIK

The laser refractive procedure is effective in a larger range of 1.00D–10.00D cylinder. The selection of cases, surgical procedures and postoperative care are the same as in LASIK for spherical power. The other procedures available are astigmatic epi-LASIK and astigmatic C-LASIK. Astigmatic epi-LASIK is preferred over PRK for its inherent advantage of less postoperative haze, less operative pain and early recovery. C-LASIK is claimed to be best of all the procedures available. It is a wavefront guided method.

Comparison Between PRK and LASIK

Comparative features of PRK and LASIK are detailed in Table 11.5.

Advantages of LASEK Over LASIK

LASIK is most practiced laser procedure, yet it has some disadvantages. The advantages of LASEK over LASIK are:

Table 11.5: Comparison between PRK and LASIK

Features	PRK*	LASIK†
Instruments Laser Microkeratome Suction ring	Frequency-doubled ND:Yag Not required Not required	Excimer Essential Essential
Postprocedure patching	Required	Generally not required
Postoperative pain	+++	±
Period of topical steroid use	6 month	2–3 week
Visual rehabilitation	Late	Early
Stromal haze	++	±
Time taken to stabilize refraction	4–6 month	Less than 1 month
Visual predictability	Low to moderate	Very high
Range of correction	1D–12D	1D–30D
Regression	Common	Few
Long-term regression	More	Less
Range of correction	1D–12D	1D–30D
Repeat surgery	After 1 year	After 2–3 week
Learning curve	Prolong	Short
Flap complications	Nil	Present

*PRK, photorefractive keratotomy; LASIK, laser-assisted in situ keratomileusis

1. No flap-related complications.
2. LASEK can be performed with ease on thin cornea.
3. No chance of postoperative corneal ectasia.
4. LASEK can be applied on a larger zone.
5. Additional myopic correction by ablation is possible.
6. Chances of dry eye are less in LASEK.

Management of Latrogenic Astigmatism

Astigmatism can be primary when only corneal curvature in two meridians differ for which no cause can be detected in the eye. This the commonest type of astigmatism. If some disorder present in the eye that can be related to astigmatism, it is called secondary astigmatism. It could be:

1. Non-iatrogenic.
2. Iatrogenic.

The common causes of secondary astigmatism are keratoconus, keratectasia, pterygium, limbaldermoid, orbital tumors, traumatic iris prolapse, tilting of lens, tilting of IOL. Sometimes, secondary causes can be iatrogenic, i.e. keratoplasty, conventional lens extraction, small incision cataract surgery (SICS), postoperative iris prolapse, trabeculectomy scar, squint surgery, encircling for retinal detachment.

Out of all of them, most distressing astigmatism is seen following penetrating keratoplasty. There, in spite of successful surgery, the vision remains subnormal due to irregular astigmatism caused by multiple sutures. Generally the astigmatism is compound, which can be corrected partially by spectacle. Contact lenses are difficult to fit in the postoperative keratoplasty.

Management of Postkeratoplasty Astigmatism

The options available to correct postkeratoplasty astigmatism are:

1. Selective removal of sutures.
2. Relaxing incision.
3. Relaxing incisions with compressive sutures.
4. Corneal wedge resection.
5. Ruiz procedure.

Selective Suture Removal

Selective suture removal is the most common and to some extent effective method. The postoperative sutures in keratoplasty should not be removed before 3 months after the surgery in case of interrupted sutures. The sutures in the steep meridian are removed in phased manner. The particular suture or sutures that need to be removed is best determined by keratoscopy or video keratography. Continuous sutures are not removed before 1 year.

Relaxing Incisions

Relaxing incisions are given on the donor cornea, 0.5 mm inside the graft junction in an arcuate fashion, given along the steeper meridian. This corrects up to 8D cylinder. The incisions are in pairs, opposite to each other. They are fashioned up to 60% of the corneal depth. The relaxing incisions are given only after all the sutures have been removed.

Relaxing Incisions with Compressive Sutures

After the relaxing sutures have been given, few interrupted sutures are given on the graft junction 90° away from the steepest junction.

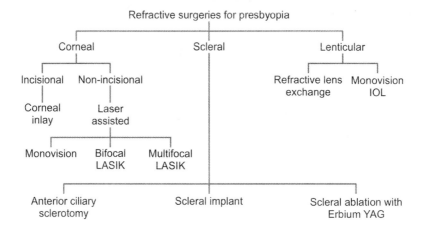

Figure 11.15: Refractive procedures for presbyopia (IOL, intraocular lens; LASIK, laser-assisted in situ keratomileusis; YAG, yttrium aluminum garnet)

Corneal Wedge Resection

Corneal wedge resection is tried only on very high astigmatism, i.e. 10D–20D cylinder under retrobulbar or peribulbar anesthesia. The wedge is created in the recipient cornea. A triangular piece of corneal wedge is fashioned. The outer width of the wedge is 1–1.5 mm wide. The depth of the wedge is about 60%–70% of the corneal thickness. The length is about 90° arc. The ends of the wedge are sutured by interrupted sutures of 10 zeronylon.

Ruiz Procedure

Ruiz procedure is mostly used in correcting postkeratoplasty astigmatism that may be as high as 10D cylinder. In this procedure, five to six horizontal parallel keratotomy incisions are made by diamond knife in a ladder fashion along the axis of the steepest meridian. The horizontal incisions lies tangential to the optical zone. Two radial incisions are given on each side of the horizontal incision. Care is taken that the radial incisions do not touch the end of the horizontal sutures, because this may result in poor wound healing.

REFRACTIVE PROCEDURES FOR PRESBYOPIA

Presbyopia is not an error of refraction. It is an aging process where initially the accommodation is subnormal. This deficiency progressively increases to a stage when there is no accommodation available. The presbyopia can easily be corrected by hassle-free near vision correction like bifocal contact lenses or monovision, in persons who do not like to use spectacles.

Still there are some persons who will not like to use a contact lens even. The only choice left to them is refractive surgeries. The refractive surgeries available for presbyopia are relatively newer developments and have not proved to be as effective as errors of refraction, hence it is not practiced as frequently as in errors of refraction. The present-day surgery available is based on well-known presumption:

1. Relentless growth of the lens throughout the life.
2. Accommodation is due to inherent elasticity of the lens.

The lens is kept taught by tension of suspensory ligaments. The increase in curvature of the lens is brought about by contraction of ciliary muscles. This has been challenged by the present-day concept, which presumes that the size of the lens increases in all dimensions including the equator with age. This decreases the distance between the lens and the ciliary body resulting in poor function of ciliary body. Thus, it is postulated that if the working distance can be increased by scleral expansion, the accommodation can be brought back. The surgeries can be done on the sclera over the ciliary body or at the limbus (Fig. 11.15).

REFRACTIVE SURGERIES FOR CORRECTION OF NEAR VISION DEFECT

Types of Near Vision Defect

The near vision defect can be divided into two groups, i.e. phakic near vision defect and aphakic near vision defect. The near vision defect in presence of lens is known as presbyopia, which is fully accommodation dependant. The accommodation is brought about by lens and ciliary body. Presbyopia sets in round about 40 years and gradually increases up to 60 years of age when it gets stabilized. The near vision defect in aphakia is stationary. There are two sets of surgical procedures available to correct the two entirely different conditions. The aphakic near vision defect is easy to correct without possibility of reverting to the original status. This can be done by:

1. Leaving mild to moderate myopia: This gives sufficient good distant vision as well as near vision.
2. Monovision: Correct one eye for distance and the other eye for nearby IOL.

Correction of Defect

The refractive correction in phakic near vision defect should be done only when the presbyopia has stabilized. The various options available are given below.

Surgical

Surgical correction can be on the following ways.

Sclera expansion surgery on cilio-scleral complex: Scleral expansion bands and radial sclerotomy. The surgery can either be done on the sclera, over the ciliary body or at the limbus. The former is simpler, done under topical anesthesia, where four radial incisions are given in four quadrants in between the four recti. In the latter, the surgery is done under retrobulbar or peribulbar anesthesia. The conjunctiva is reflected toward the cornea in four quadrants. Four scleral tunnels are made 2.5 mm away from the limbus and segments of PMMA sclera implants are placed one in each tunnel and the conjunctiva reposited.

Lens: Correction can be done as follows:

1. Clear lens extraction with bifocal IOL and pseudoaccommodative IOL.
2. Refractive lens exchange.

Cornea: In cornea the correction can be carried out as detailed here.

Corneal inlays: Implants are put just under the superficial layer of the cornea. It is 1.5 mm in diameter and ultrathin; almost half the thickness of a sheet of paper. The second type of inlays is an ultrathin circular disk 3.8 mm in diameter and 10 micron in thickness with a circular hole of 1.6 mm in diameter in the center. The hole placed in front of the pupil. This reduces the size of the pupil and increases the depth of focus as in a pinhole.

Laser Based

Laser-based corrections can be:

1. Monovison LASIK.
2. Monovison conductive keratoplasty.
3. Bifocal LASIK.

Monovison conductive keratoplasty: The procedure is a modified form of conductive keratoplasty used in hypermetropia. As the name suggests, it is used in one eye only. The eye operated is the non-dominant eye. The procedure takes very short time and the near vision is stabilized in few weeks.

Bibliography

1. Agarwal LP. Principles of Optics and Refraction, 2nd edition. New Delhi: CBS Publishers; 1979.
2. Appleton B. Clinical Optics, 1st Indian edition. New Delhi: Jaypee Brothers Medical Publishers (P) Ltd; 1990.
3. Badrinath SS, Prema Padmanaban (Eds). Refraction in Shankara Nethralaya Clinical Practice, Pattern in Ophthalmology, 1st edition. New Delhi: Jaypee Brothers Medical Publishers (P) Ltd; 2004.
4. David Abrams. Duke Elder's Practice of Refraction, 10th edition. New Delhi: Elsevier India (P) Ltd; 2006.
5. David Middleman. In: Pyeman, Sauders, Goldberg (Eds). Geometric Optics and Clinical Refraction in Principle and Practice of Ophthalmology, vol. 1, 1st Indian edition. New Delhi: Jaypee Brothers Medical Publishers (P) Ltd; p. 213.
6. Davson H. Physiology of the Eye, 2nd edition. London: J & A Churchill Limited; 1963.
7. Duke Elder S, Smith RJH. In: Duke Elder S (Ed). Clinical Methods of Examination in System of Ophthalmolgy, vol. VII, 1st edition. London: Henry Kimpton; 1962.
8. Fraunfelder FT, Roy FH, Joan Randol. In: Fraunfelder FT, Roy FH (Eds). Refractive Disorders in Current Ocular Therapy, 5th edition. Philadelphia: WB Saunders Company; 2000.
9. Goldberg MF. In: Pyeman GM, Saunder DR (Eds). Optics and Refraction in Principle and Practice of Ophthalmology, vol. 1, 1st Indian edition. New Delhi: Jaypee Brothers Medical Publishers (P) Ltd; 1987.
10. Goldmann H. Applanation Tonometry. Transactions of the Second Glaucoma Conference. New York: 1957.
11. Grover AK. In: Gupta AK, Krishna V (Eds). Refractive Corneal Surgery in Current Topics in Ophthalmology, vol. VII. New Delhi: Elsevier India (P) Ltd; 2004. pp. 185-94.
12. Gupta AK, Krishna V. Low Visual Aids in Current Topics in Ophthalmology, vol. VII. New Delhi: Elsevier India (P) Ltd; 2004. pp. 672-90.
13. Harley RD. Refraction in Children in Pediatric Ophthalmology, 2nd edition. Philadelphia: WB Saunders Company; 1983.
14. Hunter DG, West CE. Last Minute Optics, 1st Indian edition. New Delhi: Jaypee Brothers Medical Publishers (P) Ltd; 1997.
15. Khoo CY. 101 Questions and Answers about Contact lens, 1st edition. Singapore: PG Publishing; 1985.
16. Khurana AK. Low Vision Management in Theory and Practice of Optics and Refraction, 2nd edition. New Delhi: Elsevier India (P) Ltd; 2008. pp. 293-305.
17. Khurana AK. Refractive Surgery in Theory and Practice of Optics and Refraction, 2nd edition. New Delhi: Elsevier India (P) Ltd; 2008. pp. 306-48.

18. Lalit Verma. Guidelines for glaucoma investigation. AIOS Journal.

19. Levinson BA, Rutzen A. Surgical Options for Correction of Hyperopia in Highlights of Ophthalmology, vol. 35, Indian edition. pp. 9-11.

20. Markiewitz HH. The so-called Imbert-Fick law. AMA Arch Ophthalmology. 1960;64(1):159.

21. Michelle Pett, Herrin. Ophthalmic Examination and Basic Skills, 1st Indian edition. New Delhi: Jaypee Brothers Medical Publishers (P) Ltd; 1990.

22. Mukherjee PK. Examination of the Eyes Requiring Optical Correction in Clinical Examination in Ophthalmology, 1st edition. New Delhi: Elsevier India (P) Ltd; 2006. pp. 213-31.

23. Mukherjee PK. Ophthalmic Assistant, 1st edition. New Delhi: Jaypee Brothers Medical Publishers (P) Ltd; 2013.

24. Mukherjee PK. Pediatric Ophthalmology, 1st edition. New Delhi: New Age International (P) Ltd; 2005.

25. Mukherjee PK. Physiological Optics in Ophthalmic Assistant, 1st edition. New Delhi: Jaypee Brothers Medical Publishers (P) Ltd; 2013. pp. 54-86.

26. Mukherjee PK. Physiology of the Eye and Optics in Ophthalmic Assistant, 1st edition. New Delhi: Jaypee Brothers Medical Publishers (P) Ltd; 2013.

27. Murillo-Lopez FH. Anisometropia in Current Ocular Therapy, 5th edition. Philadelphia: WB Saunders Company; 2000. pp. 585-9.

28. Nathan P. Handbook of Optometry and Eye Disorders, 1st edition. New Delhi: Jaypee Brothers Medical Publishers (P) Ltd; 2006.

29. Paul Riordon Eva. In: Vaughan D, Asiry (Eds). Optics and Refraction in General Ophthalmology, 15th edition. Appleton and Lange; 1999. pp. 355-60.

30. Rakow PL. Contact Lens, Ophthalmic Technical Skills Series. New Delhi: Jaypee Brothers Medical Publishers (P) Ltd; 1989.

31. Rammurthy D (Ed). Refractive Surgery in Ready Reckoner in Ophthalmology, 1st edition. New Delhi: Jaypee Brothers Medical Publishers (P) Ltd, AJR Medi Solution (P) Ltd; 2010.

32. Ritu Arora, Krishna V, Gupta AK. In: Gupta AK, Krishna V (Eds). Laser Refractive Corneal Surgery in Current Topics in Opthalmology, vol. VII. New Delhi: Elsevier India (P) Ltd; 2004. pp. 195-221.

33. Roy M, Bhartiya P, Vajpayee RB. In: Saxena S (Ed). Refractive Surgery in Clinical Practice in Ophthalmology, 1st edition. New Delhi: Jaypee Brothers Medical Publishers (P) Ltd; 2003. pp. 82-104.

34. Shrinivasan V, Tulsiraj RD. Ophthalmic Instruments and Equipments, 2nd edition. Madurai: Arvind Eye Hospital; 2003.

35. Singhal NC. Low Visual Aids in Principle and Practice of Optics and Refraction. New Delhi: Jaypee Brothers Medical Publishers (P) Ltd; 1996. pp. 209-13.

36. Singhal NC. Principle and Practice of Refraction and Optics, 1st edition. New Delhi: Jaypee Brothers Medical Publishers (P) Ltd; 1993.

37. Singh MD. Theory and Practice of Goldmann Applanation Tonometry. A video. 2012.

38. Sorsby A. Butterworth. Ophthalmic Optics in Modern Ophthalmology, vol. I. London; 1963.

39. Sukumaran N. Practical Guide on Refraction, Revised edition. Madurai: Arvind Eye Hospital; 2000.

40. Surbhi Arora, Singh G, Uma Sridhar. Presbyopia and Recent Modalities of Treatment Ophthalmology Today, vol. XI. pp. 113-6.

41. Vander JF, Gault JA. Optics and Refraction in Ophthalmology Secrets, 1st edition. New Delhi: Jaypee Brothers Medical Publishers (P) Ltd; 1998.

42. Vaughan D, Taylor Asbury, Paul Riordan, et al. General Ophthalmology, 15th edition. USA, Connecticut: Stanford University; 1999.

Index

Page numbers followed by *f* refer to figure, *t* refer to table and *b* refer to box.